MEDICAL OVERKILL

DISEASES OF MEDICAL PROGRESS

RALPH C. GREENE, M.D.

GEORGE F. STICKLEY COMPANY 210 W. WASHINGTON SQUARE
PHILADELPHIA, PA 19106

About the Author

Dr. Ralph Greene is clinical professor of pathology at Northwestern University Medical School. A board-certified pathologist, he received his M.D. degree from Washington University in St. Louis. He has held teaching appointments at the University of Tennessee Medical School and Oakton Community College and was a visiting professor of pathology at the University of Massachusetts Medical School. Dr. Greene has made numerous contributions to the medical literature and has published articles for consumers on medical subjects.

DEDICATION

To all those members of the medical and allied professions and their patients who question dubious assumptions which result in iatrogenesis, unnecessary intervention and unbearable costs.

ACKNOWLEDGEMENTS

Most of the material for this book has been derived from standard medical periodicals and texts which are listed in the bibliography. My personal experience and that of unnamed colleagues played a significant but smaller role. I take pleasure in thanking Ann Weller, Laura Mueller and Micaela Sullivan of the American Medical Association Library and Rose Slowinski of Northwestern University's Evanston Hospital Library for their efficient and unselfish help in literary research. I am also grateful to those members of my family who endured my demands on their time and patience particularly my daughter-in-law, Corrine Greene, who rendered invaluable assistance with the preparation of the manuscript.

ISBN-0-89313-065-6
Library of Congress Card #82-050527

Printed and Manufactured in the United States and published by the George F. Stickley Company, 210 West Washington Square, Phila., Pa. 19106.

CONTENTS

COMMON ABBREVIATIONS AND ACRONYMS

AABB	American Association of Blood Banks
ACP	American College of Physicians
ACS	American College of Surgeons-American Cancer Society
AHA	American Heart Association
AJCP	American Journal of Clinical Pathology
AJM	American Journal of Medicine
AMN	American Medical News
BP	Blood Pressure
CABP	Coronary Artery Bypass
CAD	Coronary Artery Disease
CAP	College of American Pathologists
CAT-CT	Computerized Axial Tomography
CCU	Coronary Care Unit
CDC	Center for Disease Control
CPR	Cardiopulmonary Resuscitation
D&C	Dilatation and Curettage
ECG-EKG	Electrocardiogram
ER	Emergency Room
FDA	Food and Drug Administration
HAV-HBV	Hepatitis A Virus-Hepatitis B Virus
HHS	Health and Human Services
HMO	Health Maintenance Organization
ICU	Intensive Care Unit
IM-i.m.	Intramuscular
IV-i.v.	Intravenous
JAMA	Journal of the American Medical Association
JCAH	Joint Committee on Accreditation of Hospitals
MGH	Massachusetts General Hospital
MI	Myocardial Infarction (Heart Attack)
MLO	Medical Laboratory Observer
MMWR	Morbidity and Mortality Weekly Report (from CDC)
NEJM	New England Journal of Medicine
NIH	National Institutes of Health
OR	Operating Room
OTA	Office of Technology Assessment
PDR	Physicians' Desk Reference
PSRO	Professional Standards Review Organization
PR	Pulse Rate
SC-s.c.	Subcutaneous
T&A	Tonsillectomy and Adenoidectomy
TSS	Toxic Shock Syndrome
TUR	Transurethral Resection
USPHS	United States Public Health Service

Preface

There has been an insidiously increasing epidemic of iatrogenic illness in Western countries for several decades. And YOU could be a victim. IATROGENIC is a word best known by doctors. Derived from the Greek *iatros*, meaning physician, and *genesis*, meaning production, it is broadly applied to mean any adverse condition produced in a patient as the result of diagnostic procedures or treatment by a physician or hospital. Paradoxically, this increase is occurring despite and because of the growth in medical knowledge, improvements in medical technology and the development of new drugs to treat previously incurable conditions.

Prior to 1880, a random patient, with a random illness, meeting a random doctor could expect more than a 50-50 chance of being *harmed*. Between 1880 and 1912 his chances were even; and after that year the odds were in his favor, stated Dr. Alan Gregg, Director of the Rockefeller Institute for Medical Research in 1953. For these improvements we can thank Louis Pasteur, who proved the germ origin of infectious disease; Lord Joseph Lister, who, acting on Pasteur's discovery, developed sterile techniques which saved millions of lives; and Wilhelm Roentgen, who discovered x-rays. Thus diagnosis became more precise, and surgery safer.

"Any rational individual will agree that, on the whole, modern medical practices have done vastly more good than harm," wrote David M. Spain, M.D., Professor of Pathology, State University of New York, in his 1963 book *Complications of Modern Medical Practices*, the first comprehensive account of adverse results. However, some current critics argue that the newer advances in medicine have done more harm than good. Ivan Illich, the philosopher-author of *Medical Nemesis* and *Disabling Professions*, Rick Carlson, who wrote *The End of Medicine*, and Robert Mendelsohn, author of *Confessions of a Medical Heretic*, affirm that doctor and hospital-induced illness cause more disability and death than can be counter-balanced by the obvious benefit of many diagnostic and therapeutic procedures.

Although these anti-doctor diatribes provoke thought, they lose much of their validity by making broad generalizations from very few cases (anecdotism). They fail to recognize the positive aspects of appropriate medical and surgical intervention. In response to my question regarding treatment of severe trauma, during a recent seminar at Northwestern University, Illich remarked that neurosurgical management of head injuries would be largely unnecessary if we did not have mechanized transport and industry! And Mendelsohn advises against the immunization of children, even with polio vaccine.

The purpose of this book is to promote the good and diminish the harmful effects of modern medical practice. It will provide consumers with accurate information on "diseases of medical progress" which comes from research and long observation of colleagues, hospitals, and patients.

1.

MEDICAL CARE AND THE RISK OF IATROGENESIS

Most diagnostic and therapeutic procedures are necessary and effective. On balance the good exceeds the harm. Our life expectancy is at an all-time high and continues to rise. Americans and West Europeans born this year can anticipate a life span to 72-76 years, 25 years more than in 1900. We have more relief from pain, shorter hospital stays and less time lost from production because of illness. During the first 30 years of this century, the progress was due to greatly improved living conditions, hygiene, nutrition and immunization. In the past 50 years, advances in diagnosis, treatment, and especially lifestyle have added to longevity, despite the deterioration in our environment. Our greatest killers, in descending order, have been coronary heart disease, cancer and stroke. Although cancer has increased, coronary disease and stroke have shown almost 30% *decrease* in mortality in the United States since 1968. Most investigators attribute this saving of almost a million lives to improved nutrition and physical fitness, and early diagnosis and treatment of high blood pressure. But under certain circumstances, medical intervention can be a two-edged sword.

High Technology And High Risk

In the decade of the '70s, chemical, electronic and nuclear technology produced space-age procedures of extreme complexity and cost which can cause severe adverse effects and sometimes fatal complications. Even when these mysterious tests provide answers to diagnostic riddles, they often penetrate the body with some danger and do not help to cure a disease or reduce the patient's suffering.

Every body-invasive procedure and every drug carries the risk of adverse results—those from medication are called "side" effects or reactions. (The founder of one of the largest drug firms in the world once remarked, "A drug without toxic effects is no drug at all.") Modern diagnostic methods, pharmacology and surgical procedures are much more powerful and invasive than older techniques. They therefore produce more frequent and more severe adverse effects—just as automobiles cause more accidents with more serious consequences than did horse-drawn carriages. Physicians must calculate the harm-benefit ratio before undertaking any diagnostic or therapeutic maneuver—remembering their Hippocratic Oath, "Primum non nocere" (first, do no harm).

Several years of clinical trials precede the release of new instruments and drugs by the Food and Drug Administration (FDA). Despite this scrutiny, adverse effects are sometimes not noticed, recorded, and/or published until drugs have been used for many years in hundreds of thousands of patients. Unfortunately, many doctors and hospitals frequently adopt new techniques of unproven efficacy and safety, repeating medical blunders of the past while accelerating their cash flow. The investment pays off for the doctor and hospital, but not always for the patient.

Lewis Thomas, president of Memorial Sloan-Kettering Cancer Center in New York and a prolific and thoughtful medical philosopher-researcher, recently scrutinized the alleged benefits of high technology in medicine. He concluded that it has been oversold. Except for spectacular changes in the management of some (non-hospital-acquired) infectious diseases, only a few significant advances have been made and these entail relatively simple techniques. We now can effectively treat some cases of acute childhood leukemia and other cancers, replace hormone deficiencies caused by diabetes and reproductive organ disorders, prevent and/or treat anemia and jaundice of the newborn, and perform better surgery because of advances in anesthesia and in our understanding of body chemistry. He concluded that "we are left with the same roster of common major diseases which confronted the country in 1950 . . . we have accumulated a formidable body of knowledge about some of them . . . not yet sufficient to permit either the prevention or the outright cure of any of them."

New treatments are not necessarily better than old. Multiple tests do not assure better diagnosis; however, staff review committees have encouraged doctors to over-order such tests to ensure thoroughness, and approval by the Joint Commission on Accreditation of Hospitals (JCAH). However, a reversal of this trend began in 1981 when Blue Cross/Blue Shield withheld payment for many routine "shotgun" tests and obsolete procedures.

"Diagnostic overkill," the performance of more and/or costlier tests than are actually needed for patient benefit, occurs for various reasons. Many of these unnecessary procedures are dictated by hospital by-laws. (Physicians who have personally experienced hospitalization frequently complain about "diagnostic overkill" when they are on the receiving end.) Also, attending doctors, like Caesar's wife, wish to appear above reproach by avoiding even the suspicion of carelessness. Errors of omission as well as commission can lead to malpractice litigation. Some wish to impress their patients by their thoroughness. They need to confirm an uncertain diagnosis or test the reliability of a new procedure.

As a practicing pathologist, I observed that the younger, least-experienced physicians ordered the most tests. This has been confirmed by studies in several prestigious hospitals. Scattergun screening procedures (in baffling cases, in routine preventive "health" examinations, or in so-called cancer prevention examinations in asymptomatic persons) frequently disclose unexpected, doubtful or borderline chemical abnormalities. A slightly elevated blood sugar level can create the suspicion of diabetes, and elevated urea nitrogen level can suggest kidney disease. These simple automated tests are then repeated, and if the results are the same, more sophisticated, costlier, and perhaps invasive tests are ordered. The original out-of-line results might now revert to normal, but other tests may show new irregularities. Now both doctor and patient are distressed and frustrated. The patient is launched into an exhaustive search for an underlying disease, a maelstrom called the "Ulysses Syndrome."* The mental and physical disorders which follow a false-positive result are reminiscent of Ulysses' torturous 20-year voyage home from the Trojan War. During his travels he was involved in a series of needless, often hair-raising, and sometimes dangerous adventures. The healthy and sick alike make a long journey through a medical morass and, like Ulysses, experience a number of unpleasant adventures along the way.

There are at least ten syndromes which stem from relying on laboratory tests rather than on the patient's history and physical exam, according to a 1980 report in the *American Journal of Medicine*. One of these is the "Chicken Little Syndrome," which is described as: "The false-positive result (acorn) which strikes the physician (Chicken Little), causing great excitement about the fascinating case of Addison's disease (adrenal failure), or pheochromocytoma (adrenal tumor)." The author concluded that physicians, like Henny Penny, must be wary of false-positive results and misinterpretation of laboratory data. The patient becomes apprehensive and neurotic, and the physician frustrated, while expenses escalate. Rarely is an actual cause disclosed, and still less often can medical intervention alter prognosis favorably.

It is important to know that all treatments for cancer, chiefly chemical and radiological, and even some surgical procedures, can induce other cancers. Also, antibiotics can cure certain infections, but frequently have undesirable "side" effects and may provoke other infections. All drugs have dangers in varying degrees. Know the names of the medicines you have taken and are now taking, and advise your doctor of past and present adverse reactions such as rash, nausea, vomiting or dizziness. Each of us responds differently to treatment, whether medical, surgical or radiological.

Be wary of your physician's eagerness to try new techniques which he

---

*So-named by Dr. Mercer Rang, in 1972.

has just read about in a journal, heard of at a meeting or learned about from an equipment or drug salesman who dispenses free samples. Although the Food and Drug Administration and pharmaceutical companies urge doctors to report untoward reactions, many adverse effects and even large-scale disasters like the thalidomide tragedy which resulted in monstrous defects in newborns have at least temporarily been covered up. Physicians and drug companies have feared the consequences of unfavorable public response and resultant malpractice suits.

You must question the necessity for any surgery. Don't let yourself be subjected to complex, sophisticated procedures performed by small hospitals and laboratories which do not do them often enough to acquire expertise. Be sure your doctor fully informs you of the rationale and risks of all your diagnostic procedures and treatments, especially if they are new.

Be aware that childbirth is not an illness. Unless there is a serious problem such as pelvic disproportion or a medical complication such as toxemia, home delivery in some areas is even safer than that done in a hospital, where infection and emotional trauma reside, despite the recent development of homelike "birthing" rooms.

Throughout history, many medical thinkers have understood that serious damage could be caused by drugs and surgery. Actually, until 100 years ago, there was no proof or logic behind most medical practices. Medical mistakes were notorious—Molière, in the 17th century, added doctors to his long list of impostors in his satirical plays which still rank among the most scathing literary condemnations of fakery. In the 18th century, Voltaire scoffed, "Doctors pour medicines about which they know little, for diseases about which they know less, into people about whom they know nothing." Our third President, Thomas Jefferson, had great respect for science and believed in the importance of medicine to the national welfare. But "physicians," he said, "should not substitute presumption for knowledge. . . . we may safely affirm that the ignorant and presumptuous band of medical tyros destroys more of human life in one year than all outlaws do in a hundred."

In the 1840s, Dr. Oliver Wendell Holmes, father of the Supreme Court Justice, claimed that childbed fever was caused by infection carried on doctors' hands from autopsies to the patient. His views were violently opposed by his colleagues. A few years later, in Vienna, Dr. Ignatz Semmelweis discovered that the death rate of women delivered by hospital physicians was 1 in 8, by hospital midwives, 1 in 40, while those delivered at home seldom became ill at all. Incredibly, of the 183,955 newborns admitted to the Vienna Children's Hospital between 1784 and 1838, 146,920, or almost 80% died. Because Dr. Semmelweis urged doctors to wash their hands he was ridiculed even more furiously than was Dr.

Holmes and was driven insane. Dr. Holmes is also remembered for his caustic remark, "If all the materia medica as used today were thrown to the bottom of the sea it would be all the better for mankind and worse for the fishes." Millions of lives were needlessly lost until surgical cleanliness and asepsis (antiseptic or sterile conditions) were generally adopted towards the end of the 19th century.

Before the Victorian era was over, science and scepticism had caused most of the futile treatments of the past to be abandoned: opening the skull to release demons thought to cause headaches and insanity, "bleeding" for a variety of ailments, the outdoor treatment of pneumonia, cold tub baths for typhoid, violent catharsis to eliminate unhealthy "humors," starving fevers and withholding water for cholera. Sir William Osler, Chief Physician of Johns Hopkins Hospital and later Regius Professor of Medicine at Oxford, found only about a dozen drugs to recommend to his students. "Man is distinguished from the animals," he said, "by his desire to take medicine."

Where Does Iatrogenesis Lurk?

Although your life expectancy exceeds your grandfather's, your iatrogenic risks also exceed his. During the past 25 years, our chances of surviving catastrophic illness or accidents have been improved by techniques for dialysis; kidney transplants using potent drugs to suppress rejection; intensive and coronary care units (ICU and CCU) with dehumanizing life-support and monitoring equipment which looks like a cross between an airplane control tower and an updated version of Dr. Frankenstein's laboratory; burn units and trauma centers. Nevertheless, Murphy's Law—anything that can go wrong will—is applicable to these complex facilities.

The United States is in the midst of an unacknowledged iatrogenic epidemic little suspected by the public. A few figures will illustrate its dimensions. One-and-a-half million (3.5%) hospital admissions in this country are due to reactions to prescribed drugs. Once in the hospital, 18-30% develop additional drug reactions, doubling the length of their stay. In fact, out of 67 deaths in one hospital, one in four were drug-related. Hospital infections occur in 5% of patients, causing a 25% increase in mortality. Seven percent of postoperative wounds become infected. Over 20% of patients in non-surgical units of teaching hospitals suffer iatrogenic mishaps and of these, over one-fourth are due to diagnostic and therapeutic procedures. One recent report stated that over 12% of ICU admissions were for iatrogenic disease, half of which were considered preventable. And once in an ICU, iatrogenic events multiply and are associated with 10% of hospital deaths (as we shall see in later chapters).

Theodore White, in writing *In Search of History*, proposed the "Law of

Unanticipated Consequences" which he applied to social and political innovations. It is equally applicable to medicine, for it is impossible to foresee the final longterm result of any new drug or medical, surgical, x-ray or laboratory procedure. Who could have foretold that many pioneer radiologists and their patients would die of x-ray-induced cancer; or that the "miracle drugs"—sulfonamides, penicillin and their antibiotic successors—would result in the evolution of resistant strains of bacteria (chiefly pus-formers and intestinal organisms) which withstand current treatments? Some of these bacteria exist primarily in hospitals and are seldom found elsewhere. They are carried by hospital personnel, including doctors and nurses, and have the potential for infecting patients and visitors.

Not all iatrogenic damage is preventable, but some is caused by ignorance, error and carelessness. Too often greed (perhaps subconscious) is the motive for unnecessary surgery, diagnostic tests, and consultations which compound risk. No specialty is immune. Sometimes four or more doctors collaborate on a single case. This may lead to divided, overlapping responsibility and incompatible treatment.

Surgical mishaps, although not as numerous as those due to drugs, cause more dramatic damage. Historically, many blunders have occurred which were not recognized until years later. I remember the fruitless tying of the breast arteries to relieve and prevent heart pain (angina), started and discarded in the 1930s. Postoperative and post-delivery patients were confined to bed for two weeks until the 1940s, delaying recovery and enhancing the possibility of fatal blood clots in the lungs. The wartime shortage of doctors and hospital beds prompted earlier discharge with the discovery that earlier mobility hastened healing. An expensive and dangerous freezing technique was used in the 1960s to "cure" stomach ulcers. Radical mastectomy for breast cancer is currently under attack, led by Dr. George Crile, Jr., of Cleveland. Although standard since 1895, it has a higher death rate, causes more mutilation and emotional trauma, and produces no more cures than simpler operations. When I suggested to several powerfully entrenched surgeons that they reconsider the radical operation, I was subjected to personal and professional criticism. My opinion was confirmed by a recently published 30-year study at the Princess Margaret Hospital of Toronto, which proved that as many patients survive with removal of the tumor only (lumpectomy) and follow-up x-ray therapy as with the radical operation.

Chemotherapy and radiotherapy are more powerful now than ever. Catheters invade the heart and even the coronary arteries. Flexible fiber-optic and illuminated cylindrical instruments permit visualization of the digestive tract, bronchi, bladder, vagina and abdominal cavity. They even permit minor surgery, such as tying the fallopian tubes for sterilization. Opaque substances are taken by mouth and rectum, and dyes are injected for x-ray studies outlining the liver, gallbladder, kidneys, urinary bladder, blood vessels, spinal cord and brain. Large needles puncture the bone marrow, liver, breast, lungs, spleen, amniotic sac (bag of fluid surrounding the fetus), spinal fluid space and kidneys to remove samples for chemical and microscopic study. Air injections accentuate x-ray examination of the brain and adrenal glands.

None of these invasive manipulations is without hazard. Accidents occur even with the best management and without ignorance, carelessness or willful misconduct. The most dedicated, experienced doctors who would never use unacceptable methods cannot completely shield their patients from risk. Moreover, if a hospital performs less than 100 of a given invasive procedure annually, the percentage of deaths will be eight times greater than in a hospital doing at least 400 annually.

Adverse drug reactions are the most frequent iatrogenic mishaps. They generally are less spectacular, disabling or fatal than surgical, radiological or invasive casualties. However, hundreds of deaths, mostly of children, occurred in the late 1930s, when toxic diethylene glycol (a component of anti-freeze) was used to put sulfonamide, an early antibiotic, into liquid form because youngsters have difficulty swallowing tablets or capsules. The thalidomide tragedy of the '60s is another striking example of iatrogenic disease.

Unconscious pecuniary motivation rather than overt greed may influence an apparently ethical surgeon to perform unnecessary and more extensive operations than required. I have known incidents in small community hospitals where influential surgeons have tried to institute sanctions against members of the watch-dog committees mandated by the Joint Commission on Accreditation of Hospitals to determine the justification for certain operations. One Chief Surgeon, informed that 22% of his appendectomies were unnecessary, as were 30% of his gallbladder removals, became enraged. (At that time the JCAH considered 5% a reasonable limit.) He attempted to induce the Board of Directors and the Staff Executive Committee to fire or force the resignation of his fancied enemies!

The grim history of radiation injury began early in this century, when scores of pioneer radiologists and their associates contracted and died of cancer. Others were disabled by the scars of internal and external burns. Despite these forewarning calamities, learned by all medical students, excessive radiotherapy continued. Hundreds of thyroid cancers, many fatal, have developed in young adults who may have forgotten or never have known that they were subjected to x-rays 20 to 30 years ago for minor ailments such as enlarged tonsils and adenoids, acne, and ringworm. Standards for x-ray equipment and usage have recently improved, but only after FDA inspectors found many new devices faulty and capable of causing excessive doses. This is particularly dangerous for pregnant women because it may cause birth defects in the fetus and later, cancer.

Even a blood test in a doctor's office can result in a local or general infection, including hepatitis, if the needles and skin are improperly sterilized. Last year I had a cortisone injection for tennis elbow. This resulted in a nasty, painful, red, hot, swollen "staph" infection which extended down my right forearm and required two large incisions to drain the purulent material. I became quite ill with a fever of 103 degrees and generalized debility. The antibiotics my orthopedic colleague later prescribed may have controlled the infection, but they caused violent abdominal cramping, pain and diarrhea. This mishap could have been ample cause for a malpractice suit.

Blood sampling for multiple tests by daily vein puncture can result in anemia during a prolonged stay in a hospital. Although unusual, some patients have required transfusion, with added risks.

In recent history many thoughtful American physicians have been concerned about iatrogenesis. In 1914, Dr. E. A. Codman, of the Massachusetts General Hospital, was the first to assert that medical and surgical *results* should be monitored. He felt that hospital efficiency should be rated by the outcome of patients' illnesses rather than by the quality of the doctors' and nurses' notes. Records of behind-the-scenes departments such as laundry, dietetics, and maintenance were even less important at that time. Although Dr. Codman knew the aftermath of treatment in his small private hospital, he agreed that it would not be possible then to do the same in larger, mostly public institutions.

Is such monitoring possible—and performed—today? Despite technological and administrative progress, hospitals now are still rated and approved by the JCAH, specialty societies, and governmental agencies on the basis of paper performance, such as having the proper committees and staff organization by process instead of outcome.

Many critics have felt that iatrogenesis would decrease if difficult or unusual operations were performed primarily at specialized centers. However a 1979 study showed that this would be true only in such technically difficult cases as transplants of organs, heart and vessel surgery, and neurosurgery. The more common operations on the intestine, uterus, gallbladder and lungs are as successful in low-volume hospitals with approved staffs.

How Much Has Iatrogenesis Increased?

There are instances in the course of a serious illness when the attending physician must decide that risky diagnosis or treatment action must begin immediately and that "the buck stops here." Calculated risks regarding the harm/benefit ratio must be taken and accepted; adverse effects may be unavoidable. Despite such careful consideration, physician and hospital-induced complications have multiplied in the past 25 years.

The first authoritative and prophetic modern warning was made by Dr. David P. Barr, Chief of Medicine at Cornell University's New York Hospital, in his address to the AMA convention in 1955. "Unfortunate sequelae (results) and accidents," he said, "attributed to well-intentioned diagnosis and treatment, were noted in 5% of patients admitted to medical wards." Dr. Barr was particularly concerned with the dangers lurking in the then budding high technology.

In 1964, Dr. E. M. Schimmel of Yale's Grace-New Haven Hospital found that 20% of patients studied had complications in an 8-month period. He felt that the increased use, potency and complexity of drugs, invasive diagnosis and the aging of the patient population were the most important reasons for this new epidemic. And in 1966, Dr. L. G. Seidl showed that 17% of Johns Hopkins Hospital admissions suffered one or more *drug reactions* alone, increasing with patient age. It is likely that data from these large comprehensive (tertiary) care hospitals will differ from that of smaller, less sophisticated community hospitals. In 1971 Dr. Oscar Thorup of the Mayo Clinic added that 20% of hospital admissions, have at least one medical or hospital-induced complication before discharge. The risk is intensified, he feels, by multiple procedures. For example, most patients have 20-40 tests and frequently are given many different drugs.

Dr. N. P. Couch of Harvard's renowned Peter Bent Brigham Hospital studied mishaps in large bowel surgery alone during 1978. In 16 incorrectly treated patients, the mortality was increased ten-fold, the cost seven times, and the length of hospitalization four times. In 1981, Dr. Couch published another paper about mishaps at the same hospital: of 5,600 surgical admissions in one year, he studied only the 2,500 general surgery cases, omitting orthopedics, thoracic, cardiac, urologic, neurologic, ear, nose and throat, and eye surgery. Thirty-six *avoidable* errors were discovered, twenty-three of which were initiated in another hospital from which patients were transferred. Surgical "misadventures" occurred in one of 156 patients about once every ten days. Twenty of these 36 patients died in Peter Bent Brigham Hospital, 11 directly due to surgical errors. Of the 16 survivors, 5 were permanently impaired; only 11 fully recovered. The average time spent in the hospital was 42 days, and ranged from 1 to 325 days. The costs of hospitalization varied from $3,400 to $342,000—and the *total* cost came to $1,703,402. Those who died had incurred charges averaging $1,400 and the survivors, "only" $700 per day. It is the futile attempt to maintain life by extraordinary means that doubles cost.

The total *excess* cost was $1,300,000 or $40,000 per patient and $1,000 per patient day. "These 36 patients represent a very low proportion of the total, but it's a complete disaster for the patient and his family," said Dr. Couch.*

In 1981, Dr. Knight Steel studied 815 consecutive medical cases at the Boston University Medical Center, excluding cancer, which bears a large risk of adverse results from chemotherapy. *Thirty-six percent* of these, or 290, developed iatrogenic illness. Nine percent of the 815 had life-threatening complications or were left permanently disabled. Two percent died. These 290 patients suffered 497 adverse incidents; in 305 of these patients lives were threatened or they risked permanent impairment. Patients who were transferred from nursing homes or from other acute care hospitals had more *unavoidable* iatrogenic mishaps than those admitted directly from their homes, as were those sent to the intensive care unit and coronary care unit. Older patients, those given multiple drugs, and those who remained in the hospital for longer stays also had an increased number of mishaps. Patients with major complications averaged 19 hospital days, eight days before the incident and 11 after; patients without complications averaged 5.6 days.

Dr. Steel defined as iatrogenic any illness resulting from diagnosis or therapy and including incidents such as falls and bedsores, which are not natural consequences of disease. He added that iatrogenesis is not necessarily due to culpability of the physician or hospital, nor are all mishaps preventable. They are natural hazards of modern medicine.

Causes of iatrogenic events, according to Dr. Steel's study:

Drugs	208
Diagnostic tests and treatment	175
Diet, nursing, transportation	79
Heart catheterization	45
Intravenous treatment	34
Arteriography and dialysis	30
Urinary catheterization	10
Miscellaneous	114

It is evident that over a quarter of a century after Dr. Barr's original report, and despite, or *because of*, all of the advances in equipment, pharmacology, and diagnostic techniques, medical (non-surgical) risks have increased up to seven times. Patients now admitted to hospitals are routinely given urinalysis, blood counts, multiple blood chemical tests and frequently, x-ray examinations of the chest and electrocardiograms. Attending physicians may prescribe other less common and more compli-

*The precise nature and causes for these mishaps will be discussed in the chapter on surgery.

cated tests, depending on hints from the patient's history and physical examination. This "probing for causes" may lead to early diagnosis and treatment with new drugs, devices or surgery, which may be dangerous. In some cases, sufficient evidence is not yet available about their adverse effects. There is also scant evidence of increased effectiveness.

In 1979 a Canadian Task Force reported the most comprehensive evaluation of the periodic health exam. Packages were developed for various age groups and for individuals at high risk, rather than applying all tests and examinations indiscriminately. Great savings and increased efficiency were found also by the American College of Physicians by tailoring programs to the apparently healthy individual's history, age and sex.

Hospitals now have utilization committees which attempt to reduce unnecessary admissions and prolonged stays. Thus, admissions are now more inclined to include the more seriously ill patients, and the likelihood of medical or surgical intervention is enhanced, which increases the risk of iatrogenesis. These risks generally are not manifest during the first day but may become evident after the first week. It must be presumed that the benefits outweigh the risks, given the severity of the illness, its natural progress, and the value of alternative, perhaps safer therapy.

The attending physician must often take a calculated risk in choosing his handling of each case. To complicate the duties of the staff doctor, the JCAH sends inspectors every year or two to check results of surveys by surgical, tissue, infection control and other committees, which may rob members of the medical staff of valuable time. Processing records is emphasized rather than patient outcome. Therefore, we need new methods to monitor the real values of hospitalization *to the patient*. This must be accomplished continuously with a minimum of costly outside interference.

The late Dr. Franz Ingelfinger, an independent and respected thinker, editor of the *New England Journal of Medicine* and Professor of Medicine at Harvard, emphasized the role of iatrogenesis in 1977.

> Let us assume that 80% of patients have either self-limited disorders or conditions not improvable, even by modern medicine. In slightly over 10% of the cases, however, medical intervention is dramatically successful . . . But, alas, in the final 9%, give or take a point or two, the doctor may diagnose or treat inadequately, or he may just have bad luck. Whatever the reason, the patient ends up with iatrogenic problems. So the balance of accounts ends up on the positive side of zero.

Medical and hospital care costs rose an unprecedented 15.1% in 1981 over 1980—almost 10% of the Gross National Product. *Usual and customary fees* have exploded under the permissive regulations of Blue Cross/Blue Shield and governmental payers such as Medicare-Medicaid.

The impersonal third-party bureaucracy dispenses seemingly unlimited funds.

Medicine is now the nation's largest industry, far exceeding Defense.

2.

MEDICAL RIP-OFFS: PAIN IN YOUR POCKETBOOK

The soaring cost of medical care is one of the greatest problems now facing American consumers. The average family's medical bill, even without catastrophic illness, is staggering. The medical industry has made a tremendous effort to justify this huge national expense by pointing to the scientific advances made in curing disease by early detection through new diagnostic techniques; larger, better equipped facilities; costly, intricate instruments; and better trained and paid hospital personnel. All of this is supposed to save thousands of lives annually.

While medical economists estimate that the U.S. has spent $287 billion on "health" care in 1981, 24 times more than in 1950 when only $12 billion was spent, there is growing evidence that this added expenditure is not the reason Americans are now living longer and enjoying healthier lives.

Information (apparently largely ignored by the public) shows that we make great sacrifices to pay for needless tests and treatment in the name of "health" care, while doctors and health institutions are generally aware of the great waste involved in many of these procedures. For example, while almost all doctors subject their patients to regular check-ups to "prevent" illness, or more precisely, to detect disease in its earliest stages, physicians do not subject themselves or their families to regular check-ups. They know what recent studies have shown: the outcomes of most illnesses are not influenced by the number or types of tests performed. Thus, if a person has no signs or history of disease, only a few inexpensive tests are diagnostically useful.

The medical establishment advocates many procedures to cater to the national obsession with extensive medical care. Respected critics within the profession have written many articles stating that this dependency has been spawned by the over-selling of diagnostic procedures and tests.

Medical costs, like those of other industries, rise with demand. The public is enthralled by sophisticated equipment for "prevention," detection, and cure; however, most will not take the time or responsibility to maintain their own health. Many of us have learned to rely on the medical establishment, with all of its impressive apparatus, instead of leading sensible, healthy lives. And we do not even follow the practice of our own doctors of avoiding unnecessary examinations and tests.

In 1978, more than 200 physicians attended a symposium at Northwestern University. When asked how many submitted to routine check-ups, only three raised their hands. Most felt that they would rather not know if they were going to die of some rare hidden disease in fifteen or twenty years! They recognized that a "clean bill of health" gives a false sense of security. When asked why they recommended periodic check-ups when they knew such check-ups don't improve health or longevity, several replied, "You know it and I know it, but the public doesn't know it. And if I don't do it, they'll go to someone who will."

During 1977 and 1978, I served as Consulting Physician to a Cancer Prevention Center in Chicago, which has been in operation since 1937. Who knows how many hapless thousands have endured its comprehensive, 2-day testing? All receive the same tedious tests, regardless of age or risk factors. The clinic had a zealous public relations department which actively solicited TV and radio time, extolling the value of its head-to-toe examinations. Every human orifice was probed, peeked into, and sometimes swabbed. Youths were subjected to the same examination of the lower bowel (sigmoidoscopy) as middle-aged men and women, although their risk of cancer is negligible. And, of course, all women received Pap tests for cervical cancer even if they were virgins or had no cervix because of previous surgery.

But despite warehouseloads of data, the Clinic had never conducted any surveys to determine whether or not people who have been examined annually over a period of years have had longer or better quality lives than a similar population who did not undergo this ritual. Despite several attempts by its physicians to conduct examinations tailored to fit high or low-risk individuals, the Clinic's Board of Directors refused to modify its methods. And so indoctrinated were some of its clients that many thought a dire disease would strike them if they skipped an annual session. One affluent lady in her 60s told me tearfully that her husband was now helpless because of a stroke: "And I know it happened because I didn't insist that he have his examination last year."

The Life Extension Institute was created by Dr. E. L. Fisk in the early 1900s. Insurance companies were quick to subscribe to his belief that periodic examination could not only detect, but prevent and lead to the cure of chronic, unseen disease. If true, this would enable them to achieve greater profits. But there was no evidence to support the "curative component," or alter the outcome of the hidden diseases. This "bottom line" would not be tested and found to be fallacious for 50 years.

THE MYTHOLOGIZING OF THE ANNUAL PHYSICAL

"Prevention" has been growing in importance since the 1920s, when periodic examinations were endorsed by the American Medical Association and the U.S. Public Health Association with the slogan, "Have a Health Examination on Your Birthday" which aimed at a goal of 10 million examinations during the first year. There were few dissenters who wondered how the "inroads of certain progressive chronic diseases" could be influenced by the therapy available at that time. The Depression halted this movement, but the myth that asymptomatic adults, harboring hidden disease, could be benefited by the annual physical was revived with greater enthusiasm after World War II.

What is prevention? Despite growing skepticism and recent contrary evidence which has appeared in media available to the consumer, the annual or semi-annual "physical" has been optimistically promoted as a deterrent to disease, a prolonger of life, a saver of money, and a profitable enterprise. Tailoring examinations to fit the needs of different age groups and individuals with various risk factors is seldom considered. Its merits continue to be proclaimed by many doctors, clinics, cancer prevention centers, health spas, hospitals, labor unions, businesses hoping to reduce their health insurance expenditures, insurance companies, and governmental agencies. Advances in electronics and computerization have been accompanied by increases in the number of blood and chemical tests, EKGs, and Pap smears.

All this detection is supposed to reassure us that we will attain well-being, prevent disease and perhaps be rewarded by a "clean bill of health." The only bill you get, however, will be from the clinic or the doctor. A 1965 University of Pennsylvania report told of 350 executives who died between annual examinations done by 10 different clinics. Only half of the diseases causing death, including coronary heart and blood vessel disease, cancer, and depressive suicides were diagnosed or anticipated by "check-up" (only 43% of the fatal cancers were detected). And even if all of the fatal diseases had been detected, it is probable that their outcomes could not have been altered in most cases.

The largest of the group health organizations—the Health Insurance Plan in New York and the Kaiser Permanente Foundation in California—have studied the longevity of hundreds of thousands of their members who were subjected to annual physical examinations over the past 25 years. The studies indicated that individuals who had routine examinations did not have longer or better quality lives than did similar numbers of people who were not given examinations.

Check-up costs for the well or worried well vary from $150 to $400, to which may be added the expense of hotel and hospital, travel, spa facilities, and loss of work time. The national bill of health was estimated at $20 billion annually in 1975 (it is much greater now) by Dr. James Fries in his book *Take Care of Yourself.* In some cases the apprehension caused by early diagnosis merely lengthens the period of lessened quality of life—while treatment, which may prove ineffective, is prolonged and more costly.

Often, a routine check-up will elicit a slightly abnormal result in one of many tests. These variations demand repeated tests plus elaborate and more costly procedures for confirmation. Thus the spiral ascends, and the hapless victim is subjected to expensive, possibly invasive diagnostic procedures, including unproductive biopsies. With rare exception, this quest ends up finding nothing, or worse, finding an incurable, untreatable disease. During this time, the patient and his family are beset by anxiety, expense, loss of time, referrals to specialists, and frustration.

A real-life example of the "Ulysses Syndrome" is embodied in the trials of a healthy athletic, 40ish attorney I know who, despite his usual skepticism, was brain-washed by the slogan "Fight Cancer with a Check and a Check-Up." During his first examination, he had a complete physical, x-ray tests, urine analysis, and multiphasic screening (multiple blood chemical analysis).

Then,

> several weeks later, Joe was upset by a letter informing him that his blood urea nitrogen (BUN) was slightly elevated and that he should consult a doctor to rule out serious kidney disease. A prominent kidney specialist re-examined him and ordered additional tests. Joe now developed anxiety and insomnia. More intricate, expensive and time-consuming kidney function tests of the blood and urine were conducted. All were negative, except for the continued mildly high urea nitrogen. Next, the doctors injected his arm vein with a dye which concentrates in the kidney. (Within seconds, the dye outlines the kidney so that clear x-ray films can be viewed.)
>
> Joe's right kidney was found to be distorted, suggesting a tumor and he was admitted to a hospital for an arteriogram. While tests and examinations were repeated, Joe was stricken with fear and slept poorly, despite the sedatives he now required. In the morning, he was given a copious enema, high in the bowel. He was placed on a litter and once more wheeled into the x-ray department. After novocain was injected into the skin of his right groin, a scalpel incision was made to expose the femoral artery, the main artery of the leg. A long, flexible, slender tube (catheter) was inserted upward into this artery from groin to the approximate level of the lowest rib. It entered the main artery from the heart (aorta) and under fluoroscopic observation it was thrust higher and manipulated into the artery of the right kidney. A dye was now injected (painfully) through the catheter to fill the branches of this kidney artery.
>
> The dye outlined the blood supply to the kidney, and the radiologist's pic-

tures showed only a harmless extra branch of the artery which was compressing and distorting part of that organ. It had no relation to any disease, nor did it cause the elevated urea nitrogen. The doctors conferred and told Joe that his elevated urea was purely "incidental" and was probably caused by his high protein diet and strenuous exercise. He was discharged the day after he entered, with only a slight pain in his right groin to remind him of his ordeal, and doctor and hospital bills that came to $958.36.

Two days later, Joe found a tender, throbbing lump, an inch and a half in diameter, under the skin, at the site of the sutured groin incision. He promptly called his specialist, who arranged for him to meet with a blood vessel surgeon within the hour in the emergency room. He was re-examined and re-admitted, this time to determine whether he had blood clot from a minor leakage of the injured artery or a more serious complication of the procedure—an aneurysm. (An aneurysm is a thin-walled, sac-like ballooning of an artery which can readily rupture, causing massive hemorrhage and possible death.)

After even more complicated tests, the verdict was that the damage was merely a pulsating blood clot which would heal spontaneously in six to eight weeks, while he limited his activities. And for this new misadventure, all he would have to show would be a residual lumpy scar and an additional bill for $536.42.

Joe returned home, his week in shambles. Several important clients could not wait, and took their problems elsewhere. His doubts about the value of routine examination were confirmed and enhanced. He and his medical advisers had embarked on a futile, quixotic quest—a blood chemical abnormality in search of a disease! He had joined the ranks of the victims of iatrogenesis caused by "scattergun" testing.

After healing, Joe has continued his strenuous physical activities, including the completion of several marathons. Recently, out of sheer curiosity, he had a blood urea test again. It was still slightly elevated, but this time the doctor did not hazard any further suggestions.

A colleague told me about Martin,

a 50-year-old active food wholesaler, a non-drinker and non-smoker who was an enthusiastic skiier and mountaineer. At a club where he played racquetball four times weekly, he became acquainted with a physician who learned that he had never had a "check-up" since discharge from the army 25 years previously. Martin was persuaded to undergo this costly ceremonial. And thus, a vigorous, symptomless "jock" was transformed into a neurotic patient by abnormalities that showed up in the lab tests. Two blood chemical components with jaw-breaking names, abbreviated SGOT and SGPT, were slightly elevated, suggesting the possibility of liver damage (which has risen to become the seventh leading cause of death in the U.S.). The tests were repeated and the same elevations of the chemicals were found. Multiple referrals to specialists, x-ray examinations and consultations followed, with much personal and family distress. Martin was then sent to the famed medical mecca, the Mayo Clinic, with more probing for causes. The second time, under local anesthesia, a wide bore needle was inserted through skin and muscle into his liver and a cylinder of tissue was removed. Microscopic examination revealed old, healed scarring (cirrhosis) of the liver, with no sign of active inflammation. The specialists concluded that at some time in the past, perhaps while in the army, he had contracted mild, symptomless liver inflammation (hepatitis) which had "burnt out" but left knobby scars.

There was no reason to do anything about this old, healed liver condition. No treatment of any kind or restriction of activity was indicated, nor was it expected to alter the quality or length of his life. He has only a few months of anxiety, insomnia, discomfort, a waste of several thousand dollars, and time lost from his business as a lingering memory of his chance encounter with an over-zealous doctor.

Of course, not everyone goes through so many specialized tests during a routine physical. Some of the most publicized and widely recommended screening tests are considered unnecessary in nonsymptomatic individuals by many renowned medical experts. Today, fewer tests are considered worthwhile, and these are generally not needed annually. *Time* magazine, in 1976, carried the first article to appear in the mass media criticizing routine examinations. The most abused annual tests include the "Pap" smear for cervical cancer, multiphasic blood screening, the EKG and stress tests for heart disease, the x-ray examination of the chest for cancer and other diseases, and the rectal and colon cancer tests, all of which do not lead to better or longer lives *unless the subject is at high risk*. The following section will explain the purpose of each test, who needs them, and when.

The Pap Flap

One of the most overused procedures in medicine is the annual or semi-annual "Pap" test for cervical cancer. The "Pap" test is named for its founder, Dr. George Papanicolaou, who discovered that cancer cells could be identified in smears taken from vaginal mucous secretions, the sputum, urine, and stomach fluid. Although it is simple, harmless, and relatively inexpensive (to the doctor), and it may detect precursors of malignancy, it is not necessary to have one every year after the first two negative tests. While the "Pap" test helps to detect precancer, which can be treated and cured, many of those promoting the test are in a position to capitalize on its overuse. The so-called cancer prevention clinics and entrepreneuring physicians, particularly gynecologists who play on women's natural fears, have helped create the high demand for this test.

After two negative "Pap" tests, the chance of women developing cervical cancer is exceedingly slight. In the first smear, abnormalities, not necessarily cancer, but possibly precancer, occur *five times per 1,000* women tested. However, this includes women at highest risk, those who have had repeated unhygienic sexual contact with multiple partners, usually beginning in their teens. This group is the most likely to contract genital herpes and other conditions which can be precursors to cancer. Monogamous women with monogamous husbands have much less chance of having a positive "Pap" test. Virgins are at least risk.

If the first smear is negative, the chances that the second smear will be positive decline to about five cases per 10,000. In lower risk women, the chance of a positive result declines to about one in 15,000. In succeeding tests, the chance of getting a positive result on the "Pap" test is negligible.

There is no hard evidence that links the "Pap" test to the decline in cervical cancer. Although there has been more than a 50% decline in deaths from this cancer (which kills 7,400 American women annually, or seven per 100,000), half of this decline occurred in the 1930s. The "Pap" smear did not come into general use in the U.S. until the 1950s. Similar pre-Pap declines have been noted in New Zealand and British Columbia. There is tremendous geographic variation in the annual occurrence of *new cases* of cervical cancer. It ranges from 180 per 100,000 in Colombia, South America; to 12 per 100,000 in Israel (including Arab women); and 90 per 100,000 in El Paso, Texas; to 23 per 100,000 in Connecticut. In the more affluent or hygienic areas the greatest number of Pap smears are performed, but the least number of new cases of cervical cancer are found.

In a 1977 article in *Preventive Medicine*, Drs. John W. Gardner and Joseph L. Lyon concluded that "on the basis of all evidence, a causal relation between cytologic screening (the "Pap" test) and the declining mortality and incidence of cervical cancer cannot be established." Better hygiene, birth control, improved gynecologic care, circumcised partners, and an increased number of complete hysterectomies (removal of the womb and cervix) all take part of the credit for reducing the deaths from cervical cancer.

Many critics add that approximately 7% of "Pap" smears have false-positive results. In these cases, the women are told that they may have cancer or precancer, leading to needless mental anguish, repeated testing, and sometimes unnecessary surgery. Conversely, 20 to 30% of women who have atypical or cancerous conditions are erroneously told that they have normal results, permitting potentially curable cancers to spread widely throughout the body until they become incurable.

The recommendation that American women have an annual "Pap" smear has also been challenged by public health researcher Anne-Marie Foltz and Yale epidemiologist, Jennifer Kelsey. They charge that the test became entrenched as a yearly health measure before its merits could be established. At best, they say, institutionalization of the annual "Pap" test has been a "dubious policy success." They add that the cost of mass annual screening, including office visits for women seeing their gynecologists for the annual test, runs into millions. Almost unbelievably, women who have had complete hysterectomies, and those with no sexual experience, are still often urged to have annual "Pap" tests.

Evidence from all developed countries shows that "Pap" tests should be performed less frequently on those in low-risk categories. Over 70 reports in the medical literature have suggested reducing their number and frequency for most women. For the best and most cost-effective results, a Canadian study recommended a smear soon after the first sexual intercourse, and another a year later. If both tests are negative, they should be repeated only every three years until age 35, and every five years thereafter. It generally takes eight to ten years for a pre-cancer (dysplasia) to become a cancer confined *(in situ)* to the lining of the cervix, and a similar period for this *in situ* cancer to spread. The Canadian study also found that the routine pelvic examination, which generally accompanies the smear, was unproductive, since it had not reduced the incidence of death from hidden gynecologic conditions such as ovarian cancer.

In 1980, The American Cancer Society (ACS) revised its guidelines for the cancer-related check-up, recommending that all procedures be done less frequently than in previous years. They still tilt towards conservatism, although I admit there is room for differences of opinion.

Despite the evidence and advice of the carefully documented reports, extensive testing continues. An informal study of physicians found that opinions regarding the desired frequency of the Pap smear varies directly with expected income. Many doctors, especially gynecologists, still recommend semi-annual tests.

A 1975 estimate of the annual cost of Pap tests in the U.S. by Dr. L. W. Copleson of the University of Chicago was put at $1.25 billion, if all women over 23 were screened annually. For the individual, this translates into current figures of about $30 an office visit. The laboratory that examines the smear, incidentally, charges the physician only $2.50 to $4, depending on the volume of work the doctor sends in. If you are billed separately by the laboratory, as you should be, you should be paying from $6 to $8 in lab fees. Actually, a nurse-clinician can obtain the smear as well as a doctor and send it to the same laboratory, and your total bill will be greatly reduced. New methods are now being developed that will allow you to take the smear yourself, saving you everything but lab fees. These are two illustrations of much-needed fundamental changes in medical care delivery on a national level.

The Blood Pressure Test

As recently as 1975, medical skeptics thought that the simple, inexpensive test for high blood pressure was one of the few valuable annual screening procedures. This asymptomatic illness predisposes the individual to heart disease and stroke, our leading causes of premature death. Since it is relatively common and can be effectively treated by weight loss, exercise, salt-free diet and inexpensive medication, annual mass screening for high blood pressure was considered essential.

While this is true of some patients who comply with instructions after being tested, two recent reports have questioned the benefits of mass screening. A 1973 National Institutes of Health survey and another by Dominion Foundry and Steel, Ltd., in Canada showed that when employees learned they had hypertension, their absenteeism doubled, compared to those with normal blood pressure. Absenteeism increased whether or not treatment had begun or was effective. The blood pressure of many patients actually increased following instructions regarding diet, exercise and weight loss, since they generally did not comply with the instruction or take the medication prescribed. Hypochondria and apprehension increased among those who were informed of their hypertension, so the program at Dominion Steel was discontinued because production fell, at great cost to the company and without beneficial effect on general health.

Even motivated patients may not comply with treatment for high blood pressure because of deeply entrenched poor living habits. Businessmen feel they must entertain clients with high-caloric, highly seasoned meals, and social pressures call for similar displays.

It is nevertheless prudent to check the blood pressure of those who may be expected to comply with instructions. Dr. Lester Breslow of the University of California and Anne R. Somers, a New Jersey expert on medical economics and health education, have suggested schedules for blood pressure determination. Since sudden changes in blood pressure are unusual, these determinations need only be performed twice between the ages of 20 and 30, three times between 30 and 40, four times between 40 and 50, five times between 51 and 60, and annually thereafter. In 1976, the Mayo Clinic concurred with this schedule.

When should you become concerned about your blood pressure? If you are under 65, pressures of 150/90 (systolic-expanded/diastolic-contracted), or higher should be reported to a primary care physician for possible treatment. In 1981, the National Heart, Lung and Blood Institute announced that they are considering dropping to 80 the level of diastolic pressure in adults that would indicate concern. This means that one may be at increased risk for heart, stroke and kidney disease. This new definition would add 15 million Americans to the 60 million adults who already have hypertension of varying severity. It is likely that in borderline cases, weight loss, exercise and a salt-free diet will eliminate the need for medication. After 65 or 70, pressures up to 170/100 may not need treatment, but would still require a reliable physician's interpretation. The average case of moderate hypertension can be controlled with only three or four visits per year to a doctor.

Multiple Blood Chemical Screening Tests

Multiphasic testing (for numerous blood chemical components—not blood counts) has become so ritualistic that it may be a substitute for a physician's evaluation. Although it may be of great value in helping to diagnose an illness in those exhibiting symptoms, the now-automated process is of no proven benefit for the nonsymptomatic. It is true that testing of blood samples taken during a periodic check-up may detect unapparent disease. However, there is no evidence that this can in any way affect the outcome.

What good is the discovery that you have a serious but not manifest illness if this knowledge does not increase your chances of improved well-being or recovery? Although it may be of interest to insurance companies or employers, what will it do to the quality of your own life? On February 26, 1980, the *Wall Street Journal* commented "A simple blood test . . . is leading to the diagnosis and treatment of people who didn't know they were sick and, often after evaluation and treatment, neither the doctor nor the patient knows whether the patient is better off."

One of the specious reasons some give to justify multiphasic screening is that among the 12 to 18 chemical tests, the unexpected finding of a high blood calcium level points to overactivity of the parathyroid glands (four small, button-like nodules attached to the thyroid in the lower neck). Severe skeletal softening, digestive tract ulcers and kidney stones may be caused by this excess hormone. Not surprisingly, since these automatic procedures have become standard, there has been a four-fold increase in the diagnosis of overactive parathyroid glands at the Mayo Clinic, half of this in people without symptoms. At the Mayo Clinic 142 persons with symptomless high blood calcium levels were studied; 32 underwent surgery to remove parathyroid tissue. None of these persons, with or without surgery, showed any evidence of bone, digestive or kidney disease after five years and most were well after ten years. They did not have an increased death rate. There was nothing in the original report of high calcium levels to predict which people should or should not undergo surgery. Medical follow-up with multiple chemical tests is costly in time and money, and generates extreme anxiety. These asymptomatic people would have been far better off if the tests had not been done until symptoms appeared.

A University of Utah survey of 574 families, done over a span of years, recently found no difference in health between groups of persons who had been subjected to multiphasic screening and groups not tested. The only difference between screened and non-screened subjects was an increase in time hospitalized for the screened subjects because of test results which suggested the possibility of diseases requiring further investigation. Similar studies in Connecticut, Ohio, California, England and Canada failed to reveal any advantage to the public from such a well-intentioned program.

Despite this evidence, over *12 billion* of these procedures are still performed annually in this country, at a cost to subjects of $4.5 billion. But the monetary aspects are only part of the cost. False-positive and borderline results, mostly involving such chemicals in the blood as sugar, urea nitrogen and uric acid, require repetition to eliminate the possibility of diabetes, kidney disease or gout. This results in needless worry and expense, and the "Ulysses Syndrome" becomes epidemic.

It has been shown that almost 40 percent of true abnormal results found by multiphasic testing, in or out of a hospital, are overlooked by the attending physician, often because finding these figures is a "needle in a haystack" search amidst the welter of paper work the doctor must examine for each patient.

> A sturdy 16-year-old, whom I shall call Fred, was admitted to my hospital several years ago because of morning "dazes" in which he failed to recognize his parents or articles of clothing. After the usual work-up, including multiphasic screening, his attending physicians found no evidence of organic disease. A tentative diagnosis of schizophrenia was made and he was transferred to a nearby psychiatric hospital. There it was observed that his mental lapses, called fugues, occurred only in the morning and disappeared after breakfast.
>
> His blood sugar was found to be low. A diagnosis of an overactive pancreas, possibly caused by a tumor of the cells producing insulin, was considered and Fred was readmitted to the original general hospital. There, a review of his records revealed that the first multiphasic screening had also shown a low blood sugar, which evidently had been overlooked. An abdominal operation revealed that the pancreas was normal. However, a massive tumor, hidden beneath the intestines, was found and removed. His blood sugar returned to normal the next day, and his confusion disappeared.

The correction of high levels of blood cholesterol, which is among the constituents determined by multiphasic screening, possibly may reduce the risk of coronary heart disease in young people who are willing to change their diet and lifestyle. To be really effective, cholesterol testing should be done on children prior to entering grade school. After age 65 the test is pointless, because there is no evidence that any hardening or narrowing of the arteries can be reversed after this age.

Multiphasic screening is not only a fraud for healthy, asymptomatic adults but its cost is highly inflated: rarely do the findings indicate any disease whose outcome can be altered by medical intervention. The usual battery of 12 to 18 chemical tests of a single blood sample costs the physician $4.75 to $6, but the patient is charged from $20 to $37.

The first medical billionaire was Edwin C. Whitehead, the founder of Technicon, principal manufacturer of the SMA 12/60 (Sequential Multiple Analyzer), the automated machines that perform the multiphasic screens. These electrochemical devices can perform 60 groups of 12 different tests in one hour upon a single small blood sample. Newer models operate even faster and perform a greater variety and number of tests. The whole operation is virtually untouched by human hands.

The Routine EKG and Stress Test: A Waste of Time and Money for Most

If you have no symptoms that may indicate heart disease, "baseline" electrocardiograms are pointless. And if your EKG shows a minor abnormality due to disturbed rhythm or old heart muscle damage, how will learning about it from your doctor help you? He must tell you, because if he did not, he may face a future malpractice suit if trouble develops later. Most people become needlessly apprehensive and may become cardiac neurotics, restricting the physical activity which may actually help their condition.

A case was made public of a bus driver who developed chest pains diagnosed as angina (heart pain) caused by narrowing of the coronary artery, on the basis of an allegedly abnormal EKG. As a result, he lost his job and despite numerous attempts to find work, remained unemployed. The thought of being unable to support his wife and four children finally drove him to suicide. Tragically the autopsy revealed that his heart and coronary arteries were entirely normal. The bus driver's suicide must be considered a result of iatrogenic depression.

Conversely, the EKG may give false-negative results, presenting persons with genuine heart problems with a spurious "clean bill of health." When I was coroner's physician, I performed an autopsy on a firefighter. One afternoon while off-duty, this robust 50-year-old went to the aid of his buddies; using great force, he tried to open a rusty hydrant with an elongated wrench. He dropped dead from the exertion while his friends watched in dismay. Although he had had a normal EKG several months previously, at autopsy his coronary arteries were slit-like and narrowed by yellow fatty cholesterol deposits. Frequently an EKG will not indicate narrowing of the coronary arteries unless the heart muscle is damaged. Because of the suddenness of his death, there was no time for his heart muscle to show deterioration.

Shortly after this incident, the body of a newlywed 38-year-old man was brought to our morgue. He, too, had had a normal EKG several months previously. It was St. Valentine's Day and his wedding night. While in bed with his new bride, he gasped, "I'm going," and fell lifeless. This tragedy caused understandable fright and emotional shock resulting in longstanding frigidity in the young widow. Postmortem examination revealed extensive coronary narrowing and heart muscle damage with rupture—literally, a broken heart on St. Valentine's Day!

Unfortunately, these cases are not unique. Even the more elaborate exercise stress test, during which the EKG is taken during carefully measured treadmill or bicycle exercise to determine capacity for exertion, may be abnormal in persons who have no cardiac illness and normal in those who have underlying disease, with or without symptoms.*

In a recent study the Air Force found that 60 percent of aircrew men who had EKG abnormalities were actually free of heart disease. The flip side is that false-negative results occurred in patients who had symptoms of heart disease due to coronary artery narrowing. But, because their EKGs were normal, management of their illness was delayed.

Even if there is evidence from the medical history, physical examination and testing that a patient has heart damage which is causing no present threat the doctor should try to avoid converting a happy extrovert into a depressed, anxious worrier. I have seen many cases of closed arteries and healed heart muscle damage in autopsies of elderly people who died of other causes and never experienced chest pain or shortness of breath. These oldsters were lucky to have escaped costly batches of fruitless testing with the accompanying pain and anguish of trying to adjust to a once hidden condition that caused them no unpleasantness.

Despite this evidence, EKGs are performed on patients without symptoms or with diseases unrelated to the heart on a mass scale each year, at a cost of billions of patient dollars. Many hospitals require an EKG for all adult admissions, a waste of time and money.

Almost everyone who wishes to begin jogging or other strenuous exercise after a sedentary existence is advised by doctors to have a treadmill or bicycle stress test. This is a time-consuming torture costing an average of $200. A physician must be in constant attendance to monitor the EKG, the heart rate, the blood pressure and the examinee's reactions. After the exercise is completed, the subject must be observed for 10-15 minutes or until all signs have returned to their pre-test level. Then the continuous EKG record must be carefully analyzed for minor changes in pattern.

Honest, competent physicians prescribe these tests in order to predict the possibility of sudden death due to narrowing of the coronary arteries by fatty deposits and calcium (arteriosclerosis). If the heart muscle is

---

*In 1818, William Coffitt, a British civil engineer, devised an elongated stepping wheel on which dozens of prisoners were made to walk side-by-side, a form of punishment regarded at that time as cruel and unhealthy. Today we pay a sizable sum to undergo the same type of torment.

already damaged, further defects may be prevented. Of course another consideration is the avoidance of malpractice litigation should a cardiac "accident" occur. But many people have varying degrees of coronary narrowing, from minimal to complete, without symptoms of chest pain or shortness of breath. It is a lot less costly to avoid a heart attack by proper diet, exercise, and not smoking than to go through a gamut of tests or treat a heart attack after it has occurred.

Autopsies reported in the medical and lay literature have been performed on famous athletes who exercised vigorously for many years. Dr. Paul Dudley White, President Eisenhower's cardiologist and bicycle advocate, reported on Clarence De Mar, who ran in the Boston Marathon for 50 years, and Dr. Peter H. Gott reported on champion oarsmen. These athletes died of non-cardiac causes in their 70s or later. It was found that their coronary arteries had twice the average diameter, which would tend to prevent obstruction from any cause.

Many studies have been done on the effect of strenuous exercise upon the heart. One of the first followed the discovery by the London Transport Company in the early 1950s that the active conductors on their double-deckers had much less heart disease than the sedentary drivers. Col. Kenneth Cooper of the U.S. Air Force, now Director of the Aerobic Institute in Dallas; Dr. R. S. Paffenbarger of Stanford University who studied 17,000 Harvard graduates; and a recent study of British civil servants, have all confirmed that strenuous exercise reduces the risk of heart attack by 50 percent. No instance was found in which death was due to the effect of exertion on a previously healthy heart. And prior exercise tolerance tests did not decrease the risk of death in any of the groups studied.

In 1966, Dr. David Redwood of the National Heart and Lung Institute was one of the first to express concern because his group, like the doctors at the Air Force Academy, found abnormal stress test EKG responses in persons who were not found to have coronary obstruction. This was demonstrated by x-ray visualization (angiography). Although these people may have a greater chance of later developing heart disease, there is no evidence that anything medically can be done to prevent this outcome. Other researchers agree. A report by the AMA Council on Scientific Affairs, late in 1981, stated: "Because of the relatively high percentage of false-positive tests in the healthy population, as well as false-negative tests in patients with symptomatic heart disease, the value of the test has come under attack. . . . There seems to be little purpose in subjecting young, asymptomatic subjects to this test . . . (and) because the prevalence of coronary disease is much lower in women than in men under 60, this is particularly true in women . . . It has little use in the healthy population as a case-finding device."

In a sample of 2,400 asymptomatic men, clinical examination failed to discover the 1 percent who could be expected, on the basis of an abnormal exercise test, to have 33 times the expected risk of developing symptomatic coronary artery disease during the next five years than those at lowest risk. There was no predictable gain unless four or more risk factors were present: family history of heart disease, smoking, sedentary lifestyle, high blood pressure and elevated blood cholesterol.* Yet, once discovered, can the lifestyle of these people be changed and, if changed, will it prevent further progress of the disease? Only the most motivated, and these are few, can be expected to comply with instructions.

Recently, the Chicago Police Department, concerned with the high heart attack rate and negative image of its fat, flabby officers, instituted a voluntary fitness program which, unfortunately, was not utilized by most policemen. No expensive equipment was required—only a bench or high step had been used (the bench-step or Kasch Pulse Recovery Test) by their medical advisers. It was considered adequate to evaluate their capacity for exertion and endurance.

When ex-President Carter collapsed during a foot-race a few years ago, the White House physician, Dr. Lukach, was criticized because he had not advised a stress test. Dr. Lukach replied that as the President had no symptoms of heart disease and no risk factors, such as high blood pressure, diabetes, high blood fat levels, and insufficient exercise, the test would be of limited value. There is, of course, considerable controversy regarding stress-testing for asymptomatic persons over 40 with or without risk factors if they plan to undertake a vigorous exercise program.

The real purpose of the test is not to determine whether exercise will cause angina, but whether the subject is at risk for sudden death from irregular heart rhythm with or without exertion. Therefore, it is sensible to test airline pilots and others who hold many lives in their hands in the performance of their duties.

For most of us, mild progressive exercise which does not cause chest pain or undue shortness of breath will suffice, with attention to the pulse rate.† When the equivalent of two miles of running four times a week is attained, the pulse rate may be allowed to become faster. You must proceed at your own rate and not compete with your fellow fitness trainees. Dr. Kenneth Cooper's paperback book *The New Aerobics* is one of the best guides to an individualized fitness program.

The controversial Nathan Pritikin of the longevity institutes treats persons who have suffered coronary disease with gradually increasing

---

*Although it is generally true that exercise is the most important protector of the heart's health, four sudden heart deaths were reported in 1979 in South African marathoners. However in these cases, smoking and a family history of heart disease appeared to be the primary predisposing factors. The autopsies all showed evidence of coronary artery disease.

†Pulse rate during exercise should not exceed 80% of 220 minus your age: at age 40, 220—40=180, and 80% of 180 is 144, which should be your maximum training pulse.

exercise and a low-calorie, less-meat, and high-fiber diet, free from fat, sugar and salt. Although the evidence is not conclusive, he claims that his patients achieve a reversal of coronary narrowing due to fatty deposits, thus avoiding costly (average $25,000) and dangerous bypass operations. Many patients report cessation of chest pain and shortness of breath, loss of excess weight, and the ability to jog and play racquet ball. Some former patients have completed 26-mile marathons. Dr. C. Richard Harper, Medical Director of the Aviation Insurance Agency, which writes disability policies for 10,000 pilots, believes that Pritikin's program has saved the careers of 13 commercial pilots who were grounded for cardiovascular disability but regained their flight privileges after his regimen. The insurance company has saved $500,000 in disability benefits.

The charge for the Pritikin regimen is at least $4,200 for a month's stay. Although it seems costly, this includes all expenses except travel. (Though rigorous, it is less expensive than a coronary bypass.) However, it has been questioned by investigators at the University of Alberta in Canada. They say that there is evidence that the extremely low fat and low protein intake may lead to reduced resistance to infection and poor wound healing, and that the low intake of iron and calcium makes the program unsuitable for pregnant women or those of child-bearing age. This followed a study of 50 patients with arteriosclerosis by Dr. Gordon Brown, who believes that the more moderate American Heart Association Diet (available as a paperback book), with exercise, would be just as effective, more palatable and less hazardous. For those with sufficient will-power, the cost of the Pritikin program can be avoided since the simple measures can be undertaken anywhere with the guidance of a knowledgeable physician.

The stress test has been widely abused as a profit-making enterprise by entrepreneuring directors of fitness and health centers and even YMCAs. They have all joined in believing in the American dream of a better life through technology. Iatrogenic danger, although slight, is not completely absent, since death can occur to 1 in 10,000 persons undergoing the test.

There are no figures for the total cost to the nation of the futile exercise stress test in the asymptomatic population. At an average fee of $200, it must be in the range of tens of millions from overselling to the gullible public. Since there is no evidence that it enhances the quality or length of life and since it can be replaced by inexpensive pulse rate observation with a gradual increase in activity, it should be relegated to the garbage dump of medical history.

The Overuse of X-rays

Studies by the Food and Drug Administration (FDA) warn that each year too many people are exposed to unnecessary damage from radiation. The FDA has found that one-third of all diagnostic exposures are unnecessary, a waste of millions of dollars. In 1977, 30% of all new x-ray equipment was found to be defective, sometimes delivering larger doses than required. And 10% of x-ray tests had to be repeated, increasing the exposure time for examinees.

There are, of course, financial incentives for the overuse of x-ray tests. Patients are not always referred to more competent, specialized radiologists when doctors own their own equipment and therefore can include this procedure in their office bill. But the fear of malpractice litigation is also partly responsible; doctors do not want to omit any test whose absence might later imply carelessness.

Around 250 million diagnostic x-ray procedures are performed each year in the U.S. at a cost of $6 billion. Several studies have shown that the ability to detect and effectively treat disease would not be impaired by reducing the number of x-ray examinations. A study of x-ray examinations of the arms and legs at the Yale-New Haven Hospital has shown that up to 19% of these could be eliminated without harm to patients. In national terms this would save $80 to $140 million. A large Washington hospital found that it could reduce the number of x-ray examinations of the chest following head trauma by 50% by having a clear statement of when to x-ray prepared by a hospital staff committee.

The FDA has determined after a 3-year comparative study in two hospitals in Seattle that 40 to 60 percent of x-ray examinations of the skull performed on patients with head trauma could be safely eliminated. Doctors in one of these hospitals used rigorous criteria (such as unconsciousness, blood in the middle ear, spinal fluid draining from the nose) for selecting patients for the skull x-ray examinations—resulting in a 40% reduction in these tests. In the other hospital no controls were imposed and there was a 64% *increase* in skull x-ray procedures during the same 3-year period. No differences in the outcomes of the head injuries were recorded in the two hospitals.

Excessive use of skull x-ray procedures and CAT scans is common in the hospital emergency room, where practically all patients with any history or signs of skull trauma, convulsions, headaches, or disordered thinking are subjected to these examinations. In 1977 the FDA estimated the cost of emergency x-ray procedures at $250 million; eliminating 40% could save over $100 million.

The Medical College of Pennsylvania studied 6,000 asymptomatic men over 45 for ten years with chest x-ray exams twice yearly. Cancer was discovered in 121 and they were treated immediately. However, only eight of these men survived five years—the same survival time as in cancer victims who have symptoms. The National Institutes of Health conducted a more extensive survey of 30,000 heavy smokers. They too discovered that screening for lung cancer by x-ray or sputum examination does not result in lowering of the death rate.

Lung cancer will kill 111,000 Americans in 1982, 9,000 more than in 1981, and 129,000 new cases will be diagnosed, according to the American Cancer Society. The death rate from lung cancer is increasing, especially among women (striving for equality unfortunately includes smoking). Once detected, its cure rate is negligible. Lung cancer will kill 25% of the 430,000 cancer victims expected in 1982. For those without symptoms, lung cancer screening by x-ray or sputum examination does not lower the death rate.

It has been standard practice to do routine chest x-ray studies and EKGs before instituting treatment for high blood pressure, which exists in 17% of American adults and predisposes to heart disease and stroke. But in a recent study of 107 patients at the University of Arizona College of Medicine, it was found that unless there were other chest or heart symptoms, these tests did not help to determine the outcome—and never influenced the management—of their hypertension. The researchers concluded that such routine studies added only to cost, loss of time, and unnecessary x-ray exposure.

By simplifying or eliminating excessive pre-treatment studies, physicians will be able to devote more time and thought to treating the millions of Americans whose high blood pressure is not yet controlled.

Intensive Care As Routine

The increased iatrogenesis associated with Intensive Care Units (ICUs) will be discussed in later chapters; their cost alone concerns us here. Many physicians send their patients to the ICU because they believe the monitoring and supportive care in an ordinary hospital room is inadequate. But ICUs are intended only for acute (but reversible) life-threatening conditions. Dr. William DeMuth of the American Cancer Society Committee on Cost Containment warned this year that "if terminally ill patients are treated [in ICUs], not only will massive expenditures result, but patients requiring this care for survival will be denied it. Our obligation is to identify those patients who would do as well in less expensive accommodations . . . Daily charges range up to $1,200 and we have witnessed expenditures of thousands of dollars in a single shift. Therefore we must evaluate the requirements for this care on a daily basis."

As few as 1.3% of the population consumes about half of the hospital resources available in a single year. But only a small fraction of patients who have severe underlying chronic disease, surgery of extreme magnitude, or unanticipated complications really need the ICU for long periods. Many doctors feel that most patients, except those with severe traumatic injury and certain heart and lung complications, will do as well in standard room settings. The ICU is not a postoperative recovery room, although I have witnessed its use for that purpose.

CANCER SCREENING

Breast Cancer

During 1982, breast cancer will occur in 7% or 1 out of 11 American women. Over 112,000 new cases are diagnosed annually in this country. Its occurrence increased 18% from 1935 to 1965 and 50% from 1965 to 1980. The mortality (death) rate has remained the same for 50 years despite the increase in the number of cases—approximately 27 out of 100,000 or 37,000 total deaths (1% in men)—as better treatment balances the increased incidence. As the birth rate decreases, the breast cancer rate increases, because women who become pregnant before the age of 25 are at lower risk. Breast cancer is the leading cause of cancer death in women, as well as the leading cause of deaths from all causes in women 40-44 years old.

Despite the billions of dollars spent in research, early diagnosis of breast cancer is not precise. In 1978, the National Cancer Society reported the results of a joint national cancer detection project covering 250,000 women. There were mistaken diagnoses in 48, of whom 37 had needless surgery. The principal methods now used to detect early breast cancer are thermography, mammography and monthly self-examination. Thermography and mammography (x-ray examination of the breast) cost approximately $50 in most clinics. Thermography, the detection of heat produced by the tumor, may actually cause harm as many false-positive results cause needless anxiety and fruitless biopsies. Conversely, false-negative results may delay treatment.

Mammography is controversial. Dr. John Bailar of the National Cancer Institute thinks that because mammography must be repeated annually to be effective in women under 45, the danger of radiation-induced cancer is considerable. The Health Insurance Plan of New York found that breast x-ray examination reduced the death rate slightly, but only in women over 50. Mammography also produces many false-positive results. After the mastectomies (breast removals) performed on Betty Ford and Happy Rockefeller, my laboratory was swamped with requests for biopsies (microscopic examination of tissue) of the breast which were all negative for cancer following false-positive mammograms of understandably anxious women. Out of 2,000 asymptomatic women who undergo mammography, only one will be truly positive for cancer. The dosage and rate of error is high, although cancers as small as 1/20 of an inch in diameter, too small to be detected by manual examination (palpation), may occasionally be visualized. But this is detection, not cure. Some experts believe that there is scant evidence that an annual mammogram is any better than one every three or four years for improving survival.

It is my opinion that the test should be applied only to women at high risk. Those with tuberculosis have more breast cancer as a result of frequent chest x-ray exams and fluoroscopy. Women who have been treated with x-rays for acne or breast inflammation, or who have had multiple fluoroscopies for any reason; a family history of breast cancer (mothers and/or sisters); childlessness or first pregnancy after 34; previous cancer in one breast; other organ cancers, especially of the lining of the uterus; a high fat diet; abnormal breast conditions such as certain types of cysts; estrogenic hormone intake, or obesity, high blood pressure and diabetes in combination are all at a much greater than normal risk. However, the risk-benefit ratio must be carefully weighed before advising mammography in all of these cases. Researchers have found that women whose mothers and/or sisters have had breast cancer are more sensitive to the cancer-producing effects of x-rays. How the added exposure of mammography will affect the life expectancy of those subjected to previous x-rays has never been determined. Cancers, like people, have different personalities. Some are incurably malignant even if discovered early when they are very small. Others are indolent, grow slowly and may never spread to other organs. But generally, treatment of smaller cancers leads to better cure rates than those of larger cancers.

One of the most effective methods of detecting early, small cancers is free, riskless, and does not involve traveling to see specialists or technicians. In 1978, the Vermont Breast Cancer Network Demonstration Project reported a study of 335 patients with breast cancer. One-fourth of these women practiced monthly breast self-examination. It was found that the size of the tumors removed at surgery averaged less than one inch in diameter compared to almost two inches in those who did not do so. Other studies have confirmed these findings. Dr. Peter Greenwald, who headed a New York State Health Department team, estimated that breast cancer mortality could be cut 19 to 25% if this safe and free practice were universal. It is obviously now impractical for every women to visit a physician for this purpose each month. (Men should also practice self-examination of their testicles, since early diagnosis can result in an almost 100% cure rate of some testicular cancers).

Other relative risk factors for breast cancer are: age over 50, when more than 80% of breast cancers occur; living in the Western Hemisphere or a cold climate; being white and living at an upper socioeconomic level. It is interesting to recall that Japanese women of the past generation who generally had three children by the age of 25 have only one-sixth the rate of breast cancer as American women or their Japanese-American descendants who have become fully Westernized. Other significant demographic findings are those of a study of 13,000 French Canadian nuns who had the highest breast cancer rate of any group analyzed (and the lowest rate of cervical cancer). This reinforced the results of a survey of the cancer mortality in 32,000 U.S. nuns from 1900 to 1954 who also had high rates for breast cancer and low rates for cervical cancer.

It is possible that with lower doses and new techniques, diagnostic breast x-ray procedures will improve in accuracy and safety. At this writing, a combination of annual mammography (for high-risk women) and monthly self-examination for all bring the best results. During a meeting of breast cancer specialists in 1981, it was reported that mammography still produces 15% false-positive results and 10% false-negatives. It is hoped that new techniques using lower and less dangerous voltages will improve its accuracy.

Colon Cancer

Rectal and lower bowel cancer is the second highest killer, after cancer of the lung, among malignant tumors. There will be 57,000 deaths and 123,000 new cases of colon cancer in the United States in 1982. It is primarily a disease of affluence and Western culture, common wherever a high-fat, low-fiber diet is the rule. In this respect it resembles coronary heart disease. There is tremendous geographic variation, the extremes being 52 cases per 100,000 population in Connecticut and Scotland and 3.5 per 100,000 in Uganda. Many investigators, following the pioneering work of Dr. Denis Burkitt in Africa, agree that it is associated with other large bowel diseases such as colitis, appendicitis, diverticulitis, benign tumors and even hemorrhoids.

Early detection by proctoscopic or x-ray examination was thought beneficial in reducing the death rate from this disease a decade ago. But for a disease which is commonly considered curable, the 5-year death rate, generally in excess of 60%, continues to be disappointingly high. Surveys by the Mayo Clinic, where 3,000 proctoscopic examinations failed to reveal a single case, and by the National Institutes of Health have found these tests generally ineffective in reducing mortality rates. Another study of 1,700 elderly people found only two cancers while 30 false-positive results were obtained. But a much less expensive check (about $5), the hemoccult test for invisible blood in the stool, is much more practical.

If the hemoccult test is positive, proctosigmoidoscopy (examination of the rectum and sigmoid colon with a lighted instrument) should follow to find the source of bleeding. Unfortunately, while 20 years ago 80% of colon cancers were within the reach of this 10-inch instrument, there has been a recent shift, for unknown reasons, to a higher position in the bowel, so that only a minority of cancers (40%) are now visible by this method. X-ray studies by barium enema have so many false-negatives that a more refined but costly technique, colonoscopy, in which a fiberoptic instrument can examine the entire large bowel, has been found useful following negative barium enema test results.

Two reports have documented that after normal findings during barium enema examination, colonoscopy can locate a source of blood loss in 20% of patients with occult (hidden) blood and more than 40% of patients with visible blood in their stools; 25-30% of these abnormalities or 5 to 10% in patients with blood in their stools, were cancers. Another advantage of colonoscopy when the occult blood test is positive is that it will detect small benign tumors (polyps) which may later become malignant and are easily removed with this instrument.

The Fallacy Of Testing

The evidence is overwhelming that most diagnostic tests are performed too often, while many should not be performed on symptom-free adults at all. Mass screening of people who are not sick is not successful because the few tests that might be useful are not given as often as is necessary to those who are maximum-risk cases. Many tests turn up too many false-positives in the absence of disease and too many false-negatives in the presence of real disease. The costs of the needless tests which usually follow such results constitute a large proportion of the national expenditure for medical care. Furthermore, early detection of an unsuspected disease seldom affects the outcome of that disease.

The evidence indicates that the routine or annual "physical" is unjustified despite its advocacy by reputable doctors and health institutions. Conscientious physicians will be glad to explain to their patients the meaning of, and need for, the tests they order. They use sophisticated and expensive tests only to obtain information that will increase the quality and length of life by favorably influencing the outcome of an illness that is discovered.

Experience has shown that there is no patient benefit from the routine order in many hospitals that every new adult admission—even for the most minor complaint—have an EKG, chest x-ray exam, blood test for syphilis, complete blood count (CBC), urinalysis, multiphasic screening and, for adult women, a Pap smear. The average charge for this is $65 and rising. Recently, in several states, Blue Cross/Blue Shield stopped paying for these tests unless they are individually justified by the attending physician. It is to be hoped that this signals the beginning of the end for this wasteful practice which causes needless annoyance and expense.

Necessary Tests

Now that we have seen that most tests are useless for symptom-free persons, which tests *are* useful and how often should they be performed? Determination of blood pressure, blood cholesterol, eyeball pressure for glaucoma, occult blood in the stool, and self- or doctor- examination of the female breast and mammography in high-risk women may detect unapparent disease which can be favorably influenced by treatment or change in lifestyle. But only the glaucoma test is devoid of *all* criticism at this writing. The verdict on the proctosigmoidoscopic test for lower bowel cancer is still not final.

If you are over 18 and under 65, visiting a doctor or having annual examinations is needless unless you feel ill, are pregnant, have a visible abnormality, or are injured. If you are between 18 and 30, you should have a single "baseline" physical and blood cholesterol test and blood pressure determinations evey five or six years, and women should have two annual Pap smears after the first intercourse. If the Paps are negative they should be repeated every three years until age 35.

Everyone aged 40 to 50 should have blood pressure determinations every two or three years, and after 35, women should have Pap smears every 5 years. From 50 to 60 the blood pressure should be taken every 2 years and annually thereafter. Eyeball pressure tests for glaucoma should be done annually after 40. Despite the controversy, it would be wise to have a hemoccult test each year after 40. And that is all you have to do unless you have symptoms.

The Wasteful Autopsy

The TV personality, "Dr. Quincy," has presented the public with a false portrait of pathologists. Solving crimes, bringing criminals to justice, and resolving personal problems appear to be his main concern. But the average pathologist does not have these legal duties. In smaller cities where certified forensic pathologists are not available, the local coroner may however call for his services in deaths suspected of being due to unnatural causes.

The impressive slogan, "The dead teach the living" is often prominently displayed on the walls of hospital morgues. Although autopsies are extremely valuable when crime, compensable disease, accidents or malpractice is suspected; in the training of medical students and residents; and in determining the effectiveness of drugs or surgery, the vast majority are not performed for these purposes.

As presently performed in community hospitals, most autopsies are a waste of time and money. The usual case is that of accurately diagnosed coronary heart disease, with repeated attacks and abundant laboratory, EKG and x-ray study confirmation. Or, the patient died of cancer of the lung, colon, breast or stomach which spread to other organs. A fruitless operation has been performed and the disease confirmed microscopically. Even if an unexpected brain tumor or kidney abnormality is disclosed, it is difficult to understand how any future patient can be benefited by this gory ritual whose function is to impress the hospital accreditation committee. The cost to the hospital will be $600 to $1,200. This is not assessed to the family of the deceased, but is part of hospital overhead which is added to all patients' bills.

MANDATORY CONTINUING MEDICAL EDUCATION FOR YOUR DOCTOR

Because of accelerating technological advances in the art of medicine, physicians must constantly keep up-to-date on new developments. For years, conscientious doctors have attended local meetings, in and out of their hospitals, and have made efforts to learn from others in their special field. But for the past few years there is a mandatory continuing medical education (CME) requirement for relicensure in 35 states. Twenty-two specialty boards, organized and administered by doctors, also have a CME requisite for recertification, generally 50 hours of attendance at approved classes annually.

Once voluntary, lifelong learning is now mandated by state law and medical organizations. Many physicians resent the regulation of their continuing education by external agencies. Over two-thirds of this nation's doctors must partake of CME in a formal, accountable way or face penalties such as loss of membership in a specialty society, a state medical association or, in some states, loss of license to practice.

Medical educators organize these programs, for which considerable fees are charged, ranging from $100 to over $2,000 for tuition. This creates monetary incentives for the instructors, generally medical school professors who have smaller incomes than the practicing doctors in their audience. Travel expenses average $980; lost income from practice is approximately $1,900; seminar dues, $536; books and journals, $540; miscellaneous expenses, $105. Most think the costs excessively high and the time spent unreasonable, averaging 13 days annually in formal courses, in addition to six hours weekly in medical reading. Most physicians believe that in-hospital meetings and programs, consultations and discussions with colleagues, and reading current journals and books are more useful than formal courses requiring sometimes extensive travel.

How does CME affect the quality of care rendered to the public? It seems logical that exposure to new knowledge would improve physician efficiency and favorably affect patient outcome. However, data from several investigations of family practice reveal no improvement. For example, an evaluation was made of a 20-minute lecture on the use of a new test for screening women for immunity to rubella (German measles). (The 20% of women who are *not* immune may bear deformed children unless protected by vaccine, if they should contract rubella while pregnant.) It was found that although there was a 30% increase in requests for this test from the instructed class, the same increased demand came from doctors who did *not* attend the lecture. Therefore, this increase reflected a general trend rather than the effectiveness of the teaching. Studies of instruction in listening to heart sounds and a workshop in improving responses to abnormal urine and blood tests also showed no beneficial result. A doctor's habits may not realistically be expected to change after a single CME encounter. Physicians assimilate and confirm new knowledge gradually, from many sources, formal and informal, such as reading and peer contact. Individual curiosity and desire to advance one's ability will lead to self-improvement without legal compulsion.

In 1980, six papers were published by the American Society for Health Manpower Education and Training. All discussed methodology and management, but none mentioned the outcome in terms of patient improvement and survival. The reports did not suggest that hospitals should inaugurate community programs for teaching behavioral changes to promote health and fitness and thus reduce health costs, a topic which seldom appears in CME sessions.

According to Dr. William Ruhe, the American Medical Association's leading expert on CME, there is no evidence that accreditation of CME courses guarantees their quality or relevance to patient care, the chief concern of the consumer.

Before it became mandatory, specialty societies voluntarily organized teaching programs for their members. But now, medical schools see a ready-made source of cash and income for their faculty. They enjoy their slice of the $1 billion that doctors expend each year. But who is actually profiting?

CME has become big business. Industry has joined the quest for profit. Health Learning Systems of Bloomfield, N.J., packages multi-city radiocasts using educational grants from drug firms and says only that it is making "very big money." Drug firms also promote CME programs with free tuition as public relations gestures. There is now a booming business in mail order self-assessment tests. Doctors can check themselves on new medical information, mail the answers back and receive CME credit. The largest subscription, 40,000, is from the American College of Physicians. Says Dr. Robert Moser, its vice president, "A well-informed physician is apt to be a better person to take care of a patient—but the bottom line is *improved patient outcome* . . . and the most well-informed physician may be the worst applier of that knowledge at the bedside."

Dr. Robert Geake, a Michigan Senator, sponsored a bill in 1977 making CME mandatory. But, paradoxically, he acknowledges that "it is possible to accumulate the required 50 CME credits yearly and learn virtually nothing." I must agree. After years of meetings and short courses, I cannot recall a single procedure for patient benefit that could not have been more easily and inexpensively acquired by staying home and reading journals, attending local meetings, and participating in hospital staff interchange of ideas.

Doctors, being human, may take advantage of the pleasurable opportunities associated with CME programs, which are often held at exotic vacation retreats. After all, a session on obstetrics is of little benefit to a pathologist. Attending irrelevant meetings creates incentives for socially and professionally accepted cheating.

The dilemma of CME is that there is no documentation that it benefits patient care. Do improved quality of life, better or less expensive treatment, relief of pain and suffering, and superior survival statistics result? CME attendance imposes a financial outlay of over $1 billion annually, passed on to you, the consumer. New developments, especially those hastily presented and involving high technology, are often of dubious value to the patient and may generate iatrogenic illness even if applied skillfully. Lectures and short courses on complex procedures, diagnostic or surgical, cannot make already incompetent physicians proficient; but following this instruction doctors may attempt procedures beyond their capacity, to the patients' detriment. Proficiency can be acquired and retained only by day-by-day practice and monitoring by one's peers. There are sufficient journals and medical texts to keep the conscientious practitioner abreast of new developments. Failure to use knowledge already possessed can cause substandard care which cannot be remedied by CME. In 1981 at the Convocation of the American College of Surgeons, its new President, Dr. G. Tom Jones, Chief of Surgery at Cornell University, stated that despite all efforts, "an estimated 20,000 of the 70,000 U.S. physicians who perform surgery are either inadequately trained or unqualified."

THE MALPRACTICE MANIA DEFEATS ATTEMPTS TO CONTROL COST

In this litigation-conscious country, suits against physicians have been increasing at an alarming rate and astronomical sums have been awarded to plaintiffs. Many insurers have gone out of business, and doctors have found it necessary to develop their own protective plans, generally through their state societies. In San Francisco a strike by physicians protested the high insurance rates. In New York, as in California, certain specialists—orthopedists, plastic surgeons, neuro-surgeons—must pay premiums of up to $40,000 annually, which increases patient charges. Another response to the rising number of large malpractice awards has been the increased volume of costly laboratory tests to avoid any possible imputation of negligence. During 1975, 10% of the total medical care funds, or $12 billion, was spent for laboratory services. Since the annual national growth rate is 15%, the outlay will be $48 billion in 1985, all coming from consumers' pocketbooks.

Some lawsuits are the result of animosity caused by the collapse of the traditional doctor-patient relationship. When the relationship was close and trusting, the patient, even when damaged, would not sue his physician but would "ride along." Dr. Christian Barnard, although trained in Minnesota, stated that he would never have dared to perform the first heart transplant in the United States. Malpractice suits are unheard of in South Africa, and in Canada and Great Britain they are severely limited. The physician-patient relationship has been eroded in the United States because of the constant intrusion of third parties, such as insurance and government agencies. And there has been a proliferation of specialists whose relationship is impersonal and who too frequently display insensitivity to apprehensive patients.

Many liability suits against doctors are spurious, frequently filed because an overeager lawyer encourages the patient or family. These may be more difficult to defend than more meritorious cases which are frequently settled out of court. Hospitals, like doctors, must also be insured for astronomical liabilities. Depending on location, this adds many dollars to the average daily bed charge.

PIRATING PHYSICIANS—A DISGRACE TO MEDICINE

The last cause of inflated medical and hospital bills is outright fraud. There is, unfortunately, a small percentage of dishonest members of the medical industry. These include laboratory operators, druggists and doctors who feel that if there is money in Medicaid and Medicare, they might as well enrich themselves.

These doctors bill the government for surgery not done or unnecessary. For instance, one sent statements for two abortions on the same woman in one month. Another billed for an abortion on a woman whose womb he had previously removed. Low-grade hospitals have sent vans to Skid Row areas to collect alcoholics (who are Medicaid recipients) for two weeks of so-called group psychotherapy—at taxpayers' expense. I have known many doctors who charged for hospital visits that were not made or merely for saying, "How are you today?" and then not making any notes on the chart until the patient was discharged.

Some medical laboratories do blood and urine testing, Pap smears and even anatomic diagnoses on surgical (including abortion) specimens, then kick back money to the doctors who referred the tests to them. Others do free private work for doctors in exchange for Medicaid and Medicare work sent to them. Thus the patients are billed for work that cost the doctor nothing. This practice has also been common in work done gratis by state laboratories—premarital venereal disease testing, for instance. One state laboratory did even the most complicated test without charge, *if facilities were not available in the local community;* the doctors would simply dun their patients for the procedures.

Pharmacists fill prescriptions for expensive brand-name drugs by substituting generic drugs costing a fraction as much and billing the federal government for the higher priced item.

Dentists charge for work that is not done. One billed for 14 fillings in the same tooth, another for the extraction of 92 wisdom teeth from 23 patients on the same day.

The FBI has investigated Los Angeles hospital officials who accept favors from laboratory owners which do not show up as income, such as weekends at Palm Springs. The health care industry is like any other.

Although there are periodic investigations by governmental agencies resulting in loss of licensure or the closing down of some of the worst offenders, medi-fraud, like other corrupt practices, continues. These acts are not only unethical but illegal. Federal statutes define them as felonies, punishable by prison terms. However, I know of no medi-fraud crook being jailed, except in Detroit, where of 42 convictions, nine received short terms of confinement. The rest were given fines or probation. Less than one percent of the FBI's crime fighting effort is devoted to medi-fraud. The problem is much greater than the investigative capacity to cope with it. Like the fee-splitters of past generations, the perpetrators of Medicaid and Medicare fraud have accepted this chicanery as a way of life and a necessity for survival in business, to be discussed openly and without shame.

Medicare will pay out $48.3 billion and Medicaid $38.2 billion in 1982. Crooked medical care providers are expected to skim a total of over $11 billion in federal and state taxpayers' money from this $81.5 billion bonanza. Senator John H. Heinz of Pennsylvania remarked after listening to an FBI witness: "You have described an almost unimaginable number [of] instances and types of unethical and illegal conduct . . . a pestilence of cheating of both the elderly and the taxpayers . . . a growing epidemic of payoffs and kickbacks. You have proved, in sum, that fraud is endemic among the providers that you investigated." Can this potentially fatal disease of our government medical program be eliminated or even palliated without changing the fee-for-service system? This is the foundation stone of free enterprise medicine in our country. It is also a blank check on our Treasury for those who wish to exploit opportunities for swindling that legislators, presumably with the best of intentions, have offered them. What motivates these licensed professionals to steal from us? Most doctors achieve a high income level (67% over $50,000 a year and 16% over $100,000). I am reminded of the immortal words of the late Willie Sutton, who, when asked why he robbed banks when he was of superior intellect and ability, answered, "That's where the money is."

WHAT IS TO BE DONE?

Under the Carter Administration a tentative beginning was made towards lessening the burden of overpriced medical care by placing a ceiling on hospital charges, limiting them to a 9% increase each year. Seed money was provided to encourage Health Maintenance Organizations (HMOs), a form of prepaid group medical care which provides more efficient use of resources. Yet the cost-push of higher salaries for personnel, new equipment, expanding physical plants, and the demand-pull of "miracle" technology continues to dispel incentives for thrift. Medical insurance actually raises costs because it motivates doctors to over-order and hospitals and patients to accept without question the validity and quantity of new procedures.

What must happen is the elimination by doctors and consumers of the demand for *useless* medical care and the encouragement of true *preventive* medicine. This would require intensive public education, starting in the first grade, stressing the responsibility for individuals to maintain their own health. It has been estimated that such a program would cost approximately $9 billion per year, but would save far more from our total expenditure of $287 billion. If preventive measures, focusing on cancer of the lung, cervix, colon and breast were followed, we could eliminate 15,000 cancer cases and 17,000 deaths annually among industrial workers alone, saving industry almost $1 billion and workers $2.8 billion in lost earnings. This would be only a minor fraction of the savings for our entire population.

Smoking-related illness costs us over $15 billion in medical and hospital bills; loss of income another $3 billion. "This does not include the loss from fires caused by smoking nor the tremendous but difficult-to-calculate monetary loss from [over] 320,000 deaths from smoking-related causes," said pioneer smoking foe Dr. Alton Ochsner at the annual meeting of the American Association of Family Physicians several years ago. The cost to us must be greater in 1982, and far exceeds government income from tobacco production.

Children must be taught the fundamentals of good health, and parents, doctors and teachers must set an example by exercising, not smoking, eating and drinking less, taking fewer harmful drugs and driving more carefully. Americans must not be brainwashed by "health" or cancer prevention agencies who have a vested interest in performing over $20 billion-worth of useless and frequently harmful examinations each year. The national effort to clear the environment of industrial and automotive pollutants must be expanded. These common sense measures are hampered by the public relations and lobbying efforts of giant corporations, particularly the tobacco, petroleum, and food industries whose products contribute to our destructive lifestyle.

There is a recent trend, encouraged by Blue Cross and Blue Shield, to perform as much surgery as possible without an overnight stay in the hospital (ambulatory surgery). This may be achieved in hospital outpatient departments or in one of the many centers constructed for this purpose. Since 21 million inpatient surgical procedures are performed annually at a cost of over $30 billion, with an average charge of over $1,500, the elimination of room charges alone could save 30 to 50% or $10-15 billion. There will also be less time lost from family and job and less risk of iatrogenic consequences from hospitalization.

Some of the most frequently performed operations do not usually require hospitalization: biopsy, dilation and curettage (D & C), tubal closure for sterilization, some breast operations, cataract and cosmetic surgery, tonsils and adenoid (T & A) removal, and hernia repair. These amount to approximately one-sixth of all operations done in hospitals or over 3.4 million each year. A recent study of 13,500 non-hospitalized patients, 83 percent of whom received general anesthesia, showed only 106 complications, no cases of shock and no deaths. There were only 74 cases of excess bleeding and 10 infections, which is far less than might be expected in a hospital. Only 16 patients were transferred to a hospital, none under life-threatening conditions.

Patients with severe infections of bone, joints, heart valves and kidneys, have been hospitalized for the administration of intravenous antibiotics for six weeks or longer. It has been found that these drugs could be given at home, saving at least $142 per day—the cost of a semi-private room. In approximately 200 patients in a study of outpatients given intravenous antibiotic therapy, there have been less complications than in hospital treatment.

"Let the buyer beware" may be a cliché, but it is time for this caveat to be applied to unnecessary, unproven, risky and overpriced medical care, the consumer's greatest financial and health hazard.

3.

RADIATION: THE UNSEEN PERIL

Radiation—silent, invisible—pervades our environment and our bodies. It creates numerous health hazards, but because so much of it seems unavoidable, it is accepted as a fact of life. We can do nothing about cosmic rays striking the earth from space, nor about background radiation from thorium-rich soils or bedrock. Fifty percent of our exposure comes from these natural sources. Man-made radiation can be harmful or beneficial, too. Three percent comes from fallout from nuclear weapons testing. Lesser quantities are emitted by the waste from nuclear power plants, by radar, or by consumer products such as color television, the luminous wristwatch, certain smoke detectors, and microwave ovens. Living or flying at high altitudes increases the dosage. Planned exposure, medical and dental, accounts for forty percent.

Near disasters at the Three Mile Island nuclear power plant in 1979 and Windscale, England in 1957 have caused general concern. The incidence of leukemia among residents of Utah and Nevada who were exposed to high levels of radioactivity following nuclear weapon testing has ominously increased. But public alarm is fleeting. Governmental and industrial agencies have convinced most of us that the benefits outweigh the risks. Only a major catastrophe with tens of thousands of victims would cause us to accept a lifestyle based on a reduced power supply.

The discovery of x-rays by Dr. Wilhelm Roentgen, a German physicist, in 1895 permitted more accurate diagnosis and therefore more effective treatment of many diseases. The new specialty of radiology played a large part in this improvement; but it simultaneously created the greatest planned source of damaging radiation. Much information concerning death and illness from this exposure never reaches the public but is buried in medical journals and unpublished hospital records. Authorities agree that this risk can be significantly reduced without delaying diagnosis by decreasing unnecessary use and improving the quality of equipment and personnel. Medical and dental radiation is the largest block of radiation subject to human control.

Unlike background radiation, the 40% of all radiation we receive from medical and dental sources, including diagnostic and therapeutic procedures, is not evenly distributed, although seven out of ten of us are x-rayed each year. In 1978, we were subjected to 661 million exposures, an average of about three per person. The General Accounting Office and the Food and Drug Administration, in separate studies, have argued that at least one-third of the more than 250 million diagnostic x-ray studies were unnecessary and therefore 3,000 untimely deaths due to cancer could have been avoided. The FDA found 30% of new equipment defective, causing x-ray overdosage. Also, one-tenth of the operators used faulty techniques requiring repetition of exposure; miniature films, used in screening for lung disease, required larger doses but failed to detect one out of four early cases of tuberculosis.

From 60-80% of older medical and dental equipment lacked safety screening, causing scattering of rays to other parts of the body and to the operators and resulting in higher doses than were actually needed. An unknown number of doctors who have had little or no formal radiological training own x-ray machines which they use in their private offices and clinics. I have seen the poor diagnostic quality of these films and the necessity for repetition. But these doctors have a vested interest here, since they can derive more income from taking their own x-ray pictures than by referring the patient to a certified radiologist. The chief physician and owner of a local clinic, complaining to me that a vacationing doctor did not order enough x-rays (and lab tests), said "We can't make any money that way."

The FDA reported that most hospitals have standing orders for chest x-ray examination on each new admission, regardless of the reason for entrance. These tests are often repeated because of technical errors. Blue Cross/Blue Shield have now cancelled payments for these routine reports. On several occasions I have rejected routine chest x-ray exams while being treated for minor ailments having no relation to the chest or its contents. These refusals engendered alarm and indignation among the hapless technicians who were only "carrying out orders." A firm stance, however, saved me unneeded exposure and expense.

Diagnostic x-rays are only part of the radiation that the average consumer is exposed to each year. The treatment of cancer constitutes the greatest dosage, but until recently, x-rays were used in many minor ailments, such as enlarged tonsils and adenoids, oversized thymus (a gland in the upper chest), birthmarks and acne, with sometimes long-delayed tragic results. Radium and isotopes (radioactive elements such as iodine, carbon, cobalt and phosphorus) are used because they concentrate radiation in selected tissues such as the thyroid, muscle or bone marrow not only for treatment, but also for the detection of disease (by measuring the radiation emitted by these organs).

Radiology is not an exact science. A negative chest x-ray test does not rule out lung cancer. From 20 to 50% of these malignancies are missed on the first diagnostic film. In 1981, Drs. John Forest and Paul Friedman reported in the *Western Journal of Medicine*, that early x-ray examinations did not detect the disease in 22 of 27 cases known to have lung cancer. In five cases, the findings were misinterpreted. Failure to diagnose the problem in 23 patients delayed treatment and lessened what little chance of cure might have been possible.

The Threat From Exposure

There is agreement that high-dose radiation to treat advanced cancer presents a risk of immediate radiation sickness and the development of other cancers. However, there is controversy surrounding the health hazards of low-level radiation, such as diagnostic x-rays and isotopes. To dispel myths, it is important to understand how radiation affects body tissues. Most experts believe that there is no absolutely safe level of exposure to any form of radiation. Once you have been subjected, the effects of a dose, however minimal, remain and if the dose is repeated, the effects will be cumulative.

Cancer can take from 10 to 35 years to develop. We are only now fully realizing the grim costs of early x-rays to patients and the incidental exposure to radiologists and technicians. Although there has been a recent decline in the use of x-rays for therapy, diagnostic x-ray exposures continue to increase and will account for a large percentage of the expected 70,000 to 200,000 *additional* cases of cancer that will appear by the year 2000, according to an ongoing National Academy of Sciences study. The FDA has put an arbitrary danger point at twice the yearly average that the public is exposed to from normal, background radiation plus medical uses. One diagnostic x-ray examination of the chest, however, is almost 25% of the so-called safe level. But is this realy safe? In 1979, Dr. Irwin Bross, of the Roswell Park Cancer Institute in Buffalo, New York, surveyed 500 men who were exposed to standard diagnostic x-rays. He reported that their risk of leukemia was ten times higher than expected. Dr. Bross also stated, in testimony before a government Environment and Health subcommittee, that over 250,000 American women "have been marched through the radiation fields [of mammography.] In 15 or 20 years they will become victims of the worst iatrogenic breast cancer epidemic in medical history." Dr. John Goffman, in his 1981 book *Radiation and Human Health*, argues that these figures are underestimations; that 94,000 of our annual 400,000 cancer deaths are due to x-ray exposure and that doses vary widely from the same machines.

How does radiation cause cancer? Radiation creates electrically charged particles called ions, which can be imagined as tiny bullets. Ions strike and alter body cells and DNA molecules which carry the genetic codes that determine our physical destiny. This damage changes the code to produce cancer. Some people are more sensitive to radiation than others. After a long period of repeated exposure, even at low doses, cancer, cataracts and deformities in the newborn may develop, along with weakness and shortened life-span. Several generations may elapse before genetic defects, in addition to the small percentage caused by natural background radiation, become apparent. Large doses will cause severe burns and radiation sickness. This is manifested by anemia, infection, generalized hemorrhages and severe pain. Death will occur in 50-100%, depending upon the extent of the ionic attack. The Atomic Bomb Casualty Commission, which maintains facilities and staff in Hiroshima, has amply documented these tragic consequences.

Diagnostic X-rays

Since 1925, it has been known that many pioneer radiologists died of cancer or developed deforming skin tumors, as did dentists who held films with their own hands. Leukemia is nine times, and other cancers 70% more frequent in radiologists than in other physicians. The average lifespan of the previous generation of radiologists was four years shorter than were those of their unexposed colleagues. However, since 1960, radiologists have had normal death rates because they now merely read the films and use fluoroscopy (continuous x-ray visualization) less than they did before. Their technicians actually handle the equipment and take the pictures and the risks.

A 1981 Johns Hopkins study traced 6,500 radiologists for the past 70 years. Their death rate from heart disease was almost 30% higher than a comparison group of ophthalmologists. Perhaps with faster film and newer, better-shielded equipment, the current generation of workers in this specialty will have better odds. At present, however, x-ray technicians, despite protection by lead shields and aprons, have a greater chance of being stricken by cancer than other people do. Their fertility is decreased and miscarriages are more frequent than expected. Unfortunately, they operate equipment for thousands of x-rays and cannot escape stray ions.

The fluoroscope was invented by Thomas A. Edison in 1896. With it, the beating of the heart, its size and shape, and defects in the lungs, stomach and intestines could be studied without actually taking pictures. Soon doctors, their assistants, and patients were being ignorantly overexposed. Clarence Dally, an assistant of Edison, was one of the first to die as a result of cancer which developed following x-ray burns. Many pioneers of radiology who met the same fate had tested their machines by using their hands to see how clearly the bones appeared. Shielding by lead screens was done rarely and everyone in the room was exposed.

Despite the documentation of damage by the turn of the century, overexposure continued. Children, including those still unborn, were fluoroscoped and their insides displayed to their parents. This accounts for the increase in leukemia and other forms of cancer which occurred in the 1920s. Cancer of the breast and thyroid occurs more frequently after repeated fluoroscopy of the chest. The Bureau of Radiological Health of the FDA followed 1800 women discharged from tuberculosis sanitoria between 1930 and 1954. During a period of several years, 1050 were examined fluoroscopically an average of 100 times. These women were compared with a group of 700 with tuberculosis who did not receive fluoroscopy. Twice as many cases of breast cancer as expected were detected among patients who were fluoroscoped; there was no excess in those not exposed. The greatest risk occurred between the ages of 15 and 19. After 30 there was no excessive risk, suggesting that young women are particularly sensitive to radiation injury. The risk increased with dosage. Cancer did not appear until 15 years after the first exposure. Some cases were not detected until 40 years later. Now that tuberculosis has been largely conquered, mammography presents its peril to the breast. An Oxford University study recently estimated that the chances for contracting all forms of cancer increased 50% after multiple diagnostic x-rays.

Pregnant women, especially those in their first trimester pose a special problem, because they and their unborn children are at serious risk from any exposure. In the United States, 23% of women having their first baby receive x-ray measurement of the width of the pelvis (pelvimetry), to determine the space for the baby to pass through. Diagnostic x-ray procedures for abdominal, gynecological and urinary conditions are performed on pregnant women, greatly increasing the risk of miscarriage, stillbirth or congenital abnormalities. The chances of fetal abnormalities occurring from these diagnostic x-rays are up to three times greater than in women who did not have x-rays during pregnancy. Women in the childbearing years are at particular risk during the last two weeks of the menstrual cycle, when they might have become pregnant. X-rays of the abdomen (gallbladder, kidneys, stomach and bowel), pelvis, and hips should be deferred until the first ten days after the onset of menstruation.

Our obsession with testing induces the U.S. to have twice the per capita rate of diagnostic or screening x-ray exams as England, without improving our health statistics. In a previous chapter I described how routine x-rays may fail to disclose the presence of serious disease. Fatigue and boredom, a result of reading many negative routine films, may cause the most competent radiologist to overlook small shadows. The converse can occur when a small "spot" is discovered which may be an early cancer, a benign tumor, or other harmless condition. Physician and patient are now confronted with a dilemma. Shall they take a calculated risk and "wait and see"? Or should a major operation opening the chest and exploring the lungs be undertaken at considerable risk? The false-positive or doubtful x-ray joins other tests in generating the "Ulysses Syndrome" with its aftermath of lifelong neurosis. Unfortunately, when a lung cancer is large enough to be discovered by x-ray, it is, with rare exceptions, incurable.

The risk of leukemia is especially increased when heavy doses of x-rays are applied to the spine, as during a bowel examination with a barium enema. The bone marrow, where blood cells are formed, is most sensitive to radiation damage. Twice as many children who were irradiated while in the womb, incidental to diagnosis, die of leukemia as those who have not been exposed.

Treatment With X-rays

The first use of x-rays for the treatment of cancer occurred in 1896, a year after its discovery. Many varieties of non-malignant disease, such as arthritis, bursitis, hemorrhoids, enlarged thymus, endometriosis (misplaced lining of the womb), tonsillitis as well as skin problems such as acne, eczema, warts, moles, and ringworm, were also subjected to large doses. Radium, discovered in France in 1898 by Marie and Pierre Curie, offered another source of radiation.

By the early 20th century great hopes for the effective treatment of cancer by x-rays and radium were aroused. Cancer of the cervix was first treated by x-rays in 1905. With experience, dosage was increased, and improved equipment concentrated rays on the affected part while shielding the operator. But despite widespread knowledge of the destructive effects of radiation, it was common practice in the 1920s, '30s and '40s to use x-rays for many minor disorders. It was considered an almost universal panacea.

The first clear alarm was sounded in 1950 when the Sloan-Kettering Institute in New York reported ten cases of thyroid cancer in adolescents who had been irradiated in infancy for enlarged thymus. Soon after, 704 such cases were collected from 27 countries. A report by the National Cancer Institute (NCI) summed up the disaster: Thyroid cancers develop an average of 20 years following irradiation, up to 100 times more frequently than in those not exposed, especially in young adults; of all new cases of thyroid cancer, 40% carry a history of childhood irradiation. Many patients do not remember their treatment. They are alarmed at being recalled by hospitals for examination when their records of x-ray therapy to the head and neck are found. However, it is difficult to find those who were treated in doctors' offices because old records have been lost or discarded. Since millions of such dubious treatments were administered in the U.S. up to the 1950s, it is predictable that a great increase in thyroid cancers will occur in the next 10 or 15 years, and that many of these cancers will result in death.

If radiotherapy is applied to a localized area, a kidney, bowel, lung, cartilage, ear or skin inflammation may result. Bones may be weakened and fractures are common. Radiation treatment after surgery on the breast, lung, stomach or esophagus may result in inflammation of the heart or its surrounding membranes (pericardium), which become densely scarred, leading to heart failure. A National Institutes of Health study in 1981 revealed pericardial damage in 15 of 16 patients who had had radiation treatment 5 months to 12 years earlier. The other chest organs also suffer great damage, which sometimes causes fatal hemorrhaging from the large blood vessels. To illustrate:

> An otherwise healthy, 55-year-old dean of a local college noticed a minute, painless lump in his left breast in 1975. Biopsy revealed cancer and a radical mastectomy was performed. (Male breast cancer comprises 1% of the total.) To reduce the risk of recurrence, heavy radiation treatment was administered postoperatively. The patient regained his vigor, but three years later began to experience chest pain and shortness of breath. He could barely manage to walk the three blocks from his home to his office. Examination revealed that he was suffering cardiac compression because his pericardium was thickened and scarred as were his lung coverings (pleura). Instead of being thin and elastic, they were almost of shoe leather consistency. A lengthy and risky surgical removal of his heart covering (pericardiectomy) was performed. Over two quarts of fluid were removed from his pleural cavities. After several months of convalescence he was able to resume his administrative tasks. Shortness of breath, however, recurred two years later. X-ray and other tests revealed that his lungs had lost their spongy, elastic quality. His capacity for breathing was greatly reduced to 35% of normal. The walls of his air sacs were thickened and scarred, destroying his capacity to allow sufficient oxygen to enter his blood stream. Various medications, including steroids and inhalation treatments, had no discernable effect. His condition is progressive, and now he must be driven to his office and can work only a few hours each day.
>
> Since his respiratory deterioration will continue, the outlook is ominous and his life expectancy, although not precisely measurable, will be reduced, as is the quality of his life. Over one-half pint of fluid remains in his chest. It is impossible to be certain that the destructive radiation was necessary to prevent recurrence of his cancer. The dean estimates the total costs of his medical encounter at between $30,000-$40,000, excluding the time lost from work. The cost of the x-ray damage alone is about $25,000.

Patients who have received pelvic radiation for cancer of the uterus, cervix, ovaries, kidneys, bladder and prostate frequently develop acute inflammation of the bowel and/or stomach. This causes severe cramping, nausea and diarrhea. Chronic intestinal inflammation (enteritis) may remain, with permanent damage leading to obstruction, rectal bleeding, ulceration, and chemical changes in digestion which cause difficulty in food absorption. Weakness and weight loss follow.

These complications occur in one to 17% of patients receiving x-ray treatment to the abdomen or pelvis or both. Six months to ten or more years may elapse after the exposure before they occur. The attending physician must make a decision based on a calculated risk here. Are the chances of cure greater than the danger of these distressing and occasionally fatal iatrogenic events?

When x-ray treatment is given to the mid- or upper abdomen or chest for cancers of the lung or adjacent organs (esophagus, stomach or intestine), the patient will experience difficulty in swallowing, loss of appetite, nausea, diarrhea, and abdominal cramping. There may be severe pain in the chest or upper abdomen. The underlying damage is similar to that described above in the lower abdomen. The symptoms will depend on the location of the destruction. The mortality for this higher assault from x-rays will vary from 15-37%. Another operation may be necessary to at least temporarily relieve ulceration or obstruction, even without recurrence of the cancer.

As an example of direct local injury by x-ray treatment:

> A patient had visited his doctor because of diarrhea. Rectal examination disclosed a stony hard lump about half an inch in diameter in his prostate gland. Biopsy revealed low-grade cancer and he was referred to a local clinic for intensive radiation therapy. After receiving multiple high dose treatments for three years, his penis and scrotum began to swell, with extreme itching and redness of the overlying skin, preventing sexual relations. He was reassured by his radiologists that these distressing complaints were a "normal reaction." Treatments were continued for another nine months during which his swelling, itching and tenderness worsened. Dismayed, he sought a second opinion and was told for the first time that his injuries were the result of his radiation therapy. He brought suit against the radiologists and the jury awarded him $500,000.

The Mayo Clinic reported 78 cases of bone sarcoma in 1982 which were observed an average of 15 years after irradiation for malignant or benign tumors. Sarcomas of the lung have also appeared following radiation for other causes. Most of these victims died from metastasis to the brain and/or liver.

X-ray therapy may even enhance the development of coronary artery disease. Experimental animals have shown increased arteriosclerosis after exposure to six months of radiation.

Medical radiation in massive or repeated doses can cause the same radiation sickness as fallout from atomic bombs, but is of lesser intensity. The patient develops nausea, vomiting, diarrhea, headache, general weakness, and rapid pulse. These symptoms will subside within a few hours. If the exposure is of lesser degree but more prolonged, there will be anemia, cessation of menstruation, cataracts, loss of hair, skin thinning with underlying bleeding, and later, cancer of the skin. The underlying organs—muscles, heart, lungs, bowel and spinal cord—may all be damaged, as will the cells of the testis and ovary, causing future defective offspring. Leukemia may develop later. No part of the body is spared. The extent of the damage depends on the dose and its location.

The children of the survivors of the atomic bombings of Hiroshima and Nagasaki are serving as a test population for the genetic effects of radiation. Thus far they display only an increase in the number of male offspring. The increased rate of leukemia in their parents is now diminishing. But new cases of other cancers continue to exceed that expected. Their future, as well as that of millions of persons overexposed to medical radiation, is still speculative.

Because they are silent and invisible, x-rays do not arouse awareness of their danger. Patients should not hesitate to seek information on the hazards of x-rays from their physicians. They should learn the full physical and emotional costs of the treatment prescribed and reject any diagnostic or therapeutic x-ray procedures that are not absolutely necessary for improving their chances of survival. Although improvements in equipment have reduced the amount of radiation from *diagnostic* x-ray studies, patients should insist that x-rays in any form be used only as a last resort, when other methods of treatment and diagnosis cannot be employed.

In 1981, a Chicago survey revealed that many of the x-ray machines in clinics and doctors' offices had not been inspected for almost 20 years. (There were only six inspectors for 9,000 registered machines.) Numerous defects were found, most commonly causing overdoses of x-rays to the skull. Some of the largest and most prestigious hospitals were included in the survey, and their equipment was also found to be improperly used or defective. Although 99% of the inspected facilities had received citations for one or more violations, no fine had ever been issued. Illinois is one of the 36 states that require no licensing or special education for x-ray technicians. A physician may give perfunctory on-the-job training to anyone he hires. Technicians in some instances were office managers, secretaries, or receptionists doing double duty.

X-ray films of poor technical quality may be misread and cause a high rate of error in the diagnosis of early cancer, tuberculosis and lung disease due to exposure to industrial dust and fumes. This can delay diagnosis and treatment. When x-ray studies must be repeated because of technical error the increased dosage accumulates.

Adding Insult To Injury

In the late 1920s, a chemical called Thorotrast was first used to outline body cavities for clearer x-ray pictures. It was inserted into the nasal sinuses, fallopian tubes, branches of the lungs, and kidneys. About the same time, Lipiodol, an iodine compound, was used to delineate the bronchial passageways. It was also injected into the fallopian tubes for x-ray visualization, primarily to determine tubal blockage which causes sterility. Neither of these contrast media is used now, because it was soon found that, while aiding diagnosis, they were a threat to health. By 1932, articles were appearing which reported that Thorotrast caused cancer of the sinuses and liver. Lipiodol was found to cause inflammation and tumor-like masses in the fallopian tubes. Yet it was not until the 1950s that Thorotrast was discontinued. As late as 20 years after administration of this chemical, an increase in cases of cancer of the liver, leukemia and other blood disorders was noted in those who had received it.

Compounds used as adjuncts to x-rays today are safer than Thorotrast and Lipiodol, but the dangers remain. Patients are not always informed about the known hazards of these procedures, and even when informed, they may not understand the risks involved.

During the last generation, angiography—visualization of arteries, veins and lymph channels in all parts of the body by injecton of contrast chemicals outlining their structure and course—has become important not only for blood vessel surgery, but for the diagnosis of tumors and inflammatory disease. Arteries are disrupted by space-occupying masses which are clearly outlined. Newer contrast media, many containing radioactive elements (isotopes), are also widely used. These compounds are concentrated in a selected organ and the radiation emitted is detected by a sensitive scanner. Both procedures cause many adverse effects due to the manipulation of the instruments used for injection, the radiation, or the toxicity of the chemical.

Angiography is a difficult procedure, even in skilled hands, and the side effects can be severe. It may be harmful because of allergy to the compound injected producing hives, or more seriously, swelling of the larynx, with obstruction to respiration or shock which may be fatal. Invasive procedures are used, with catheters long enough for direct injection into the arteries (arteriography) supplying the heart, brain, legs, kidneys, abdominal organs, aorta, or lungs. The heart chambers and aorta may be directly or indirectly filled with opaque media. In special cases the veins or lymph channels may also be outlined, with similar risk of reactions.

Chicagoans will remember that the late Mayor Richard Daley had a carotid arteriogram done for repeated mental lapses. An operation to clear the channel of obstructing arteriosclerotic narrowing (endarterectomy) was performed with excellent results. Carotid arteriography is frequently utilized in cases of stroke, temporary repeated forgetfulness or other mental symptoms. It is hoped that, as with Mayor Daley, the carotid, rather than smaller brain arteries (which cannot be cleared), will be found to be narrowed and the loss of blood circulation to the brain relieved by endarterectomy.

Fatalities due to carotid arteriography occur only in four of 1,000 cases, but complications similar to those when other arteries are injected occur in 4 to 8%. There may be complete or partial blindness which spontaneously disappears in two-thirds of the cases. Often brain damage, present before the test, is increased due to further arterial narrowing or blood clotting.

The use of contrast media to fill the coronary arteries (angiocardiography) requires delicate balancing between the seriousness of the patient's illness, the dangers of the test, and the skill of the operator. The procedure lasts 1½ to 3 hours and is accompanied by pain, skipped heart beats and a burning sensation when the contrast medium is injected. The radiation exposure is equivalent to 1,000 chest x-ray examinations. The patient is stiff and cramped from lying strapped to a hard table and those with lower back pain require considerable sedation. Cost is $700-1500.

Despite serious adverse effects, coronary arteriography, a preliminary to heart bypass operations, has been the fastest growing invasive procedure in the past ten years. It is performed twice as often as cesarean section in childbirth. Invasive cardiologists are trained in increasing numbers, and they have financial incentives to prefer surgical rather than medical care.

The fatality rate of coronary arteriography varies with the experience of the radiological team. In hospitals performing 500-700 of these procedures annually, it is from one in 200 to one in 100, while in those performing less than 200 it is two or three times greater. In smaller institutions it may be as high as eight times greater. No hospital should set up a coronary angiography service if it cannot accomplish 300 per year or more. The mortality is highest when the largest coronary arteries are completely blocked and when the radiological team is inexperienced. Patients should not hesitate to inquire from their doctor or hospital administrator about rates of reactions and fatalities whenever this, or any other invasive procedure is contemplated.

Invasive cardiac radiography for the study of the heart chambers and valves is being replaced by non-invasive methods in which radioactive chemicals are injected into a vein. Fatalities occur in 1/1,500 procedures. An American Heart Association study showed that 1% of all hearts into which a catheter was inserted suffered perforation and half of these bled into the pericardial sac. In 43 cases of perforation three (8%) died. In smaller hospitals, complications, sometimes fatal, are more common (6%) than in larger centers which perform a greater number of cardiac radiology procedures and have a reaction rate of only 1%.

The largest artery in the body is the aorta. When the injection of opaque media (aortography) is required, the aorta has already been damaged by disease and is therefore vulnerable. The trauma of a large needle injection can cause or aggravate blood clotting or weaken the artery's muscular wall, which will then become thin and cause the artery to expand like a balloon (aneurysm). However, blood clotting will narrow the passage available for blood to flow, sometimes cutting off circulation to the legs and intestines sufficiently to cause gangrene. If this occurs in the legs, amputation is required, and if the intestines lose their circulation, death invariably results. The opaque medium is injected through a vein or by insertion of a catheter through an abdominal incision. When the patient already has an aneurysm, aortography should be unnecessary, since the pulsating swelling can be felt through the abdomen.

Outlining of the main leg artery (femoral) is also done to discover narrowing due to arteriosclerosis; this narrowing can be bypassed by a less dangerous operation than a coronary bypass. An injection is made into the artery under the groin. In a survey of 5,000 patients, local complications included bleeding with a surrounding blood clot, sometimes causing a hollow pulsating expansion (false aneurysm). In rare instances, internal blood clots may form (femoral thrombosis) which may prove serious or even disastrous.

Arteriograms can also be used to obtain better details of the lungs and intestinal tract. The reactions will depend on the locations of the organ and individual sensitivity. Media containing iodine can also be administered by vein. In a study of 3,000 studies of the gallbladder (cholangiography) 10% had mostly minor reactions. In 81,000 kidney examinations (urography) almost 6% developed side effects such as flank pain, fever, albumin or blood in the urine and rarely, fatal kidney failure.

When media are given by artery or vein, there is no way to predict that general reactions, as opposed to local effects from instrumentation, will occur. Prior testing is unreliable, but certain groups of people are more likely to have reactions. These include those with an allergy such as hives, hay fever or asthma, those with known sensitivity to iodine or those who have had a previous reaction. Out of 112,000 patients studied who had these blood vessel injections, 5% experienced a reaction. Generalized sensitivity reaction or local infections may occur when radiopaque material is injected into the body in any of the following radiologic procedures:

The lymph circulation which runs parallel to arteries and veins is seldom injected with opaque media, but when it is, it is done through a small channel in the instep and the dye reaches the almost invisible canals in the back muscles. In this way, lymph nodes which are covered by tumor can be outlined, especially in cases of Hodgkin's disease and similar lymphatic cancers.

The urinary collecting system may be outlined by injecting contrast media into the ureters (retrograde pyelography) while the catheter is observed by fluoroscope. This method is seldom used because of the danger of infection.

Myelograms are performed for the diagnosis of tumors about the spinal cord, observations of protruding discs, and distortion or narrowing of the bony canal containing the spinal cord. The material is injected into the space surrounding the spinal cord through a long needle inserted in the small of the back. Severe headaches generally follow, lasting one to two days.

The uterus and tubes can be filled with media, mostly to determine blockage in cases of sterility. Sometimes the fluid will enter the abdominal (peritoneal) cavity with the formation of tumor-like inflammatory masses. If leakage into a vein occurs, the media may be carried to the lungs with damage causing shortness of breath, cough and severe chest pain.

Irritation resulting in severe coughing can result from filling the bronchial tubes with contrast media (bronchography). When the joint cavities are injected (arthrography), minor pain from local inflammation may occur.

One of the more dangerous techniques has been the injection of a gas —oxygen, helium, carbon dioxide—into the tissues of the lower back (retroperitoneal pneumography) to outline suspected tumors, especially of the adrenal glands. Of 1,300 cases reported in the medical literature, 60, or one in 20, had fatal results and 64 had non-fatal results due to bubbles of gas entering the blood stream and damaging the brain, lungs or kidneys. Air can also be injected into the hollow spaces (ventricles) of the brain and under its covering membranes (meninges). Severe headache results in addition to the usual instrumental dangers of all invasive procedures. The CAT scan has now superseded this dangerous procedure.

Almost everyone knows about the most common contrast medium, barium sulfate, an apparently harmless, inert, insoluble white powder. Suspended in water, it may be swallowed, sometimes with flavoring added, or given by enema. This permits fluoroscopic examination of the stomach and small and large intestines, which are clearly outlined. These procedures are performed over 10 million times annually in the United States. Despite the relative simplicity of barium meals and enemas, the great number of performances permits Murphy's Law to operate as in more complex and dangerous tests.

Cases have been reported in which toxic substances have been inadvertently substituted because of mix-ups in the containers. Other "look-alike" white powders like barium *sulfide,* barium chloride and barium carbonate are soluble and may be absorbed into the body, causing barium poisoning. An account of an almost unbelievable error, *Radiologist on the Rocks,* was published by Dr. B. Felson in 1973. Careless storage of plaster of Paris in containers originally used for barium sulfate resulted in this hardening compound being swallowed by four patients. The plaster set, forming casts of their stomachs and causing great distress, but fortunately the plaster soon crumbled and was passed rectally!

If the patient has an ulcer, the barium may penetrate the stomach or bowel wall causing tumor-like masses (granulomas) on the peritoneum.

Over 65 cases of stomach perforation have been reported but, of course, many have not been described in the literature. If there is any interference with intestinal circulation or mobility due to arteriosclerosis, ulcer or tumor, obstruction from impaction in the colon can occur, requiring surgical removal. Appendicitis has also been caused by impaction in this narrow, worm-like structure.

Barium enemas are unpleasant, especially when administered unsympathetically early in the morning by a heavy-handed, indifferent attendant. But dangerous consequences, although infrequent, can occur. Perforation by the enema tip is possible when the bowel is already weakened by colitis or a tumor. Although this hazard occurs in only one case in 2,000 to 12,000, it is not rare because of the large numbers of barium enemas administered. Contamination of the peritoneum with feces will cause peritonitis, which has a high fatality rate and requires surgical repair.

The most lethal consequence of barium enema is leakage of barium into a vein. It will then be carried by the blood to the lungs with massive destruction, usually fatal, or to the liver, causing abscesses. Impaction may occur above a constricting tumor, forming a rock-like mass requiring surgical removal.

The Cat Scan (Computerized Axial Tomography)

Since the turn of the century, essential x-ray methods have not changed. But the English Musical Instrument Company (EMI) developed a space-age machine which takes thousands of slice-like sections of the head and body. First used in London in 1971, it made its American debut at the Mayo Clinic in 1973. There are now several thousand such scanners in the U.S. manufactured by eight corporations, costing $500,000 to $750,000 each. A CAT (or CT) scan costs approximately $400. Vying for prestige, one-third of all U.S. hospitals possess a CT scanner. There has been considerable controversy over their acquisition by small hospitals which do not generate enough volume to make them cost-effective. There is no doubt that they can reduce the number of angiograms, air injections, and other invasive procedures, and the use of toxic contrast media as well as radioactive isotopes. Their greatest utility is in the diagnosis of bleeding, shrinkage, swelling, and tumors within the skull and brain. Although they can detect tumors, cysts and abscesses of the pancreas, lymph nodes and other organs hitherto invisible to standard x-rays, their effect on outcome is still uncertain. Recently, the FDA found that almost 300 CT scanners emitted excessive radiation. Kidney failure has been reported in several cases from toxic contrast media used to enhance the images produced. Children, who require sedative premedication, may develop respiratory arrest, voiding problems, or vomiting, especially since the scans are ordered for suspected brain disease.

Isotope Indignity

Millions of Americans are exposed to new sources of radiation from varieties of existing elements. These sources are concentrated in different organs. A new specialty, nuclear medicine, has been created which can actually make an image (scan) of the organ being studied or provide a count of the radioactivity emitted. Iron enters the blood corpuscles, strontium enters the bones and teeth, and iodine enters the thyroid. For example, in the radioactive iodine uptake test (RAI), the patient drinks a "cocktail" containing I-131, an iodine isotope. Later, the physician places a counting instrument over the thyroid. If the count is higher than normal the thyroid is overactive (hyperthyroidism). Or a scanner can be used to produce a diagram of this activity. Similar techniques have been devised for the heart, lungs, liver, spleen, bones, kidney, and brain, using isotopes which are concentrated in the organ in question.

Most isotopes are used for diagnosis, but therapy is also performed. High doses of I-131 produce radiation, destroying some of the thyroid's function and reducing its activity in cases of hyperthyroidism. The problem is similar to that of diagnostic and therapeutic x-ray overdosage and overexposure. At present there is no consensus that the information gathered by these costly isotope methods, admittedly superior in accuracy and convenience, has actually resulted in greater long-term patient benefit than the standard chemical methods in which the patient ingests nothing.

A recent U.S. Public Health Service report revealed that 85% of all isotope counting studies involved I-131 for thyroid dysfunction. Many varieties of this test are in use, including the radioimmunoassay (RAI). Because any exposure increases the risk for thyroid cancer, especially in children, the potential danger is not inconsiderable. When I-131 is used for treatment, the dose is much larger and is scattered to the rest of the body, therefore increasing the risk of other cancers, including leukemia. Benign thyroid growths that require surgery also appear in greater numbers. The function of the thyroid may be depressed, requiring treatment for hypothyroidism.

Blood volume determinations using different radioactive isotopes, I-125 and chromium are used in cases of hemorrhage, severe burns, dialysis, or shock. They will generally be done many times in the course of an illness so the cumulative dose may be higher than intended. The older clinical and chemical methods, though not so accurate, are safer and sufficient for the purpose—patients benefit from decreased mortality, quicker recovery and lower cost.

Bone scans using strontium-85 and brain and liver scans using technetium-99 are performed less frequently and deliver less radiation but the effect is cumulative; children are particularly sensitive. Again, the question is: how do these procedures improve patient outcome in the long run? The same dilemma confronts us when we consider counts and scans of the heart, lungs, liver, spleen, pancreas and kidney. Even if the diagnosis is improved, will it favorably affect the disease, so often incurable?

Although the atmospheric test ban treaty with the Soviet Union was designed to prevent isotope fallout from affecting our populations, nuclear physicians have been zealously putting them into our bodies. We must always remember that there is no safe dose and that the older methods still work, with less risk. The Nuclear Regulatory Commission requires training and licensing of physicians and technicians. I do not know whether or not the regulations are enforced more efficiently than those for x-rays, which have been disregarded in many cases.

In 1972, the American Board of Nuclear Medicine was formed to raise standards. But even if dosage is reduced, the effects of earlier x-rays must still be reckoned with. Studies have been made by the USPHS on children in the Rongelap Islands in the South Pacific and on young people in Utah who were exposed to fallout in approximately the dose used in thyroid procedures. The results indicate that thyroid cancers and leukemia will significantly increase in the coming years among the exposed population.

Are governmental agencies and the corporations they presumably supervise predominantly interested in quelling public fear that the nuclear industry may, in the long-term, do more harm than good? After the Three Mile Island accident, ambiguous, contradictory and misleading statements appeared in the news media and confidence has been shaken. Profits are high and must be protected, in medicine as well as in the production of energy. It is, of course, necessary for the Defense Department to promote a general attitude that these tremendous forces can be tested, handled, and transported safely. It is willing to accept the risk of possibly tens of thousands of deaths as a price well-paid for improving our military posture. The advancement of the careers of many physicists may depend on whether or not they follow the official line and minimize the dangers.

Avoiding Unnecessary Exposure

We must remember that no radioactive dose, even the smallest, is absolutely safe, whether the source is standard x-rays, fluoroscopy or isotopes. The toxicity of the contrast media and the invasive techniques used to administer them compound the peril. It takes many years to fully discover the after-effects of exposure. Genetic changes may not be manifest for several generations. We still do not know the total cost of radiation in human life and disease-producing damage.

There is little incentive for the medical industry to reduce exposure. The chest x-ray examination still appears on standard admission orders in many hospitals. It is still required before employment by the Ford Motor Company, the Peoples' Gas Company of Chicago, and many hospitals that should know better. To protect employers, x-ray films of the lower back are commonly taken of workers who do heavy lifting.

Third parties—private insurance companies, Medicare and Medicaid—still pay for x-ray studies, thus eliminating financial incentives to reduce patient exposure. The FDA, at its facility in Rockville, Md., is now conducting experiments to reduce dosage. It estimates that $2 billion is spent in this country annually on the 30% of x-ray tests it considers unnecessary. Consumers must look after their own interests because, despite ethical considerations and governmental "watchdog" agencies, there are many ways for physicians to profit from the over-ordering of tests. Financial motivations become justified when "everybody is doing it," and doctors will indignantly proclaim that they are practicing good medicine by being thorough. They are also practicing "defensive medicine"—avoiding the risk of malpractice suits should unexpected illness occur. I have advised patients and friends to refuse x-ray and other tests unless their physician can explain that they will do more good than harm. An athletic, middle-aged long distance runner I know was sent to the Mayo Clinic for investigation of insomnia with no other symptoms. He was bold enough to reject the chest x-ray examination (and EKG) since there was no way these routines could favorably influence his problem.

If you have no relevant symptoms, you must question any suggestion that you be exposed to radiation by any means. There is no reason for x-ray screening unless there are familial risk factors. After age 50, women may consider mammography because new methods have improved accuracy and lowered dosage (although controversy persists). Many hospitals use obsolete or modified equipment. Monthly self-examination is safer and cheaper.

Those with symptoms should insist that their doctor explain how they will be benefited. Make sure the x-ray pictures are taken in an office or hospital department headed by a specialist certified by the American Board of Radiology. Do not hestitate to ask when the equipment was last inspected and if the operator was trained at an approved school or merely "on-the-job." Many paramedical assistants know little more than pushing buttons. If your dentist advises new x-ray studies every six months you had better find a new one.

If an invasive procedure such as angiocardiography preceding possible heart surgery is advised, ask how often the test is performed in the radiology department. If less than 300 times a year, the expert teamwork needed by medical, nursing and paramedical staff cannot have been developed, and you should insist on beng transferred elsewhere.

Despite the assertions of physicians that they are aware of the many hazards of exposure to radiation and its accessory procedures, and that they order x-ray tests only after carefully weighing the benefits against the risks, the use of x-rays continues to increase. Our population grew 7% between 1964 and 1970. During this time, the use of x-rays increased 20%. Since 1970 their usage has continued to increase. This suggests that only lip-service is paid to knowing about dangers which have been obvious for many years.

Until there is a change in the habits and social conscience of many members of the medical industry, consumers must learn enough of the risks of radiation to be able to protect themselves from unnecessary and too frequent exposure. It's *your life*, after all.

4.

FITNESS: DANGEROUS DIETS AND EXERCISE EVILS

Until a generation ago, most people accepted their bodies as structures sustaining their heads and minds. Stage, screen and athletic stars had contours to be admired, but only a few narcissistic fanatics tried to improve their appearance and performance by selecting their food and trimming their fat with regular exercise. I remember army basic training, when most recruits, flabby and clumsy, dismally failed to complete the easy obstacle course.

H. L. Mencken, the self-indulgent sage of Baltimore, has been quoted as saying "The only exercise I get is serving as pallbearer to my friends who exercise." Rotund Robert Benchley echoed, "Whenever I think of exercise I lie down until the urge passes." But these clever cynics may stir in their graves, because, despite environmental deterioration and iatrogenesis, the fitness phenomenon which began in the late '60s has coincided with the falling death rate from coronary heart disease and stroke and with our lengthened lifespan. There has been a rising demand for low-fat milk and cheese, and fowl and fish. Sales of eggs, butter, beef, baked goods, candy and sugar have fallen. But we are consuming more invisible fat, salt and refined sugar, since they are added to almost all packaged, prepared food.

In 1960, only 24% of adult Americans worked out. Today, 70 million, or almost half, are trying to improve themselves. A $30 billion industry has been created. Last year we spent $5 billion on health foods and vitamins, $50 million on diet and exercise books, and $6 billion for diet drinks. Health clubs and corporate fitness centers cost another $5 billion, while athletic clothes and equipment cost $8 billion (shoes alone, $1 billion). Buyers of bicycles, combining exercise with practical transportation, have spent over $1 billion, and enclosed, aerodynamic, human-powered vehicles will soon appear. No longer do we drift lazily in water. We swim laps and long distances. Add another $1 billion for pools, snorkeling and scuba gear. Skiing consumes $570 million for equipment alone, not including instruction, travel and accommodations. More of us hike, climb mountains and back-pack, often carrying 60 pounds. Podiatrists have increased their incomes and prestige and sportsmedicine is a new orthopedic subspecialty, accounting for over $2 billion. (Although it is only a cover-up for fitness, we have spent $1 billion for cosmetic surgery.)

A decade ago, 233 runners entered the New York City marathon; this year 25,000 applied for 16,000 places. Similar booms are reported for the Boston and Chicago marathons. Senior "Olympics" enlist participants from 50 to the 80s. Although I am near "retirement" age, I find pleasure bicycling to my office and on errands, averaging 60-80 miles weekly.

More Americans read package labels at supermarkets. We are suspicious of injurious additives: saturated fats, nitrites and other preservatives, sodium, salt, sugar, caffeine and saccharin. Even French cuisine has undergone a revolution (nouvelle cuisine) led by Chefs Michel Guerard, author of *Cuisine Minceur,* and Paul Bocuse, who wrote *French Cooking.* Both use natural sauces and fewer calories.

Despite these benefits, the flip side of the fitness phenomenon lies in its pitfalls and perils. Diets may be medically prescribed—there is general approval of the American Heart Association Eating Style and its prudent, lifelong modifications—or they may be fads.

Nutrition is an important political issue. It was included in nearly half the bills brought to the attention of the 95th Congress in 1978. Although many diseases are due to diet (faddish or ethnic), this book is concerned only with food that is medically prescribed and creates iatrogenic effects.

Obesity is relative. Some flabby, clumsy, corpulent people pretend to be content with their image. They are offended when "obese" or "overweight" appears on a physical examination form. But they cannot resist tempting, high-calorie food; 600,000 Americans are grossly overweight, although most of them know their extra poundage is unsightly and dangerous. Their death rate from diabetes, heart disease and stroke is 12 times greater than that of persons of normal weight. Their risk of cancer, gallbladder disease, gout, high blood pressure and various skin disorders is increased, and their life span is shortened.

Although the media barrage the public with protests against the Administration's plans to reduce food stamps and school lunches, Dr. Myron Winick, director of the Institute for Human Nutrition at Columbia University, said in 1981 that our country's major nutrition problem is "excess calories leading to obesity." *Fortune,* in December 1981, summarized some data regarding those most likely to be obese: blacks more than whites, women more than men, Jews more than Catholics, Catholics more than Protestants (Episcopalians are the leanest). Those of low socioeconomic status are twice as likely to be obese as are those of higher status, and those with low IQs are more likely to be obese than those with high IQs, especially females.

The army is too fat to instill confidence in its ability to withstand the physical demands of combat. Soldiers are being ordered to eat less. Some have been sent to Fort Eustis, Virginia for mandatory exercise sessions and nutrition lectures.

Medical treatment is notoriously ineffective. Total fasting is dangerous and can only be applied in hospitals because it may cause liver, kidney and hormonal complications along with increased acidity of the blood (ketosis). Hunger is reduced after the first few days and weight loss is rapid but one-fourth to half the loss is from muscle protein, rather than fat. Less than 5% of the patients so treated in doctors' offices lose more than 40 pounds, and the pounds come right back after treatment. Patients are disappointed with this reversal after the initial loss. Many of the obese cannot control their appetites because they have an excess number of fat cells due to overfeeding in childhood. This abnormality persists in spite of weight reduction, which decreases the size of fat cells, but not their number.

When patients or friends ask me what they should weigh, I offer no numerical figures because we all have different bone structures. Most of us have seen enough unclad bodies to be able to judge by viewing ourselves, nude, in a mirror. If we *look* overweight, we *are* overweight. If arms, shoulders, belly, and buttocks bulge or sag with flab, we are obese. The body fat percentage and skinfold measurements recorded at periodic examinations add to the futile accumulation of meaningless, time-consuming and costly data.

Medically Prescribed Processes

The Protein-Sparing Modified Fast Regime (PSMF) has been devised by the nutrition laboratory of the Harvard Medical School for treating patients who are 30% over desirable weight. Previous studies had found that if *high-grade protein*, such as egg white, meat, fish, or fowl, and mineral and vitamin supplements are added to a semi-starvation diet, muscle-protein loss and hunger are reduced. Most patients achieve a reduction of 40 pounds or more. The problem arises in maintaining this loss. Instruction in behavior modification and exercise reinforces lowering of calories.

Blood sugar and insulin levels will fall and blood acid will increase in those on the PSMF with accompanying fatigue, dizziness, skin dryness, muscle cramps, decreased sexual desire, temporary hair loss, constipation and increased sensitivity to cold. There may also be irregularity or cessation of menstruation. Patients should not swim in cold water or take hot showers or baths after exercise because this may cause low blood pressure, with fainting or dizziness.

Patients who are taking "water pills" (diuretics) for high blood pressure or medication for diabetes will have to substitute other treatment. If symptoms of a previous stroke remain, if there has been a recent heart attack, childhood diabetes, liver or kidney disease, or any serious illness, the PSMF will be hazardous. The very morbidly obese (those with weight twice that of their ideal weight) will not benefit. Surgery, such as the stomach bypass or stapling or teflon meshing to reduce the stomach's volume, involves its own dangers, but should be more successful.

The **Liquid Protein** ("Last Chance") diet is low in calories and bears a superficial resemblance to the PSMF. It has been promoted by the sale of 1,500,000 books written by Dr. Robert Linn, who operated several clinics and charged $120 for the initial, and $60 for the required weekly visit. It is guaranteed to reduce your wallet if not your weight. The protein is of poor biological value because it is derived from cowhide or other non-muscle supporting tissue. Gelatin is often added. In 1978, the FDA investigated 60 deaths associated with these unpalatable beverages. Over 100,000 individuals had used predigested liquid protein (PDLP) as their sole source of nourishment for at least one month and 37,000 of these has used PDLP for at least two months. All of the deaths were due to sudden heart rhythm irregularities and eventual heart failure. None had had previous heart disease. Autopsies on these victims revealed cadaverous muscle wasting like that seen in concentration camp victims.

Although many physicians report non-fatal adverse effects such as EKG abnormalities, fainting, nausea, vomiting, diarrhea or constipation, irritability, increased cold sensitivity, irregular heart beat, decreased libido, gout recurrence and hair loss, all such cases are not reported; the incidence is probably much greater than the FDA data would suggest. Its proponents claim that it is uniquely effective in resistant obesity and invaluable in reducing the mortality and morbidity associated with morbid obesity. But the PDLP and even the less injurious PSMF make no sense unless provision is made for subsequent maintenance of weight loss. Less than 5% of those who needed to lose 40 pounds or more were successful on these diets.

> A pretty-faced, but broad-beamed businesswoman I know weighed 176 pounds and was 5 feet 2½ inches tall in 1977, when she was 44 years old. Her doctor prescribed PDLP in powder form, with added vitamins, sometimes flavored with chocolate or vanilla and diluted with diet soda. After four weeks she noted loss of hair. At eight weeks her waistline had decreased 2½ inches but she was annoyed by "spots" in front of her eyes. She attended sessions at a health club three times weekly, but was very weak, had "gas" pains and fainted several times. At 13 weeks she had lost 46 pounds and most of her long blonde hair and her now-wrinkled skin turned yellow-green. Doctor and patient then decided that "enough was enough." She resumed her compulsive overeating and regained all of her lost weight in several months.
>
> In November 1981 she joined a weight clinic at a local hospital where a well-balanced, low-calorie diet and exercise were combined with behavior modification techniques. She has lost three pounds weekly and is determined to permanently alter her lifestyle.

Chemical Food Additives have been mandated by controversial legislation in many states. In the long run, there has been more good done than harm from these additives, for example, the addition of iodine to salt to prevent goiter, and vitamin D to milk to halt rickets. But salt and sugar in baby and breakfast foods may cause psychological addiction to harmful substances. Fortification of food with iron is a more complex dilemma. Although intended to prevent anemia in menstruating women, a recent government survey of 30,000 people showed that 20% of the *men*—but only 2% of the women—had anemia due to lack of iron. Paradoxically, 95% of the women were on a diet considered iron-deficient.

In 1970, the FDA proposed to quadruple the amount of iron added to flour despite the lack of evidence regarding its efficacy or safety. Dr. William H. Crosby, a hematologist at the Scripps Clinic in La Jolla, California, strongly opposed this move. An example of what can happen when the national diet is loaded with iron is provided by the Bantu of South Africa who prepare their porridge and kaffir beer in iron pots. This furnishes them with six times the iron in the average American diet. Not surprisingly, 80% of the Bantu carry excess iron deposits (siderosis) throughout their bodies and 4% accumulate iron so rapidly, it causes a form of cirrhosis of the liver (hemochromatosis), with accompanying heart disease which may cause death during their 20s. Diabetes and impotence are other unpleasant consequences.

Swedes have been eating iron-enriched food for over 30 years. In 1974, a survey of 350 persons revealed that 13 men had increased iron deposits; 2%, or one in 50 had early hemochromatosis. In a district with a population of 130,000, 10 severe cases were found in two years. This geographic evidence seems to indicate that we should not add more iron to our diet. We do not know how many Americans are predisposed to hemochromatosis, but the disease is rare in this country, appearing in only one of 7,000 autopsies.

Pregnant women are often given pleasantly coated iron tablets by their physicians, usually in bottles of 100. The easily opened bottles are left within reach of toddlers who may spill and swallow the tablets. Iron follows aspirin as the second cause of accidental poisoning in children. It incurs 500 hospitalizations each year and 10 or 12 deaths. The 1982 *Physicians' Desk Reference* (PDR) lists almost 50 tradenames of iron-containing substances, but most brief descriptions mention only that these preparations should be kept out of the reach of children. Several, however, warn against stomach irritation and heart failure with overdosage. A physician stated recently that there is not enough money in iron for pharmaceutical companies to develop and promote non-toxic iron products.

Total Parenteral Nutrition—Hyperalimentation (TPN). Many hospital patients are unable to take sufficient food by mouth, especially after abdominal surgery with complications or inflammation of internal organs, such as severe colitis. They may be starved because of accidental injury or because of intestinal bypass operations for obesity. In 1968, administering highly nutritive solutions by vein was introduced. This "intravenous feeding" can either supply all needs or supplement inadequate mouth feeding. The solutions can be taken through a catheter inserted in the large vein under the collarbone (subclavian), or through a vein in the armpit or leg.

Although hyperalimentation can be life-saving when used properly, it does have adverse effects especially in children. When food is taken orally it passes through the intestinal wall after digestion and enters the blood stream via the liver, which is a complex chemical factory. With TPN, the liver is bypassed and excess ammonia may appear in the blood, causing temporary brain damage and confusion, especially in a chronically starved patient. More commonly, the liver becomes enlarged, tender and fatty. Enzymes indicating liver disease appear in the blood. The patient may become jaundiced due to clogging of the bile channels. These complications can be relieved by adding certain amino acids, which are the building blocks of protein, to the solution. As with all invasive procedures, the liver biopsy, performed for diagnosis, and the catheter insertion add their hazards of hemorrhage and infection, fluid overload, and chemical imbalance. TPN at home—for people whose intestines have been removed or damaged by disease—costs up to $55,000 per year and carries the same complications, but may enable its users to resume work at a lower level.

Formula Feeding—Cow's milk, which is present whole or fat-free in most infant formulas, is best for baby cattle. It is poor fare for human infants despite the addition of various sugars, vitamins and minerals. The psychologic benefit of breast feeding to mother and child has been discussed by anthropologist Ashley Montagu. Artificial feeding fails to give the infant immune substances which prevent or lessen the severity of infectious disease. It may cause allergy, with eczema, hives or asthma. Additional cost must be considered. But it may be necessary if the mother's supply is inadequate, if the child is weak, ill, premature, or has a hairlip or cleft palate. Mother's milk may be given in some of these cases by means of a breast pump and feeding apparatus.

A quasi-medical, diet-related catastrophe must be mentioned. Although only a small minority of Caucasians cannot digest lactose, one of the milk sugars, many Africans and Asians are unable to digest this sugar because they are deficient in an enzyme called lactase. Despite this long awareness, multinational corporations are vigorously promoting formula feeding throughout the undeveloped world, aided by modern communication. Billboards and advertisements extoll the benefits of formula feeding. Sales personnel dressed as "Milk Nurses" visit village clinics to convince pregnant women that breast feeding is outmoded and that formulas are "scientifically" superior. "Cooperating" doctors and clinics receive free samples, equipment and supplies. There are also lures of free transportation, accommodations and entertainment at medical conventions.

The National Academy of Sciences has recently reported that even in poorly nourished women, "The quantity and quality of breast milk is usually surprisingly good." I found this to be true during my early experience as a physician in the most poverty-stricken regions of Appalachia, USA. Nevertheless, the "Milk Nurses" give new mothers free samples of infant formula which last long enough for the mothers' breasts to dry up. By then they are literally hooked on cow's milk products. Now the formulas are no longer free. The high cost forces the mothers to stretch and dilute the feedings. Insufficient calories, combined with diarrhea-producing lactase deficiency, polluted water, unsterile equipment, and lack of refrigeration, cause an estimated 3 million deaths each year, according to Dr. Derrick Jelliffe of the UCLA School of Public Health.

Jack Anderson, in a column entitled, "Deadly Diet," recently related that a military dictatorship in Central America employed death squads to execute rural health workers who encouraged breast feeding. Why? . . . The lucrative kickbacks the right-wing junta received from the sale of baby formula!

Concentrated Food—Multiple small outpouchings of the large bowel, resembling little bladders (diverticulosis) were rare curiosities in the 19th century. Recent autopsy studies, however, have shown that between one-third and one-half of people over 40 and two-thirds over 80 have diverticulosis, now the most common affliction of the colon in industrialized Western countries. It is still rare in Africa and Asia. Previous treatments were based on a misunderstanding of its origin. For nearly 50 years, leading authorities advocated a low residue, soft, concentrated diet of white bread, fats and meat to prevent irritation. Many patients are still undergoing this regimen, although it is now considered improper, since it has actually proven to be the *cause* of diverticulosis. A high fiber, bulky diet with bran, bananas and leafy vegetables will prevent diverticulosis if started in early childhood and will relieve symptoms of established disease. If an outpouching becomes acutely inflamed it will cause "left side appendicitis." It may perforate, frequently causing fatal peritonitis. Chronic inflammation may cause obstruction, bleeding and other symptoms suggesting cancer.

Uganda has the lowest rate of colon cancer in the world. There, the diet has been high in fiber, including bananas. Connecticut, our most affluent state, has 60 times the colon cancer rate of Uganda, and the fiber intake there is only one-tenth of Uganda's. Dr. Denis Burkitt, formerly of Makere University, Kampala, Uganda, has spent most of his life proving the fat-fiber connection. Rich, low-fiber diets are also associated with appendicitis, gallstones, hernias, varicose veins, hemorrhoids, diabetes, stroke, coronary heart disease and the most rampant disease of affluence—obesity.

DOCTORS' DIETS OF DOUBTFUL OR LITTLE VALIDITY

Low Calories Plus Hormones. Thirty years ago, Dr. A. T. Simeons, British-trained, but practicing in Rome, prescribed a 500-calorie diet with injections of a hormone, produced in the placenta, called human chorionic gonadotropin (HCG). It is prepared from the urine of pregnant women for commercial distribution. Although the Simeons regimen rapidly gained international attention and was used in an expanding chain of franchised "fat clinics" in the United States, there are no valid studies to confirm its efficacy. Even though the diet alone should be effective in weight reduction, it can lead to protein malnutrition.

The 1982 PDR warns that HCG is useless for obesity and that in addition to ovarian cysts which may rupture and hemorrhage, its use may also result in multiple births, headache, irritability, depression, fatigue, and enlarged breasts in men. The Attorney General of Michigan was the first to declare that such HCG clinics "would be in violation of Michigan's medical practice act." It is hoped that other states will follow this example.

The Complete Scarsdale Medical Diet—The ill-fated Dr. Herman Tarnower was the author of this profitable volume in 1978. Dr. Philip L. White of the AMA's Department of Foods and Nutrition warns, "This diet is extremely rigid. The dieter has few decisions to make . . . This very rigidity encourages compliance for a while. There is no 'metabolic miracle' performed, just tight control of what you eat." How can it be exactly calculated as 43% protein, 34.5% carbohydrates and 22.5% fat, limiting caloric intake to 1,000 per day, when the size of the portions is not specified? The dieter could easily put away an extra 400 to 600 calories. Sugar and alcohol are excluded. Breakfast is always half a grapefruit and one slice of dry wheat toast. The diet is expensive and unnecessarily high in protein, including steak, lamb chops, chicken and fish on scheduled days. The dieter is expected to lose 20 pounds in two weeks and then switch to a less monotonous eating style to "stay slim". Dr. Tarnower said that quantities of food are less important than the chemical reactions between them, an unproven and unlikely hypothesis. Yet he claimed that it was not a "fad" diet and was intended to modify behavior. It is likely that its compulsive ritual and snob-appeal led to its initial success.

The Save Your Life Diet, written by the prolific Dr. David Reuben (who told us all we wanted to know about sex but were afraid to ask) in 1975, capitalizes on Dr. Burkitt's findings of the value of high fiber food. There is nothing medically wrong with this regimen but its "mystical" feeling of fullness may not compensate for calorie counting. Quantities of food are not specified except for bran. Dr. Reuben claims that, "There seems to be something about a high roughage diet which induces an internal feeling of calmness and tranquility." Some critics warn that the rapid passage of food through the intestine may cause mineral deficiencies producing kidney stones. The rough fiber may cause an embarrassing passage of gas.

Dr. Atkins' Diet Revolution, written in 1972, converts the body to a fat-burning machine. All the gooey desserts and high protein meat that one desires are allowed. The AMA has pronounced it "bizarre" and "without scientific merit." There is no way that you can ingest 4,000 to 5,000 calories a day and shed pounds. We need a *bit* of carbohydrate to nourish the nervous system. The high fat and cholesterol content will contribute to arteriosclerosis, which causes heart disease and stroke. There may also be irregularities of the heart beat, diarrhea, and acidification of the blood (ketosis), which may cause gout to flare up and brain damage in unborn children. It is the most dangerous of the diets we are considering.

Dr. Irwin Stillman's Diets: The *Quick Weight Loss Diet* (1967) and the *14-Day Shape-Up Program* (1974) are 90% protein, permitting unlimited amounts of lean meat, fish, poultry, eggs and low-fat cheese. Eight to ten glasses of any combination of water, diet drinks, coffee, or tea are mandatory. Vitamin supplements are added, and bread, vegetables, fruit, alcohol, and sugar are forbidden. A modest 15-minute exercise program, not enough to really melt fat, is added. The idea is that it takes more energy to burn protein. To lose weight you must eat less or burn more calories. It takes the equivalent of *ten miles of running* to lose one pound. As with all low carbohydrate diets, these risk fatigue, nausea and diarrhea. Few stay on them long (which is a virtue) and then their weight rebounds. High cholesterol levels, with the risks already described, are encouraged.

The Pritikin Program For Diet And Exercise has received more TV publicity and generated more controversy than any of the others. Several years ago I visited Vilcabamba, Ecuador, where the inhabitants, genetically a mixture of Spanish and Indian, have been extensively studied by many authorities, including Dr. Alexander Leaf of Harvard Medical School, who wrote *Youth in Old Age*. They have many times the expected percentage of centenarians and retain their physical and sexual vigor in old age. They work hard on their hilly farms and subsist on a low fat, moderate carbohydrate and protein diet, practically all locally produced. Their cash income averages only a few hundred dollars annually. Nathan Pritikin has enlisted the aid of several physicians experienced in fitness training and heart problems, including Drs. Don Mannerberg and Joseph Goldstrich; they charge as "little" as $4,200, (soon to be increased to $5,000), to teach their affluent clients the no-frills lifestyle of the semi-primitive peasants of Vilcabamba in a 26-day program.

Adverse effects of this regimen have been reported by investigators at the University of Alberta in Edmonton in 1981. There is some evidence, they say, that the low fat, protein, iron and calcium intake may reduce resistance to infection, delay wound healing and make the program unsuitable for women who are pregnant or of child-bearing age. The diet and exercise agenda is extremely rigid and boring (resembling a version of a Soviet Gulag re-education camp). It is difficult to believe that many of its devotees will be able to maintain it once they leave the reinforcing discipline of the center and are subjected to peer pressure at home. They return to their accustomed habits with the exception of the strongest-willed disciples. The AMA has judged it "unpalatable and therefore untenable." But it works for the highly motivated, although controlled data are not yet available.

The Rice Diet must be mentioned, although it is now obsolete. It was devised by Dr. Walter Kempner of Duke University in the 1930s for patients with severe kidney disease, high blood pressure, heart disease, and diabetes. It was discovered that it also caused weight loss and began to be used for this purpose in 1945. The unsalted rice regimen is extremely monotonous and may cause excessive muscle protein loss. Constipation, with stools resembling small hard balls, is an inelegant complication. Dr. Kempner wrote in 1949: "The rice diet is either ineffective or dangerous unless it is done under rigidly controlled conditions." That is, unsuitable for self-use without clinic supervision.

Other Diets, the Beverly Hills, Yogurt, Cambridge, "I Love New York or Zen Macrobiotic diets—are not medically prescribed and therefore not within the scope of this book. They are all faddish or cultist, unbalanced, boring, cause constipation or diarrhea, or lack essential nutrients. Complete fasting, supplemented only by water and vitamins, can be fatal, as the deaths of the deluded IRA martyrs at Maze prison testify.

Dr. Alexander R. Lucas of the Mayo Clinic described in JAMA this year the fad of "pigging out" (also called bulemia) which is especially prevalent among female college students whose caloric intake can vary enormously. To maintain slimness, they compensate for overeating by purging with laxatives or inducing vomiting by gagging. This is reminiscent of the "vomitoriums" of ancient Rome; I am also told that some German restaurants maintain these unsavory facilities for disgorgement which allow patrons to enjoy unlimited gluttony. This peculiar fashion is reluctantly admitted, but can result in enlargement of the salivary glands, erosion of dental enamel, inflammation of the stomach and esophagus, irregular or skipped menses (with fear of pregnancy), and abrasions and calluses on the knuckles. When laxatives are used, change in bowel habits may occur, with severe constipation. "Water pills" (diuretics), less frequently used, will cause loss of potassium, resulting in extreme muscle weakness and even kidney and heart failure.

Successful, safe weight control is theoretically simple but extremely difficult in practice. Temptations abound in restaurants and refrigerators. The key to fitness is motivation, encouraged by awareness that it can happen to YOU. A little narcissism is needed to create the desire to improve one's physical attractiveness. Body fat can only be lost when caloric expenditure exceeds intake. To lose a pound of fat takes 3,500 calories, the equivalent of running ten miles. Although a bathroom scale is not needed to tell you that you are overweight, it is essential to follow your progress. You can develop your own eating style, based on the recommendations of the American Heart Association, which can be obtained free of charge from your local branch. Exercise twice as much as usual and you are on your way. Those who are not self-motivated will find inexpensive programs and courses at YMCAs, community colleges, and, in many cities, municipal parks and field houses. Health clubs, clinics and hospitals now offer medically supervised fitness programs which are more expensive. Their group reinforcement and behavior modification techniques are necessary for the weak-willed. Weight-Watchers, Overeaters Anonymous and TOPS (Take Off Pounds Sensibly Club) offer similar spiritual and mental support.

EXERCISE DANGERS

Although controversy exists, most researchers believe that vigorous, sustained exercise is the most important factor in the prevention of heart disease and strokes. It lowers the pulse rate and blood pressure, increases desirable high density blood lipoproteins, and releases tension. But caution is necessary, especially in the early training period. Some, like a well known fitness instructor I know, believe that exercise will do no good unless it hurts. In 1978, I attended his rigorous sessions. He had six daily 45-minute classes of business and professional men. If they survived his Spartan regime, they were awarded T-shirts labeled "Wilkin's Warriors." Bill led all his drills. He showed no mercy to neophytes or complainers and taunted those who could not maintain his pace. But under this hard crust he was solicitous of his charges' well-being and would call them at home if they were absent. His routine stressed weight lifting and developed strength and endurance, but was not sufficiently aerobic for the development of cardiovascular fitness.

When sudden demands are made on an unconditioned or overused body, as in the quick starts, stops and turns demanded by squash, racquetball, tennis and basketball, the knees, ankles and feet are subjected to extraordinary strain, with resultant painful injury to supporting structures. "Tennis elbow" is even more exaggerated in close-quartered wall games where wrist motion predominates. Striking the wall with the inner surface of the hand may cause damage to the ulnar artery with loss of circulation and resultant cold sensitivity.

Joggers strike the ground 800 to 1000 times each mile with an impact of three times the body's weight. Almost all of the nation's 30 million runners will develop a skeletal syndrome. Running on pavements will eventually cause metatarsal arch pain. Turf absorbs shocks and is more esthetic, but unseen irregularities may twist a runner's ankles. Painful "shin splints" can involve bone or its covering tissues. Its most severe form is a partial fracture below the knees. Eight such breaks have been reported at Duke University Hospital alone. The orthopedists there believe it is due to an unnatural gait with the toes pointed too far inward or too far apart. "Jogger's ankle" is an inflammation of tendons of the inner surface of the ankle, or of the heel (Achilles). "Runner's fracture" of the lower end of the smaller leg bone (fibula) is equally common. "Jogger's penis" is a painful frostbite which occurs when the pubic area is insufficiently clad in frigid weather.

"Jogger's nipple" is an inflammation promoted by the bouncing of breasts against T-shirts. Women runners also display increased blood levels of male hormone (testosterone) and frequently miss periods. Adolescent girl athletes may have the onset of their menstruation delayed as much as three years. Not enough data have accumulated to indicate what these changes will mean over the long term.

Golf has been described as "the best way to spoil a good walk," by Dr. Tom Cureton, physical education director of the University of Illinois. It is a social, pleasurable activity, but riding a cart does not raise the pulse rate. If one walks briskly and carries one's clubs, however, it is of physical benefit. "Golfer's elbow," injuries from sliced or hooked balls, and poison ivy in the rough are its only risks. Dr. Kenneth Cooper, author of the best seller, *Aerobics* says, "Many people think you have to run to get any benefit. But the only benefit running has over walking is that it can be done in a shorter period of time"—for equal distances.

Even swimming, considered the safest medically of prescribed sports, has its hazards. The butterfly stroke may cause "swimmer's shoulder." In north central U.S. lakes, "swimmer's itch" is caused by otherwise innocuous parasites penetrating the skin.

The "dunk laceration syndrome" strikes extra-tall high flyers who slam basketballs through the hoop, striking their hands against the rim. (This sport is seldom recommended for healthful exercise.)

Bicycling brings multiple benefits by combining exercise with elegant transportation, while combatting OPEC, pollution, traffic jams and parking problems. No other exercise is needed until ice or snow cover the pavement. But chronic low back pain can result from overuse of low-slung handlebars on ten-speed bikes. Dogs, skateboarders, skaters and daydreaming pedestrians require evasive action. Ice and roller-skating strain ankles, knees and leg muscles and the contusions caused by falls and contact with other people and objects are similar to those experienced by the incautious bicyclist. Helmets should be mandatory. Friends and I have been spared head lacerations or even worse injury by their use.

The only other sport that might be prescribed for improving cardiovascular and musculoskeletal fitness is cross-country (Nordic) skiing which supposedly avoids the risks of fractures and dislocations common in downhill (Alpine) skiing. A decade ago, slick ski suits were common. I remember the horror of seeing a skier fall while rashly traversing a closed, icy slope on Baldy Mountain at Sun Valley. He was unable to stem the acceleration of his steep slide and struck a tree, causing a fatal head injury.

Nordic skiing is inexpensive, can be practiced in parks, golf courses and even on city streets before snow removal and salting teams spoil the surface. It transforms northern winter into a happily anticipated season, instead of a time to flee to enervating southern climes. But wrist injuries caused by pole-pushing or by the basket-catching on protrusions are common. If one ventures onto narrow trails, a sudden descent down an unexpected slope with little room for turning or stopping can add some of the hazards of true downhill skiing.

When you are unable to continue your exercise program because of bad weather, and have no time to go to a gymnasium or ski, there is an easy solution. Dr. Paul Fardy, director of cardiac rehabilitation at St. Catherine's Hospital in East Chicago, Indiana, said recently, "Taking the stairs instead of waiting for an elevator will not only get you there faster but improve your heart function and general physical fitness." A pediatrician I know of has been climbing 90 stories to his apartment in a high-rise building almost every day for several years with great benefit, although *that* amount of exertion is not required!

Dr. Fardy put a group of 30 healthy men, aged 18 to 64, through a gradually more strenuous 3-month stair-climbing program in an 11-story building in which they worked. They had no regular schedule, but were told to take the stairs whenever they would have used the elevator and to take a couple of "stair-climbing breaks" each day instead of coffee breaks. He found that 25 flights were equal to slow jogging for 35 minutes, walking 3½ miles, or bicycling 8 miles in an hour. All developed slower pulses and stronger legs. There were no dropouts because quick results, ease of access, elimination of special equipment and approval by employers for time saved enhanced motivation.

Investigators at Northwestern and Cornell Universities found that elevations of the levels of chemicals called CPK, LDH, SGOT and BUN in the blood frequently occur after strenuous exercise. There are also minor elevations in the white blood cells and EKG changes. The heart may be slightly enlarged. If the subject were having an examination by a doctor unfamiliar with sportsmedicine, heart muscle disease would be strongly suspected. Small amounts of blood may be found in the urine, suggesting bladder or kidney disease, including cancer. Unless the examiner accounts for exertion, a healthy person could be twisted through the tortuous maze of the Ulysses Syndrome with its added iatrogenic dangers. Only his medical knowledge and skepticism prevented a 40-year old internist from being propelled into this syndrome a few years ago. For several years he had been jogging six miles five times weekly. Although like most physicians, he disapproves of the annual check-up, a required insurance examination revealed that his pulse rate was slowed to 44 per minute and there was a trace of blood in his urine. The insurance examiner then ordered tests for blood chemicals. Four were slightly elevated: the blood urea, suggesting possible kidney disease; the LDH and SGOT, suspicious of liver abnormality; and the CPK.

The doctor had a corridor consultation with several colleagues he met in the hospital lounge, including an internist and a surgeon. He was advised by these pundits to have additional tests, including the injection of a dye into a vein for visualizing the kidneys (intravenous pyelogram). However, he was knowledgeable enough to decline further investigation since he felt perfectly well. A year later, for reassurance, he had the tests repeated. The results were unchanged, as was his physical well-being.

Asthmatics who want to keep fit are discouraged by the problem of exercise-induced attacks of difficult breathing which require medication for relief. This unpleasant effect is presumably due to loss of heat and water from their airways. Experiments at the National Asthma Center in Denver have shown that simply wearing a surgical face mask will retain sufficient warm, humidified, expired air to prevent these attacks. These inexpensive masks will also add comfort to non-asthmatics who jog or otherwise exercise in frigid weather.

The Risk Of Strenuous Exercise To The Heart

Regular vigorous physical activity assists in weight control. Most investigators are certain that it also reduces the risk of arteriosclerotic heart disease. However, does it increase the danger of sudden death? In 1973, Dr. M. Friedman wrote in the *Journal of the American Medical Association* that more than half of 27 subjects who died instantly collapsed during or after physical activity. In that year, Drs. Kavanaugh and Shepard in Toronto found that one-third of 98 non-fatal heart attacks were triggered by exercise. Sudden deaths in 21 South African men who participated in various sports were reported by Dr. L. H. Opie in 1975. And in 1979, 18 deaths associated with jogging or running were described by Drs. Thompson and Stern. In all of these studies *no instance could be found in which death was due to the effect of extreme exertion on a previously healthy heart,* although exertion may place excessive stress on an *already diseased* heart. Most of the deaths occurred in heavy smokers. Age alone was not a factor.

The Sports Council in England has been sponsoring a study of the effects of a carefully designed and supervised course of gymnasium activity on 2000 middle-aged men, 400 of whom had a history of heart or blood vessel disease. They exercised at their individual pace for 15 minutes, three times a week. Over a period of 5 years, totalling 25,000 hours of gymnasium activity, there were no cases of collapse or any form of cardiac emergency.

A Dallas medical team report embraced 3000 adults who completed 375,000 hours of exercise, including over a *million and a half miles* of running and walking. Tennis, racquetball, handball and basketball were also prescribed. There were no deaths and only two cardiac events, one in a 61-year-old executive who collapsed while competing in a 2-mile run because of irregularly rapid heart beat. He had not been exercising regularly. Another man, 35 years old, had a heart attack after a fast one-and-a-half mile run. He, too had not exercised regularly for six months. In each case, *exercise tolerance tests were normal* approximately a year-and-a-half previously. Both men survived and, after gradual training, were exercising regularly.

The team concluded that there is a very small risk, even with normal exercise tolerance tests, of heart attacks occurring during or after vigorous exercise. This risk is intensified by smoking, previous coronary disease, the pressure of competition and physical unfitness because of irregularity or infrequency of exercise. But these risks are less than expected in a sedentary population, as many other studies have shown.

Dr. Thomas Bassler, California pathologist and past president of the Medical Joggers of America, has been the foremost proponent of the theory that long-distance running protects against coronary disease. This protection, however, is not absolute. In 1981, Drs. William Roberts and Bruce Waller of the National Heart Institute reported their studies in five men, 40 to 53 years of age, who died while running, including Congressman Goodloe Byron of Maryland who had completed six Boston marathons. These victims had been running up to ten years, averaging 14 to 107 miles weekly. Only one had ever complained of chest pain. Autopsies revealed severe coronary narrowing in all cases. Dr. Roberts expressed his belief that, "they would have died earlier if they hadn't run." Runners have a much lower rate of coronary fatalities than sedentary people do. Recent investigation has shown that levels of high density lipoprotein (HDL), a kind of cholesterol, are increased in the blood during sustained exercise. High levels of HDL have been linked to a decreased risk of coronary artery disease (CAD) since 1975. It is possible, however, that athletes who have symptomless coronary disease may develop abnormal heartbeat rhythms during extreme exertion which can cause sudden death. I believe that most people would prefer this to a lingering, agonizing illness.

Other evidence that the risk of dying from a heart attack while jogging is low was presented by a report from Brown University Medical School. Between 1975 and 1981, 12 men died while running or jogging in Rhode Island. This amounts to one death per 7,620 middle-aged joggers annually, or one per 400,000 hours of jogging. Autopsies and/or clinical histories revealed that there had been coronary artery disease in 11 and a stomach hemorrhage in one. It was not known which of the victims had known coronary artery disease, which were jogging for cardiac rehabilitation, how many and to what degree other risk factors were present, nor which had symptoms before death which would have led them to seek medical attention.

The number of deaths was so low that the investigators concluded that screening exercise tests would have been futile for identifying apparently healthy people who might be at increased risk for exercise-related death. From 2,000 to 13,000 tests would have to be done to find one potential victim.

This study confirms the conclusions of those previously described—that exercise carries a small but definite risk of sudden death. But, there is no way of knowing what would have been the fate of these men if they had not exercised. There is no way of resolving the human dilemma—which of those who died would have preferred longer life with lingering torturous illness? Could they have been helped by coronary artery bypasses or non-surgical treatment? This question has not been answered. Dr. Paul Thompson, who headed the research team, concluded that physicians can recommend exercise to adults without symptoms of heart disease "without great concern for possible cardiovascular complications."

PREVENTING HEART AND BODILY INJURY FROM PRESCRIBED EXERCISE

Once clothing and footgear appropriate for the chosen activity are carefully selected, the weekend athlete syndrome must be avoided. We see fathers trying to impress their families by racing towards the goal in touch football or walloping a softball and streaking for first. Then, like a 50-year-old fat and flabby surgical colleague who tried to run two miles without preparation to start his shape-up program, they are on the ground writhing with pain because an Achilles tendon or other musculoskeletal connection has snapped like an old shoelace. Each year, over 20 million Americans hobble or are carried into emergency rooms or clinics with injuries related to exercise: fractures, dislocations, ligament and tendon ruptures or inflammation (tendinitis), cartilage fractures, lacerations, bruises, or abrasions. The Aspen Clinic resembles an army field evacuation station.

Given an almost 40% death rate from first heart attacks, prevention is the only logical approach. The cardiac risks of exercise can be minimized by carefully supervised, gradually increasing activity as provided by the fitness programs I have mentioned. Smoking, and isometric exercises like weight-lifting, which raises blood pressure but does not increase oxygen intake, must be avoided. The shiny, impressive apparatus seen in commercial health clubs are not only unnecessary but may be dangerous. We are not interested in developing muscle bulk but in increasing heart and lung (cardiorespiratory) fitness. This point is well understood by modern, trained aerobic exercise instructors. Starting at very low exertional levels even for the apparently fit, paying careful attention to the pulse rate at the wrist or neck (not to exceed 80% of 220 minus one's age) during the training period, avoiding symptoms of over-exertion such as shortness of breath or musculoskeletal pain, almost anyone regardless of age can, with persistence, develop cardiorespiratory fitness. Overcompetitiveness must be avoided, and participants should proceed at their own pace and intensity.

Like radioactive elements, the benefits of exercise have a half-life, computed by physiologists as 60 hours or 2½ days. Therefore it will require three or four sessions a week, for the objective to be attained in three to six months. By that time no amount of exertion should cause anything worse than fatigue. The pulse can be raised to the target rate of 220 minus age. The various skeletal, muscular, joint and skin problems associated with each form of exercise may be inevitable, and their risks can only be diminished by prudence and by switching to another sport which uses different muscle groups until the injury heals or pain subsides. If your feet hurt when you run, try bicycling.

Although many physicians and coaches still advocate stress tests, I have presented enough evidence that its many false-positive and negative results can be misleading. It is not worth the expense and time expended and the discomfort, although it increases cash flow for the performance laboratory. Prudent, gradually increasing exertion will serve the same purpose while conditioning the body to further fitness. Once you have run two miles at your *training pulse rate,* you may gradually increase speed and distance to the *target pulse of 220 minus your age.* There will be no increased benefit over four days a week at that level for 30 minutes each session. Bicycling, swimming, skating, Nordic skiing or racquetball can be intermittently substituted to avoid monotony and sustain interest and can alternate with running to relieve monotony.

5.

"CURES" CAUSING CANCER

It has been known since the turn of the century that radiation causes or increases the risk of cancer. Other types of medical and surgical intervention have become recognized as significant hazards for promoting cancer during the past 30 years. The long delay (latent period), which may be years or decades, between treatment and tumor and the environmental, non-medical dangers to which we are all exposed obscure the prime cause, which may be forgotten or lost with the records. It is even likely that several cancer-causing agents act in unison, enhancing each other.

Arsenic: Skin cancer due to industrial exposure to arsenic has been known since 1820. Insecticides containing arsenic were extensively used between the 1940s and 1960s in France and Germany and caused tumors of the lung branches and liver in winegrowers. Earlier, many tumors had been blamed on the arsenic content of drinking water. During the last century, arsenic compounds such as "Fowler's solution" were administered for many skin diseases, anemia, epilepsy, asthma, and general "rundown" conditions. There were two-hundred twenty-six cases of cancer caused by arsenic reported in an early study in persons ranging from 22 to 75 years of age. The tumors appeared 20 or more years after treatment and occurred mostly in the skin, but 19 developed in various internal organs. No dose was small enough to be harmless, and the hazard increased with the amount and duration of medication. Most dermatologists and internists agree that there is no longer any reason to use arsenic medically, but the practice is still prevalent in Germany.

Tar: Although their use is decreasing, ointments and other preparations containing tar and tar-like chemicals are still prescribed for various skin conditions such as psoriasis and eczema and are added to shampoos to prevent itching. Some two hundred years ago Dr. Percival Potts described "chimney sweep cancer," which occurred mostly on the scrotum and other skin folds of these colorfully garbed but unwashed free-lancers. In 1967, Dr. A. Greither in Germany compiled 13 cases of skin cancer associated with the prolonged use of medically prescribed tar preparations, mostly in men but also in two women who had cancer of the breast and vulva.

The Second Annual Report On Carcinogens was issued by the Health and Human Services Department, on April 30, 1982, naming for the first time seven drugs which have shown evidence of cancer-causing potential. Reserpine, widely used for the treatment of high blood pressure and as a sedative and tranquilizer, led the list, followed by iron-dextran, used to treat anemia in children, phenazopyridine hydrochloride, used for 40 years to allay the pain of urinary tract infections, and streptozotocin, an antibiotic not used in the U.S.

Chemotherapeutic Agents: It has been known for some time that many of these drugs can cause other cancers to develop later. Newly incriminated in the government report are chlorambucil, procarbazine and thiotepa. While the drug treatment of cancer has shown increasing success, especially in childhood leukemia and localized Hodgkin's disease (a cancer of the lymph nodes), its adverse effects in stimulating the growth of new tumors have also been more frequent. Many of these chemical agents are derivatives of, or allied to, mustard gas, which has been a well known cancer-producing agent in industry. Since treatment generally includes several different drugs, as well as x-rays and surgery, it is difficult to determine which is the actual cause of the second tumor. The first cancer may cause death before the treatment-induced growth is discovered.

One of the first cases to be described (1951) was that of a 48-year-old man who was treated with a chemical called urethan for chronic leukemia for over a year, but died of cancer of the liver. The same agent caused two cases of lung cancer in 1954. Other drugs used for leukemia, breast, lung and intestinal cancer (myleran, radioactive phosphorus, bisulphan, and mercaptopurine) have caused the development of soft tissue tumors and additional breast cancers.

Although childhood deaths due to cancer have decreased by 40% in the U.S. in the past two decades, we still are 12th out of the 45 nations checked by the World Health Organization. Approximately five of every 100,000 children will die of cancer in this country annually. Cancer is the second cause of death for all age groups combined, but it is generally thought to predominate in middle and late life. It may surprise many to learn that it is also the second cause of death for children under 15, led only by accidents. Our relative success has exacted a price—the delayed consequences of the chemotherapy or radiation used to cure the original cancer. New, treatment-caused tumors have appeared in young men and women who overcame cancer 10, 15 or even 20 years previously. Before our new success, these growths were not a problem because the young patients did not live long enough to develop the induced cancer. New agents are constantly being developed. The list is too long to be detailed here but their risks are described in the PDR, which is available in most libraries and bookshops.

Estrogenic Hormones: In September, 1981, an editorial in the *Mayo Clinic Proceedings* by Dr. Kenneth L. Noller summed up our experience since 1971 when eight cases of cancer of the vagina appeared in daughters (aged 14 to 22) of women who had been given DES (diethylstilbestrol). The hormone was administered to these mothers during the 1940s and 1950s to prevent miscarriage. To date, over 400 vaginal and cervical cancers have been reported in the daughters living in various parts of the world. Of 304 cases studied by the National Cancer Institute in 1977, 83 died or had cancer recurrences after treatment. It is estimated that 4 to 6 million Americans (mothers, daughters and sons) were exposed to DES during pregnancy. The risk of cancer developing in daughters whose mothers received DES or similar hormones during pregnancy is 1.4 in 10,000, which is less than originally feared. However, they are at lifelong risk, because this cancer occurs most frequently in post-menopausal women. In addition to cancer, these young women also have increased spontaneous abortions and premature deliveries. Only slightly more than half of all pregnancies occurring in DES-exposed women go to term, compared to 75 to 80% of unexposed women.

A recent follow-up study at the University of Chicago revealed an excess of fatal breast and uterine cancers among these mothers, but this was not confirmed at the Mayo Clinic, where lower doses were generally used.

Sons too are affected, developing an excess of abnormalities of the penis, testicles, and lower urinary tract. These include undescended or undeveloped testicles (which predispose the individual to cancer), scrotal cysts, and reduced number and activity of sperm cells.

DES is no longer used in pregnancy but other estrogens are still being administered for menopausal symptoms, various vaginal and vulval diseases and inflammations. DES is also administered after removal of the ovaries and to relieve the symptoms and slow the growth of breast and prostatic cancer. It has recently been advocated to prevent softening of the bones (osteoporosis) with shrinkage, shortening, and development of "dowager's hump" in elderly women, and may prevent hip fractures in minor falls. It increases the risk of cancer of the *lining* of the womb (endometrium) from 5-13 times, depending on dosage and duration. Although endometrial cancer has been increasing in incidence since estrogens have been administered and kills over 11,000 women (48,000 new cases annually in the U.S.), its total death rate has declined due to improved diagnosis and treatment. But it has superseded cancer of the *neck* of the womb (cervix) as the most common malignant tumor of the female reproductive organs.

Contraceptives: The recent change from traditional to modern oral methods of contraception has been accompanied by a transfer of deaths from complications of pregnancy to complications of contraception. The term *maternal mortality* should be replaced by *reproductive mortality*. Although brain or heart disease due to blood clotting, and not cancer, is the chief culprit, the risk of cancer is increased. Benign liver tumors have been noted since 1973, and although precise data are not yet available, at least 20 cases of malignant liver tumors have been reported. Gallstones, with increased risk of cancer, have also been more common. Because of increased promiscuity and without the protective barrier of the condom, cervical cancer hazards are proliferating.

Immunosuppressant Drugs: When both kidneys have ceased to function, poisonous wastes will accumulate in the body (uremia), an inevitably fatal condition if not reversed. During the past 20 years, thousands of lives have been saved by artificial kidneys (dialysis) or by the transplantation of a new kidney. The latter choice, if available, promotes a higher quality of life than dialysis, but except in the rare cases of identical twin donors, rejection of the new kidney by the body as a foreign object is always possible. In 1965, the first case of cancer developing in the new kidney was reported, and since then, researchers have estimated that the risk is increased from 50 to 100 times. This may be due to dormant malignant cells being awakened by the drugs used to suppress rejection which reduce the body's defenses, or less often, to the development of a new cancer. This danger is so new that figures are not precise but these new cancers arise an average of 19 months following transplantation.

Other Drugs Causing Cancer: According to an FDA panel in 1979, evidence from experiments on animals indicated that four widely used drugs may be dangerous, since "chemicals found to cause cancer in animals are generally considered capable of causing cancer in humans." These include reserpine, commonly used for high blood pressure; methapyrilene, found in many non-prescription sleeping aids; selenium sulfide, an antidandruff shampoo ingredient, and disulfiram, used in Antabuse, an antialcoholic drug. As expected, the manufacturers deny this danger, making it all the more imperative for consumers to read labels and question physicians and pharmacists about the ingredients contained in their medications.

The National Institute of Occupational Safety and Health published a study in a 1981 JAMA, in which rats and mice exposed to formaldehyde developed increased nasal cancer. About one million six hundred thousand Americans, one-third working in medical and health services, are exposed to formaldehyde, a gas which, when dissolved in water, is used as a preservative for tissues removed at surgery or autopsy. Formaldehyde is also an ingredient in many plastic products.

Dilantin has been extensively used to prevent convulsions in epileptics. It has long been known to cause enlarged lymph nodes which are benign but sometimes difficult to distinguish from Hodgkin's disease. In rare cases, these nodes have become cancerous. More recently, the Journal of American Medical Association reported that fatal brain tumors called neuroblastomas may develop in children whose mothers were given Dilantin during their pregnancy.

Saccharin may be perceived as improving the quality of life in diabetics who must have sweet drinks. But it causes bladder cancer in rats, especially when the mother is exposed during pregnancy. Whether or not saccharin will cause bladder cancer in humans is as yet unclear. The general pattern of use of all artificial sweeteners is troublesome, according to an editorial in the *New England Journal of Medicine* (NEJM) in 1980. Women in the childbearing years, pregnant women, and young adults consume much more than others, and it is felt that this practice should be discouraged by their doctors.

Surgically Induced Cancer: Although rare, a few cases of a cancer called sarcoma have been noted at the site of orthopedic plates and nails, bone transplants, and dacron blood vessel replacements. More important are sarcomas developing at the site of operative scars after two to 20 years of dormancy. It is suspected that many such cases have not been reported, although approximately 30 have appeared in the literature. No part of the body predominates.

Various operations have been devised to remove or bypass benign stomach or upper intestinal ulcers. If the ulcer was mistakenly diagnosed as benign but was actually malignant, there should be recurrence within five years. On record are three hundred thirty cases occurring more than five years after the operation. Half of these cancers caused death within six months of diagnosis; one-third survived more than two years, but none was cured. These cancers occur in males five times more often than in women because men have more ulcers and more operations. (This beneficent disparity may change with more women executives having a larger role in business, professional and governmental decision-making positions, as has already occurred with lung cancer and heart disease.) The average free interval between surgery and diagnosis of cancer is 19 years.

Some 120 cases of sarcoma following radical mastectomy have been reported since Drs. Stewart and Treves' first description in 1948. The patient's age varied from 42 to 84 years and averaged 63. Two cases occurred in males. Death usually occurred within 16 months, and only 16 cases survived five years or more. These deadly tumors develop after swelling of the arm caused by interference with the blood circulation, a result of the extensive removal of tissue. Sarcoma may be expected to develop in one of 200 women who have radical mastectomies. This is another reason for the discontinuance of this mutilating operation in which survival statistics are no better than simpler procedures such as merely removing the affected breast or lumpectomy, where only the tumor is cut out, leaving the remaining breast intact.

When the urinary bladder is removed because of cancer, abnormal size or shape, or blockage of the long narrow tubes (ureters) joining it to the kidneys, the *ureters, until recently, were surgically connected to the lower bowel* (ureterocolostomy). This served as a reservoir for the urine, which was expelled with the feces. Twenty-five cases of tumors of the colon have been reported, occurring on the average of 20 years after surgery. Four were benign and 21 cancerous. Half of the cancer patients died within a year, the rest survived after another operation. The risk of developing cancer in these patients is 500 times that for normal persons. This operation has been supplanted by the new, more complicated, ileal conduit procedure, which is less prone to infection. Its cancer statistics are not yet available, but other distressing complications are described in the chapter relating to surgery.

Although smallpox vaccination is hardly an operation, it occasionally leaves lumpy scars. The literature describes 55 malignant tumors at these sites, but many more have probably not been reported. The average age, 52, is well below that for other skin cancers; for unknown reasons they occur four times more frequently in men than in women. Most have been of low grade and only three spread to other locations.

Any drug or blood product given intravenously, such as plasma, may bring the doctor, nurse or medical assistant into contact with the blood of the recipient who may be a carrier of hepatitis. Depending on geographic locality, 40 to 60% of the liver cancer patients have had hepatitis proven by immunity tests. Approximately 10% of this variety of hepatitis becomes chronically active and relentlessly progresses to cirrhosis. Cancer develops in cirrhotic livers three times more often than in the normal. It is relatively rare but invariably fatal. Because cirrhosis may also result from other drugs including isoniazid, used in the treatment of tuberculosis; methotrexate, an anticancer drug; methyldopa, used in Parkinson's disease; and halothane for anesthesia, cancer may follow, but enough time has not elapsed since these relatively new agents have been developed for us to have precise data.

Steroids, including testosterone, a male hormone, have been used for prolonged periods for the treatment of bone marrow suppression, impotence and male trans-sexuality. Liver cancer has been reported in 25 cases since 1965. A 29-year-old auto mechanic had been treated for many years with testosterone because of shrunken testicles. One day he was suddenly seized by excruciating abdominal pain and collapsed. An emergency operation revealed massive hemorrhage into his abdominal cavity from a ruptured liver which contained many deposits of cancer unsuitable for operative removal. Testosterone was discontinued, and several months later a "second look" operation found no evidence of the tumor.

Although as described in the chapter concerning radiation hazards, the use of *thorotrast* as a contrast medium has been discontinued because of its link to cancer of the sinuses and the liver, persons who have been subjected to this agent should be aware that due to the long latency period (which may be over 20 years after exposure), the risk of new cases developing still exists.

THE BAD AND GOOD NEWS ABOUT CANCER

First the *bad* news: In 1980, the American Cancer Society predicted that 785,000 Americans—20,000 more than in 1979 and 85,000 more than in 1978—would be diagnosed as having cancer for the first time. Only one-third of these victims will be alive in 1985. Among *major* malignancies, skin, lung, colon-rectum, and breast cancers are increasing. Lifestyle and environmental evils play the greatest role in this tragedy. Iatrogenesis is responsible only for the increase in breast cancer—birth control medication, although slowing the population explosion, increases the risk of breast tumors, which diminishes with early pregnancies. Cancer killed 403,000 Americans in 1979, and the estimated increase to 420,000 in 1981 exceeds that expected from the population growth. One in six in this country will die of cancer this year. A few years ago the risk was one in seven.

Despite these gloomy figures, offset by the decrease in deaths from heart disease and stroke, Dr. Vincent DeVita, Director of the National Cancer Institute, gave us some *good* news. In December, 1981 he estimated that 45% of the cases diagnosed in 1980 can be cured, not counting early cancers of the skin and cervix, which are nearly 100% curable. For persons under 55, the survival rate and quality of life "improved substantially in the 70s for patients with seven of the ten major forms of cancer." These include cancers of the bladder, breast, cervix, colon, uterus, prostate and rectum. But this hopeful progress for the *individual* due to better diagnosis and treatment, is nullified by the *national overall* increase in new cases and deaths.

CHEMOTHERAPY—PROLONGING LIFE OR DELAYING DEATH

Cancer has replaced tuberculosis as the most feared disease of the 20th century. The very word is often whispered. In her 1977 book, *Illness as Metaphor,* Susan Sontag described how it has become synonymous with death or evil. John Dean explained Watergate to Richard Nixon: "We have a cancer within—close to the Presidency—that's growing."

Tuberculosis, then "captain of the men of death," killed 200 out of every 100,000 Americans annually in 1900. Heart disease took second place with 148, and cancer was eighth with 70 fatalities per 100,000 of the population each year. Because of improved living conditions and the development of an effective antibiotic (isoniazid), tuberculosis is now not even among the first ten. Although heart disease, fortunately decreasing from its peak in 1968, is still the greatest killer of Americans, accounting for 40% of all deaths (334 per 100,000), cancer trails at 21% of all deaths (182 per 100,000). But dread of cancer far exceeds that of the more common heart disease.

Thirty years ago, treatment of cancer was only slightly more advanced than treatment of tuberculosis before Robert Koch discovered its bacillus in the 1880s. Some cancers of the colon, breast, uterus, stomach, prostate, and most cancers of the skin (except malignant melanoma) and occasionally of other organs could be cured by surgery and/or radiation. We don't know cancer's fundamental cause, although environmental influences such as tobacco and exposure to the skin's worst enemy—the sun—are proven triggering agents. Some cancers may be due to viruses; others may have to do with genetics and the body's immune, or defense system. When changes (mutations) occur in genes within the chromosomes of organ cells, they cause informational errors which are reproduced and multiply, assaulting the body like weeds devastating a garden. This random, disorderly, destructive growth is cancer.

Surgery and radiation are still the main methods of treatment for cancer, but the use of chemotherapy has increased in the past two decades. Only a few cancers are potentially curable by chemotherapy alone, but larger numbers can be controlled, increasing the length of life and sometimes its quality. In general, these drugs are used when cancer has spread to other organs, such as the liver, lungs or bone, rendering the disease inoperable, or when the cancer is naturally widespread, as in leukemia (blood cancer). Sometimes they are used after surgery if there is high risk for recurrence of the disease. They are most frequently administered in various combinations.

The chief drawback is that unlike antibiotics, which can focus on a specific microorganism, chemotherapeutic agents are not specific for individual types of cancer. In doses high enough to be effective they also attack normal body cells and have serious toxic effects. These can occur a few days or weeks after beginning administration and can involve the brain, heart, liver, lungs, genitalia, bones, blood and skin. The patient may experience extreme weakness, jaundice, shortness of breath, sweating, chills and fever, aches and pains, loss of hair, impotence, sterility, or cessation of menstruation. Irregular heart rhythm and sudden death have been reported. Chemotherapeutic drugs may also induce other cancers, particularly of the lungs, lymph nodes and leukemia. This distressing effect, although rare, appears to have increased in recent years, leukemia being most frequent after treatment of Hodgkin's disease and cancer of the bone marrow and ovary. For this reason, hospital pharmacists who handle anti-cancer drugs are extremely cautious. It has been found at the M. D. Anderson Hospital and Tumor Institute that samples of their urine caused considerably more mutations in bacteria than urine from their colleagues who had no contact with these substances.

A carcinogenic potential is possessed by some of the most effective anti-cancer drugs, according to Dr. Emmanuel Farber, of the University of Toronto's Pathology and Biochemistry Departments, in a 1981 *NEJM*. This would not be important in patients over 50 or 60 years old because there is a long dormant period before the new malignancy is manifested. But in children and young adults, the threat is greater. Over 25 compounds can produce cancer in animals and some of these have had the same effect in humans. This risk is increasing and in some patients varies from 7% to 12%. Another problem is analogous to the use of antibiotics—the survival and multiplication of resistant microorganisms is parallel to the similar survival and multiplication of resistant cancer cells. This has created a wide variety of new tests for possible anticipation of this resistance. Progress is far slower than that of the past generation's advance in the knowledge of the efficacy of antibiotics against specific bacteria.

Biochemists have devoted their skills to developing less toxic and more effective compounds than nitrogen mustard, as they did in the previous generation to conquer tuberculosis. By the middle 1960s, a large percentage of acute leukemias and Hodgkin's disease could be halted and temporarily rolled back, granting their victims normal lives. It is believed that certain acute leukemias in children, as well as localized Hodgkin's disease, have actually been cured, because they have not recurred despite cessation of treatment. Some testicular cancer victims have remained alive and free of cancer for several years. Other cancers could be made to regress for a few dubious months but at great cost to the patients and their loved ones. The question that confronts doctors and the victims of cancers that are inoperable or that have spread (metastasized) to other areas is whether the added months or years are worth the restricted, painful lives possible with most forms of chemotherapy, with or without radiation. There is no way of predicting which patient's cancer will respond to chemotherapy and whether the prolongation of life for a few months or a few years is worth the inevitable torment. The benefit is not absolute. The cure may be worse than the disease. Dr. Lewis Thomas, director of the Memorial-Sloan-Kettering Cancer Center in New York admits that the question is one of prolongation of life. "Is it possible to live well under the nonetheless certain and predictable prospect of dying?" The treatment of every case must be on an individual basis, the risks weighed against the possible benefits, knowing that the most informed judgment may be wrong. In recent years I have seen patients made so miserable that they and their families wish they had never begun chemotherapy. Others are carrying on bravely, able to perform their daily tasks. The increased susceptibility of patients under chemotherapy to infections will be discussed in Chapter 6 (Iatrogenic Infections).

Despite the understandably over-optimistic reports and predictions of the American Cancer Society and other agencies involved in fund-raising for this most worthy of causes, chemotherapy research has its negative aspects. New anti-cancer drugs must be evaluated on human subjects who have consented to serve as guinea pigs; 500 to 600 patients are usually required. There is no other way to determine their effectiveness and even if released for marketing by the FDA, their adverse effects, as well as their benefits, will not be fully known until they have been used for years on thousands of patients. No clinical trial can match this experience in practice. We must consider new chemotherapy from two different points of view—what is good for the public may not be good for the individual patient.

The National Cancer Institute collects data from 20 regional centers to which patients are referred for the evaluation of new chemotherapeutic agents. Around 150 drugs have been studied since the NCI declared "war on cancer" in 1971. A single drug, mitoxanthrone, derived from ball-point pen ink, has caused 22 deaths. Although it was developed to prevent heart failure caused by an approved drug, adriamycin, it actually worsened this effect. Dr. J. J. Wikich of the famed Sidney Farber Cancer Institute in Boston said, "There is a lot of brouhaha when a new drug comes out. But every drug follows the same pattern. They come out with a lot of excitement . . . from animal tests. But, it's given to 20 people and there's nothing. That's the same scenario for all of those 150 in the last five years, except for four or five."

Although Dr. Charles Vogel, director of the experimental clinic at the Miami Comprehensive Cancer Center, fully supports this program, he was quoted by the *Washington Post* in 1981 as saying that if he had an incurable cancer himself, he would never take part in a drug experiment. "I have my own views of life and death and how I would handle myself. If I reached the stage in a terminal illness and had exhausted the useful agents, it's hard to say what I would do. But I wouldn't be subjecting myself to toxic therapies. . . . I'd travel a lot. I'd go fishing." Another thought, "I'd kill myself."

Jerry McClennan, a newspaper deliveryman, had a "cigarette cough" which became worse in 1981. He had a chest x-ray exam and later told a friend, "When that doctor came out, he didn't waste no words. 'You got cancer in both lungs. You ain't got long at all.' I was 41 years old. It could make your knees buckle with a sentence like that." Mr. McClennan was sent to a Veterans Hospital where he consented to standard chemotherapy.

Soon after the intravenous injections, nausea would begin, with up to five hours of vomiting and diarrhea. He became so weak that he slept through most of the intervening time. But his ordeal was not effective. The drugs did not work. A doctor told him that he should try a new experimental drug.

Jerry was given an "informed consent" form which required his signature. Although the risks of the chemical were explained, he did not really understand. "I read the thing and was scared to death," he said. "I didn't want to do it, but it was either go on this or nothing. The doctor suggested it and I think he knows his business. He's educated. I felt this guy was a good schoolboy who had done his homework and that this was a drug that could knock this. I figured he wouldn't be in that position if he didn't have knowledge." Jerry did not comprehend that the purpose of his part of the experiment was not to establish the curative power of the drug but to learn more of its adverse effects and to determine its dosage. He later said that he would not have entered the experiment if he had realized that its purpose was not to offer him even a fighting chance of cure. "I damn sure don't feel like no guinea pig. I'm mostly worried about myself."

The new drug was given intravenously. "It ran into me for 12 minutes," he said the next day. "I felt woozy. I could feel my temperature [rise]. Two hours later I could feel it in my heart." He slept for several hours, bundled in a blanket and overcoat and woke up shivering and sweating. "My clothes were steamy. I was ringing wet. It made me deathly sick. . . . you just feel plain miserable all over. Your limbs, head, eyes, your mouth, your big toe even." Jerry died a few months later.

The question of how many human "guinea pigs" have died of true drug-related causes during experiments cannot be answered accurately. It is difficult for even the most careful autopsy to draw lines between death from cancer alone, cancer plus drug or drug alone. The *Washington Post* report charges that 620 to 1,450 terminal cancer patients have died from drugs, but Dr. Vincent DeVita, director of the NCI, admits to only 43. These trials, known as phase 1, are used to determine what happens to the body when the drug goes into it. All patients must be certified as terminally ill after standard treatment. Dr. DeVita insisted at a Congressional committee hearing, that no toxic drug is used unless there is "some ground" for believing that it might be beneficial. It is obvious that a desperate patient, clutching at straws, will have difficulty in giving rational "informed consent" and will seldom know all the risks, benefits, objectives, and alternatives when offered any treatment, experimental or standard. Dr. Fitzhugh Mullan, of the National Academy of Science, affirmed that there is "potential conflict of interest" when a medical researcher treats a patient while doing drug experiments. The cardinal principle of medical ethics, "First, do no harm," is frequently violated. The dilemma remains, for there is no other way of determining the deleterious effects as well as the benefits of a new drug.

All experimental drugs have severe adverse effects. The list is horrendous: kidney failure with uremic poisoning; liver failure with jaundice; heart failure with shortness of breath and swelling (edema) of the lower body; respiratory distress from lung damage; bone marrow failure with decrease of all elements of the blood cells causing anemia and hemorrhage; brain damage with confusion, agitation, hallucinations, tremor, dizziness, convulsions, paralysis and coma; depression with suicidal personality changes; increased growth of the cancer or the development of a new cancer. The patients, hoping for a miracle, do not anticipate the adverse effects or understand the real reason for the experiment. Without trial chemotherapy, many could be ambulatory at home.

The symptoms caused by chemotherapy for bone cancer, which is frequent in teenagers, are particularly distressing. Most of these tumors are treated by surgery, from local excision to amputation (as in the well-publicized encouraging case of the son of Senator Edward Kennedy). Radiation and various combinations of drugs follow, to try to prevent recurrence. The patients of all ages develop sores in their mouths, nausea with metallic taste, vomiting which can last for several days after each treatment, chills and fever of varying degree, dizziness, and anemia. They generally lose their hair within two weeks and frequently wear wigs. Although most find their families and friends supportive, often they are disturbed to find that some friends avoid them because they fear fancied contagion. They are saddened by the deaths of the friends they make in the treatment centers and obsessed by the thought that they may be next. But they are buoyed by hope and reinforced by a few examples of successful outcomes however uncertain their futures.

An example of a new anti-cancer drug is adriamycin, or doxorubicin. The FDA approved adriamycin in 1974, although it was developed in Italy in 1969. It has been used in the treatment of leukemia and lymph gland tumors and is the single most effective agent for breast, stomach, ovarian and some lung cancers. But it has the usual adverse effects, to which is added bone marrow destruction with anemia and bleeding. It also uniquely and irreversibly damages the heart when large doses are given, in up to one-half of the patients. This can be fatal or lead to permanent cardiac weakness, with heart failure occurring up to 200 days after the last dose. It is also believed that the effect of previous radiation damage will be enhanced by adriamycin. It has not been in use long enough for all of its complications to have turned up and it is possible that we have seen only "the tip of the iceberg."

Everyone remembers the optimism surrounding Hubert Humphrey's bladder cancer, which was diagnosed in 1973. The apparent success of his treatment became a media event, exploited by his doctors and the Memorial Hospital in New York. It was revealed that he had the best of early diagnosis when tiny, supposedly non-malignant growths were found in 1966. In 1973, the Senator received x-ray treatment and the cancer disappeared. In May, 1976, his doctor stopped treatment. A few months later the cancer was back. It was removed by surgery in October, after which he was pronounced cured at a press conference before television cameras for all the world to see and hear. As a precaution, "to wipe out any microscopic colonies of cancers cells that may be hidden somewhere in the body," the Senator was given a potent new drug. After a few months he refused further treatment because of the severe "side" effects of the medication, calling it "bottled death." He shriveled from vigorous maturity to withered old age during the next year and died.

The reader may criticize this account of Senator Humphrey as "anecdotal," a method which I have tried to avoid, as one can always select unusual cases for plausible proof. It is, however, typical of many similar instances I have seen, not only in my practice, but among some unfortunate friends and colleagues who continued to function after surgery but whose decline, although inevitable, was accelerated by toxic chemotherapy.

In September, 1980, the *JAMA* reported on a National Institutes of Health conference on chemotherapy for breast cancer. Barbara Chambers was the "consumer representative" on the panel. She had had breast cancer two years previously and had chosen to undergo chemotherapy. After two days of listening to impersonal statistics she asked whether any of the cancer therapists (oncologists) had studied the psychological and social consequences of post-mastectomy (adjuvant) chemotherapy. Dr. George Blumenschein of the M.D. Anderson Tumor Institute in Houston replied that he finds physicians to be "largely ignorant" of these effects. "Patients put their foot forward when they talk to the doctor. Then they discuss their difficulties with the nurse or social worker." Dr. Robert Frelick, president of the Association of Community Cancer Centers, agreed that many physicians cannot make close personal contact with their patients. "It hurts your ego sometimes to describe everything to the patient and then find she spends the next half-hour with the nurse trying to find out what you told her."

It would be inappropriate to list the scores of anti-cancer drugs and the combinations in which they are used. Except for their demonstrated value in acute leukemia and some types of Hodgkin's disease, most of the cancers in which they are effective are relatively uncommon: seminomas of the testicle, choriocarcinomas of the uterus, and childhood tumors such as Wilms' tumor of the bones and neuroblastoma. The major killers—cancer of the lung, breast, bowel, ovaries, uterus, stomach and prostate—seldom respond favorably. Chemotherapy becomes a gambler's choice, bolstered by faint hope that the possible prolongation of life is worth the added suffering and expense. Psychologists who have investigated the acceptability of this painfully restricted endurance of life are not all convinced that most adult patients would choose to pay the price for longer survival under these conditions. Dr. Richard J. Goldberg, a Brown University psychiatrist, stated in the *JAMA* in 1981 that "half of the distress associated with cancer is due to issues involving emotional and social adjustment." When patients are admitted to a cancer research unit, 75% have moderate to severe levels of depression, manifested by crying spells, non-compliance with care instructions and disinterest in further care, social withdrawal, apathy, and anger. It is obvious that it is difficult to distinguish a primary depression from one secondary to the results of treatment. Many of the anti-cancer drugs affect the brain and cause such symptoms, but these are generally not equivalent to the feelings of guilt and loss of self-esteem seen in depressed patients without cancer or other fatal illnesses.

One of the most distressing features of advanced cancer, according to Dr. Goldberg, is the "loss of social acceptability, isolation and a sense of abandonment. . . . Friends, relatives and employers may withdraw for a variety of reasons. . . . many people assume that cancer is contagious and avoid contact for fear of contamination. Even well-meaning family members may not be able to provide effective support because of problems of knowing what to talk about during a visit, or owing to the feelings of guilt or anger toward the patient." Chemotherapy is often given to prevent this feeling of being abandoned because the patient knows that something is being done, even though the doctor realizes it is incapable of stopping the cancer. Unfortunately, chemotherapy may exaggerate the patient's feeling of alienation because of its deleterious effects on the nervous system.

An ethical dilemma occurs when terminal cancer patients or their families ask about Laetrile, which has been convincingly proven to be without merit and has caused fatal poisoning from the cyanide it contains. Marcia Collins, 39, a heavy smoking, upwardly mobile business executive and ERA advocate, developed lung cancer for which her left lung was removed in 1978. In a few months, radioactive isotope scans revealed that the cancer had spread to her liver and bones. She was given radiation and chemotherapy with distressing effects, including loss of her hair, but the cancer continued to progress. In desperation, her husband took her to Mexico where she was given Laetrile and received a supply to take home. Re-examination on return showed that her abdomen was distended with fluid containing cancer cells. Radioactive isotopes were injected into her abdominal cavity but she progressed downhill to a sub-terminal state. Her husband asked their physician to administer the Laetrile. The doctor felt that it would have no more harm or benefit than the ritualistic radiation scans and chemotherapy to which she was exposed at great expense despite her obviously uncontrollable malignancy. It might ease her family's distress and her emotional transit through the process of dying. Since it could do no harm at this point, it was given with large doses of narcotics to relieve pain. Marcia soon became comatose and died.

The great strides that have been made in improving the survival of children with cancer by advances in surgery, radiation and chemotherapy have had a "flip side." Eight of ten children with Wilms' tumor of the bone will live over five years, as will most with acute leukemia. Half of children with all forms of cancer will live five years with no signs of cancer and all therapy discontinued. But what of the costs of cure? Not enough time has elapsed for full assessment. Many childhood cancers are rarities and survival is a new benefit, far outweighing the iatrogenic effects of treatment, but the number of cases is still relatively small. As more of these children live longer, additional iatrogenesis will develop. They graduate from pediatricians to care by family practitioners and internists. The late secondary adversities of successful cancer treatment are now becoming manifest, but although significant, they should not deny a child the chance of cure.

Dr. Giulio D'Angio, Director of the Children's Cancer Research Center of the University of Pennsylvania, has reviewed the costs of cure of children's cancer in *Hospital Practice* (1980). Some of the chemicals cause "flare" reactions by awakening dormant radiation effects long after radiation is discontinued. It is extremely difficult to determine whether the cancer, chemicals or the radiation cause late complications, and it is best to lump them as "combined treatment" effects. Although radiation iatrogenesis has been discussed in Chapter 3, it presents a special problem with children and will be discussed here in connection with chemoradiation therapy.

When infants have had radiation to the spine, there will be decreased growth and abnormal curvature (kyphoscoliosis). Facial deformities, excessive tooth decay and diminished output of growth hormone may occur if the head is irradiated, and there may be unequal growth of the legs if the tumor was in a lower extremity. These effects are enhanced by chemotherapy, which can cause loss of calcium and other minerals.

Cardiac damage may be extremely severe and progress to irreversible failure. The lungs may lose some of their spongy consistency, making breathing difficult. Chronic scarring of the liver can simulate cirrhosis and may be mistaken for spread of cancer. Urinary abnormalities, inflammation, scarring of, and bleeding from the bladder, and kidney failure are especially frequent in combined treatment. Nervous system effects range from somnolence to dementia, and facial paralysis to paraplegia. The endocrine system is not spared, with thyroid depression, temporary or permanent sterility, and ovarian failure resulting in decreased menses. Not enough time has elapsed for evaluating genetic defects.

Stimulation of a second cancer is the most feared consequence of combined therapy. The risk is greatest 15 years after treatment is begun and has been estimated as 17%, with leukemia leading the list.

Although intellectual impairment is rare in adolescents, depression and anxiety are common. In a study of 54 survivors over 18 years of age, social stigmatization was evident; 12 were rejected from employment because of their cancer history, six were not accepted by the armed forces, and several could not obtain medical and life insurance. Three of ten younger children who had received both chemo- and radiotherapy had impaired reasoning, mathematical ability and motor skills. Another study showed that 34 of 37 survivors had average or above average scholastic rank in high school. Perhaps the enforced isolation due to their disease and its treatment drives them to academic, rather than social and athletic, accomplishment.

Some chemotherapeutic drugs that have been implicated in causing new cancers have been withdrawn. Others (mephalan, cyclophosphamide, chlorambucil) are still dubiously used for cancers of the ovary, breast, lung and brain although they enhance the risk of leukemia and/or bladder cancer.

Immunosuppressive agents used to prevent rejection of transplanted kidneys also increase the hazard of malignancies outside of the urinary system. Lymph system cancers occur 35 to 50 times more than expected, half in the brain. The risk for all other cancers combined is doubled after kidney transplantation principally arising in the bone marrow, soft tissues, skin and lung.

Estrogenic hormones increase the risk of cancer of the lining of the womb. Although there is some evidence that long use of oral contraceptives adds to the danger of cervical cancer, these drugs actually *reduce* by 50% the development of the less common ovarian cancer.

When psoriasis, a common skin disease, is treated by a drug called methoxypsoralen plus ultraviolet light, skin cancer follows at over 2½ times the anticipated rate.

Common pain-relieving drugs (analgesics) containing phenacetin as A.P.C. (aspirin-phenacetin-caffeine) or fiorinal, can, in large doses, cause kidney damage. Over a hundred cases of kidney cancer and a few of the bladder have been associated with its use. Ironically, these compounds have been largely supplanted by non-prescription Tylenol.

As the use of chemotherapy increases, serious damage to the nervous system, although uncommon, has been observed, especially when multiple drugs are given in combination with radiotherapy. Meningeal and nerve irritation with localized weakness, and loss of sensation and paralysis, as well as encephalitis, causing confusion, speech disturbances, tremors, ringing in the ears, loss of balance, convulsions, deafness, blindness and final termination in stupor, have been noted in various assortments with many of the newer agents.

Hundred of thousands of compounds have been tested in the past 25 years. Of these, 150, on the basis of animal experiments, were found to be active, warranting trial on humans. But only 40 slow or stop the growth and spread of some cancers.

Clinical trials on patients start with Phase I. These are conducted on 15 to 30 advanced cancer cases which have not responded to any known treatment. Such patients must choose between no treatment except support and relief of pain; or experimental acceptance of a drug or combination of drugs whose therapeutic value and dosage are speculative. But adverse (toxic) effects are certain, although their precise nature and degree of damage await the termination of the trial. Since only a small percentage of these victims display slowing of tumor growth and most suffer appalling distress, Phase I trials are examples of human sacrifice. Supreme Court Justice Oliver Wendell Holmes has aptly remarked that progress is achieved only through "the death of men." Studies have shown that only a few patients understand that they are experimental subjects despite so-called informed consent.

If the trials are successful, Phase II and III studies follow to determine more precisely the drug's degree of anti-tumor activity. The initial sacrifice has resulted in chemical cures in many patients with leukemia, Hodgkin's disease and a few rare tumors of the lymph system, testicular cancer, unusual embryonic (chorioepithelioma) and bone and kidney cancers in children. Most other solid cancers are only temporarily arrested. A verdict that patient benefit is sufficient to justify the prolongation and increase of anguish and expense for patients and their families is still awaited.

Only when molecular biologists unravel the mysteries of changes in bodily cells (somatic mutation), and learn how to prevent or arrest cancer by developing genetic or immunological resistance, will real progress occur in this disease.

6.

IATROGENIC INFECTIONS (NOSOCOMIAL)—THE HIDDEN DISEASE

Despite their inescapable dangers, people need hospitals not for their *health,* but for diagnosis and treatment of *disease.* Often benefits exceed risks. Severe injuries including burns, major operative procedures (elective or emergency), or medical conditions where patients are unable to care for themselves cannot always be managed at home or on an outpatient or office basis. With so many sick people closely confined, germs floating about and carried by personnel, implements, visitors and patients, and the use of potent multiple drugs and complicated invasive and surgical procedures, hospitals are beleaguered fortresses. Shining stainless steel and spotless surfaces give no indication of the microscopic foes probing all defenses. As potential patients, we should all be concerned with the alarming increase of iatrogenic effects.

The most recent survey, taken in the spring of 1981 by the Boston University Medical Center, found that 36% of 815 patients admitted for medical treatment had iatrogenic complications, causing 15 deaths. Drugs played the greatest role, with infection following. *A nosocomial infection is any infection acquired in a hospital.* The expression is derived from the Greek: nosos=disease, komein=to take care of; hence a nosocomial infection is a "disease caused by being taken care of." Although nosocomial seems synonymous with iatrogenic, in practice it is applied only to hospital-acquired infections. It does not mean that the infection was preventable or that the hospital was negligent.

Nosocomial infections have existed since sick people were segregated for treatment in hospitals. Two million such infections occur in the U.S. each year, increasing morbidity and mortality and adding $1.5 billion to our $287 billion 1981 medical care bill. Five percent of all patients contract an infection while in a hospital which directly causes 20,000 deaths and contributes to 60,000 additional fatalities. Although nosocomial infections have increased only slightly during the past 50 years, there has been a drastic change in their variety. Most community-acquired infections have been dramatically controlled.

Large numbers of nosocomial infections reflect high percentages of seriously ill patients, typically those who enter or are transferred to major teaching centers. Leukemia and other generalized cancers are less often treated and organ transplants or open-heart surgery less often performed in small community hospitals. Invasive diagnostic procedures, dialysis, artificial heart valves and joints, and mechanically assisted respiration have all created new pathways for the acquisition and spread of infection. Because of age, debility, chemical treatment of cancer (chemotherapy) or radiation, such seriously ill patients have overtaxed immune systems and are highly susceptible to ever-present viruses, bacteria and fungi. Otherwise healthy people with appendicitis, hernias or injuries are not. Increased longevity and the improved management of previously fatal illnesses have resulted in a larger number of elderly patients who are particularly susceptible.

The media have not failed to publicize hospital-based epidemics due to widely distributed commercial products. Their medicolegal implications are obvious to administrators, doctors, and patients' lawyers, and add to the cost of malpractice insurance.

Infections acquired outside and inside the hospital may be related. Between 10 and 15% of patients admitted to general hospitals enter with infections contracted elsewhere. These people are at increased risk of developing new nosocomial infections and transmitting them to other patients, hospital personnel, and friends or family who visit the hospital or come into contact with them after discharge.

Autopsy data in 1959 showed that the types of fatal infections occurring in hospitals were strikingly different than they had been 20 years previously. Deaths from infections contracted before admission were less common, while those acquired in hospitals increased. Many of these were due to organisms not formerly considered dangerous. The lowest percentage of infections, 3.5%, occurred in a group of community hospitals and the highest, 15.5%, in a large municipal hospital. In 1968, it was estimated that one of every 1,500 patients admitted to the prestigious Johns Hopkins Hospital died of an infection acquired there. The financial and medical resources wasted by this excess were of major importance. International conferences sponsored by the Center for Disease Control (CDC) in 1970 and 1980 made it clear that nosocomial infections were not only a "full-blown national epidemic" but a worldwide disaster born of new treatments.

In June 1981, Johns Hopkins Magazine quoted statistics that 2 million infections, 150,000 fatal, are acquired in hospitals each year in the United States. If you're admitted, you have 7 chances in 100 of being part of this grim toll. Bacteria are even more adaptable than humans. More and more are developing strains that are resistant to antibiotics. There is a race between the development of new drugs and the resistance of the organisms they are devised to combat. The Joint Committee on Accreditation of

Hospitals will not accredit hospitals that do not have infection control committees and programs to monitor, prevent and combat infection. The struggle ebbs and flows, but victory is not yet in sight.

At Johns Hopkins, every postoperative wound infection requires $700 in extra care and every blood stream infection, $4,000. Heart operations average $10,000 but if the surrounding tissues become infected (mediastinitis), the cost more than triples to $33,000.

Death from infection is a major factor in preventing more cures of cancer. Many reports show that from 32 to 47% of cancer patients die of infection alone. Bacteria account for 70 to 90% of these deaths. Viruses, fungi and parasites, in increasing percentages, cause the remaining nosocomial fatalities in malignant disease.

Large hospitals have infection control teams headed by trained physician-epidemiologists and assisted by nurse-epidemiologists. In the smaller hospitals the nurse-epidemiologist administers the program. All infections are cultured, the germs identified by the microbiology laboratory, the patients' records studied, and a decision made regarding whether or not the infection is nosocomial. Cultures are also made of equipment used for anesthesia, inhalation therapy, physical therapy, sterilization, invasive procedures, nursery functions and all areas of the hospital. Patterns of bacterial, viral or fungal contamination are sought and recorded, and appropriate precautionary measures are advised and instituted.

In February 1981, the CDC reported nosocomial infection data fom 81 hospitals since 1970, averaging 1,160,000 patients and 40,000 infections annually. These represented a cross-section of U.S. hospitals and patients from small community hospitals of 100 beds to governmental and university hospitals with over 1,200 beds. The nosocomial infection rate per 10,000 discharges rose from 312 (3.12%) in 1970 to 358 (3.58%) in 1975. It decreased to 329 (3.29%) in 1979.

Municipal hospitals have always had the highest average rates of infection. In 1975-1979, the rate was 5%—in some as high as 15%—followed by federal (4.5%) and university (4.3%) hospitals. The lowest rate was in community hospitals (2.5%). Is this disparity expected? Is the socioeconomic and educational status of patients and personnel in governmental hospitals lower than those working in private hospitals, and is disciplined control more difficult to maintain? The sites of infection have not changed significantly during this period: urinary 41%, surgical wounds 23%, lung and bronchi 15%, skin 6%, blood 4.4%, gynecologic 2%, nose and throat 1.3% and heart and blood vessels 1.2%.

Intestinal infections are less frequently nosocomial except in cancer patients undergoing chemotherapy who often develop low white blood cell counts, making them more susceptible. Also, antibiotics administered to prevent or combat other infections destroy the normal germs of the gut. These are replaced by invading alien bacteria from the outside environment which are the most common cause of serious infection during chemotherapy. The hospital kitchen is the most important source, say Drs. Jack Remington and Stephen Schimpff, who published *Please Don't Eat the Salads* in the New England Journal of Medicine in 1981. Although these patients are placed in "protective" isolation, which involves the use of mask, gloves and gowns, they are allowed ordinary hospital food and water. Bacteriologic investigation has shown that uncooked salads are the most important carriers of intestinal infections and should be eliminated from the diets of hospitalized, high-risk patients.

Bacterial Infections

Any infectious disease may be nosocomial, but four out of five involve the kidney and bladder, surgical wounds, lungs, or blood stream (septicemia). They have in common a sterile interior but contaminated exterior environment. Once an organ or tissue is infected, bacteria grow, forming colonies which serve as reservoirs for scatter to other parts of the body. These sites are rendered susceptible by previous tissue damage, generally due to surgery or invasive procedures such as the insertion of catheters into cavities or blood vessels. Most germs are carried by the fingers and hands of patients, doctors, nurses, and other personnel who contaminate each other. Any area or equipment can be a source, including food and water. Fewer are airborne, traveling from patient to personnel and back to other patients, but these can be equally deadly.

Despite regulation, carelessness continues. Dr. Richard K. Albert reported in the *New England Journal of Medicine* that "on the average, hospital personnel washed their hands after contact with patients less than half the time. . . . Physicians were among the worst offenders." One survey showed that only 28% washed. Patients in the Intensive Care Unit (ICU) are the most susceptible. Hand-washing, however, has its pitfalls, as does the wearing of masks and gowns. Most infections in the Intensive Care Unit are not airborne but are spread by direct contact, according to Dr. James Rahal, chief of infectious disease at New York University Medical School. Although, cleanliness seems common sense, he found that bacteria thrive in soap "gunk" in dishes kept on sinks used for washing hands. Even liquid soap dispensers carry infection on their spouts. Individual powdered soap packets, although expensive, are best, and sinks should be placed between each patient bed, not just at the door, to prevent shortcutting. But there is a build-up of slime and moisture in sinks which enhances the growth of intestinal organisms, generally harmless to the healthy but deadly to debilitated patients in the ICU. Therefore, frequent aseptic cleaning should be mandatory. Gloves should be worn when wounds are inspected.

Almost any invasive procedure may be complicated by infection, in addition to other damage specifically due to the instrumentation and anatomic location. When the brain fluid pressure is reduced in cases of "water on the brain" (hydrocephalus), the site of the indwelling plastic catheter gives bacteria another opportunity to enter the body. Even oxygen administration and inhalation therapy have their perils, especially when pumps are used, tubes are inserted through the throat, or the windpipe is opened (tracheostomy) to permit breathing below an obstruction.

Urinary Infections: In 1980, Drs. Givens and Wenzel of the University of Virginia Medical Center reported that almost 1 million patients acquire a nosocomial bladder and/or kidney infection each year. These comprise 40% of all iatrogenic infections, and most, but not all, occur after instruments, usually catheters, have been inserted. Up to 75% of patients having instrumentation will become infected, a total of 600,000 from catheters alone. The bacteria may invade the blood stream, causing fatalities in 30-50% of all cases, as well as chronic prostate, bladder or kidney infections, and there are added adverse effects from the antibiotics which are administered to combat the infection. The researchers studied the effect of catheterization after cesarean section, bowel operations, coronary artery bypasses, and various orthopedic procedures such as hip replacement or spinal disc operations. These infected patients stayed in the hospital an average of two and half more days and spent $558 more than uninfected controls.

Urinary catheters, if draining into an open vessel, will always eventually cause bladder and kidney infections. They should be left in place in a closed system. But 20% of patients maintained on closed systems may also be expected to become infected. Once the kidneys are infected, the blood stream follows and if the bacteria localize on a heart valve, the mortality rate will be 50%. The common, pus-forming staphylococcus and various intestinal inhabitants have developed strains found only in hospitals which are resistant to penicillin and newer antibiotics.

A 36-year-old secretary, whom I shall call Frances Hartman, was suffering from arthritis. She was given a new drug called penicillamine, which in rare instances suppresses the blood-forming function of the bone marrow. Despite careful monitoring by blood counts every two weeks, after seven months of treatment Mrs. Hartman suddenly experienced extreme weakness, excessive bleeding during menstruation and large bruises over most parts of her body.

All elements of her bone marrow and blood count were now markedly decreased, a condition called aplastic anemia. This is a devastating disease with a 25% fatality rate, from which only 10% of patients recover completely. Mrs. Hartman was hospitalized and given numerous blood transfusions and various steroid hormones. The drugs and her low white cell count increased her susceptibility to infection and after several weeks she developed fever and burning while urinating. Cultures showed that her bladder was infected with a bacterium normally present in the bowel, where it causes no problems. The loss of her immunity, however, enabled it to invade her urinary system. A new antibiotic, gentamicin, relieved her infection. Her aplastic anemia improved but is still present, and the ultimate outcome is uncertain.

Surgical Wound Infections: Although aseptic practices, introduced by Baron Joseph Lister almost 100 years ago, have greatly reduced the percentage of operative incisions that become infected, 41,000 were reported from 80 hospitals during the 4-year period from 1975 to 1978; these constitute 23% of all nosocomial contaminations. There was a decrease from 86 to 81 per 10,000 patients discharged. The only exception, obstetric infection, increased from 75 to 95 per 10,000, a rise presumably linked to the increasing frequency of cesarean section. There was a startling variation among different hospital reports, ranging from 1% to 20% and averaging 7.5%, suggesting that conditions unique to each hospital prevail. The highest rates occurred in municipal hospitals, although they too showed a modest decrease, except for gynecology, which remained stable. In many of these patients, the blood stream was contaminated with bacteria.

Rates of infection vary with different surgical procedures. Simple mastectomy wounds are infected in 5-10% of all cases, but infection from hernia repairs (herniorrhaphies) occurs in only 1-5% of all cases. Patient resistance is a major factor. Those at greatest risk are the newborn and elderly, diabetics, patients receiving steroids or drugs to suppress immunity prior to transplants, the obese, and those having had long hospital stays prior to operation. The surgeon's skill and the duration of the procedure also play a part. The most common bacterium is the ubiquitous staphylococcus. Most patients and personnel harbor this germ on occasions, but 10% to 15% are chronic persistent carriers. One study showed that 21% of operating room doctors, nurses, and attendants carried staphylococci in their noses. Some infections are acquired in recovery rooms or when dressings are changed in the patient's room.

During the past 25 years, the role of normal intestinal bacteria in wound contamination has increased. These bacteria are carried on the hands of personnel or from the patient's own excreta to the skin or lungs, and sometimes via the blood stream to the incision.

Of the 300,000 surgical wound infections occurring in the U.S., community hospitals have a lesser incidence than large municipal and teaching hospitals. Among community hospitals, however, the smallest, from 20 to 100 beds, which perform fewer operations, particularly appendectomies, gallbladder and uterus removals, and hernia repairs, have more infections than those with greater volumes and more experience. This suggests that improved technique decreases the risk of contamination.

The much publicized toxic shock syndrome (TSS) associated with vaginal tampons has now made its appearance in cases of surgical wound infections. It generally occurs after common or minor procedures usually not considered liable to infection, or cesarean deliveries. In 13 instances, one death occurred. A JAMA editorial stated that it is probably a new disease, caused by a change in the virulence of the staphylococcus. Why the toxicity of this common bacterium has increased is unclear. If the new variety of staphylococcus becomes established in the hospital environment, disastrous infections may result.

Pneumonia: Pneumonia causes 16% of nosocomial infections. It occurs in 0.5 to 5% of patients and is increasing. A fatality rate of 30 to 50% makes it the largest killer, although it is third in incidence of all hospital infections. It is common in the ICU. Doctors, nurses and weakened patients spread many pneumonia-causing bacteria to each other. A study presented by the University of Utah College of Medicine in 1980 showed that 18% of 520 patients having chest or abdominal surgery developed pneumonia, the greatest risks being obesity, age and smoking. Widespread use of inhalation therapy equipment is partially responsible for the increase in lung infections which are spread by the use of nebulizers attached to oxygen or other respiration-assisting apparatus, especially those producing "cool mist." They are always moist, coated with germs and difficult to sterilize. Sometimes the windpipe is opened (tracheostomy) to assist breathing; 20% of these patients develop pneumonia because the defense mechanisms of the nose and throat are bypassed. Many cases are now caused by ordinarily harmless intestinal germs. Fungal and viral pneumonias are also more prevalent with massive antibiotic therapy, or lowered resistance caused by chemotherapy or drugs given to prevent rejection of transplants.

Legionnaires' Disease (LD) was first recognized in 1976 as an outbreak of pneumonia at a convention where 180 delegates became ill, with 29 fatalities. Clusters have occurred among inpatients, outpatients, employees at, or visitors to, hospitals. In 1978, ten patients from six hospitals in five states were autopsied and reported by the Center for Disease Control as having LD. They died an average of 5 days after onset, which occurred 5 to 40 days after admission. During a 3-year period, 2,756 patients in 80 hospitals died of nosocomial pneumonia; 105 of these were actually LD, proven by microscopic study of the lungs. It is estimated that almost 1,000 cases of nosocomial LD occur in the United States annually. Heavily smoking men with weakened immunity predominated.

Although LD was first identified in 1976, research has concluded that it actually originated in 1942 as "Fort Bragg Fever" and was the cause of several cases of pneumonia during the 1960s. The first nosocomial epidemic occurred in a Burlington, Vermont hospital in 1977, with 69 cases and 11 deaths in three months; 12 originated in the dialysis unit. In 1978, a Memphis hospital had 39 cases including staff and visitors. It was felt that the bacteria were windborne from water in the air-conditioning cooling tower, air currents carrying them to patients' rooms and even the main entrance. Two cases occurred after kidney transplants in Oxford, England in 1979, and a Los Angeles VA hospital had many cases until its water was chlorinated. In March of that year, a Pittsburgh hospital had 13 cases and seven deaths; and since then over 50 such nosocomial LD cases have occurred throughout all departments.

Intensive studies have shown that the bacteria causing LD are present throughout the water supply and air-conditioning systems of hospitals harboring nosocomial cases. They have been isolated from cooling towers, showerheads, potable water faucets, mixing valves, bedpan flushers and hot water storage tanks.

It is likely that LD is more common than previously thought, because of the 3,000 cases of pneumonia that occur annually in the U.S., one-third have had unknown cause, and many could actually be due to LD.

Skin Infections: These comprise 5.7% of nosocomial infections. When immobilized patients lie on their backs they develop foul, open sores over the bony protuberances of the back and buttocks called decubitous ulcers. New "third generation" antibiotics have been developed to combat the multitude of different bacteria involved. But their incidence is increased by poor nursing care which, sadly, is often the rule in many nursing homes for the elderly.

In the nursery, approximately one to five babies per 1000 develop skin eruptions due to staphylococci (impetigo, pustules). About 20% progress to pneumonia, blood stream or bone infections (osteomyelitis), with serious prolonged illness or death. About 30% of nursery personnel carry "staph" in their nasal passages and these germs are found on bedding, floors and tables. Bathing with an antiseptic called hexachlorophene (pHisoHex) can prevent much of this contamination, but this has been discontinued because hexachlorophene was found to be a brain and kidney irritant, sometimes with fatal results.

Blood Stream Infections (bacteremia, septicemia): These dreaded infections most frequently spread from common urinary, wound, lung and skin sources. They occur in 4.3% of nosocomial disease. Together they develop in 194,000 patients in the U.S. and cause 75,000 deaths, adding $860 million to medical costs. Most are related to therapy such as segregation in a special care unit (58%) and/or exposure to intravenous procedures (65%).

Over 100 million intravenous needle and catheter insertions for the administration of fluid, blood products and nutritive material are performed annually in the U.S. Because of contamination and other defects, 608 items in 43 million containers were recalled by their manufacturers between 1965 and 1975. Fifty-four patients suffered fatal infections and 410 were made seriously ill. The offending bacteria entered the supposedly sterile containers either during the process of manufacture or in the hospital. Because sampling of the material to be administered can only be random, there is no way that complete security can be assured.

Invisible hairline cracks and punctures can permit bacteria and fungi to enter the fluid. All accessory equipment, such as stopcocks, filters and connecting tubing, are vulnerable, as are many of the patients, whose illness has weakened their immunologic resistance to infection. In 1971, the CDC publicized a serious problem which occurred when thousands of flasks of I.V. fluid distributed to hospitals nationwide were found to be contaminated, resulting in epidemics of blood stream infections (bacteremia). The offending organisms actually lurked in the screw-cap closures. During one epidemic as many as 30% of the units of I.V. fluid were contaminated. This revelation promoted the use of disposable plastic bags for I.V. solutions.

Intravenous needle and catheter sites and the blood stream are frequently infected when the insertion and care is done by inexperienced interns and residents. This occurs less often when "I.V. nurses" perform these chores. Bacteria (or fungi) may lodge on heart valves damaged by rheumatic fever, causing fatal destruction. They may also grow on surgically inserted artificial valves from which they may spread to other parts of the body. Unusually located infections are the most serious complications of total parenteral nutrition catheters. Seriously ill patients are predisposed to invasion of their joints by pus-forming bacteria which circulate in the blood stream causing pain, tenderness and swelling, mostly in the knees.

Nosocomial Sinusitis

Sinusitis has not been seriously regarded as hospital-acquired, but at the University of Maryland's Division of Infectious Diseases, 34 cases occurred in 32 patients during the 2-year period from 1978 to 1980, accounting for 5% of their nosocomial infections. Most of these patients had tubes inserted in their noses to drain the stomach or trachea, or packing of their noses for hemorrhage, antibiotic treatment, high-dose steroid hormones or fractures of their facial bones. Fever was common, but only a minority had nasal discharge. Most patients recovered after removal of their nasal tubes, with some requiring new antibiotics, but five died of other diseases before the sinusitis improved. It was felt that this problem is more important than has previously been considered, especially in the ICU.

LABORATORY INFECTIONS

Bacteriology laboratory workers are dangerously exposed to germs with which they are working. Despite all precautions, these invisible attackers can get out of the test tubes. Since the turn of the century almost 3000 laboratory infections have occurred in the United States. During the past few decades, viruses have become the leading agents. Technicians can then transmit disease to their contacts, particularly their families.

To test proficiency in identifying organisms, typhoid cultures were sent to 4,500 laboratories between 1977 and 1979. During this time, 672 cases of typhoid fever were reported to the CDC. Over 11% of these were acquired in laboratories, where more people are exposed to this infection than in actual clinical practice.

In 1980, three other cases of typhoid in persons who did not work in laboratories but who had visited them were reported to the CDC. A 6-year-old child who ate half of a sandwich which her mother, a technician, had brought home also contracted typhoid. During the past three years, 32 laboratory workers had been hospitalized for laboratory-acquired typhoid fever—all due to bacteria used in proficiency tests. One in 12 died. Undulant fever (brucellosis) and rabbit fever (tularemia) have also occurred among laboratory workers. The overall mortality from laboratory infection is under 5%. Careless technique, perhaps contempt due to familiarity, must be considered the major cause of these mishaps.

Pathologists have been known to acquire many diseases from handling of surgical and autopsy specimens. In 1981, the New England Journal of Medicine reported two pathologists in California who were infected with tuberculosis after preparing frozen sections of lung tissue thought by the radiologists to be cancerous. In the past, when autopsies were frequently performed without gloves, "pathologists' warts" due to tuberculosis were common occupational hazards.

Nosocomial Viral Infections

Hepatitis: This serious liver inflammation strikes patients, personnel, and visitors. Historically known as catarrhal jaundice and in military facilities as camp jaundice, great advances have recently been made in understanding its mode of spread and classification into different types. It has been common whenever populations existed in close proximity.

Hepatitis B virus (HBV) was the first agent to be identified as a major risk to patients and personnel and as a primary cause of post-transfusion and post-dialysis (serum) hepatitis. Hepatitis A virus (HAV) is transmitted primarily though fecal contact. Now that HAV and HBV can be distinguished by clinical and laboratory methods, a new category due to unknown agents has emerged, labeled non A/non B (NA/NB). We have no tests for the NA/NB virus. Its diagnosis can be made only after infection with HAV, HBV, and the less usual Epstein-Barr (EBV) and cytomegalovirus (CMV) has been ruled out. NA/NB is now the major cause of post-transfusion hepatitis and is also spread by other blood products.

Post-transfusion hepatitis B has significantly declined in the past ten years due to elimination of "skid-row" and other paid donors known to be frequent carriers of HBV and by pre-transfusion testing of all blood. Beginning in the 1950s, patients with kidney failure undergoing dialysis also received HBV-contaminated blood and many became chronic carriers, transmitting HBV to other patients and to the staff serving them. This was documented in 1972, in a study of 11 Boston area teaching hospitals whose staff, especially those exposed to blood, frequently contracted hepatitis. Cases of nurses caring for pediatric patients with bleeding diseases, surgeons operating on HBV-positive patients, and laboratory staff handling contaminated blood specimens were cited.

Within the hospital, physicians, nurses, and laboratory and dialysis technicians are at greater risk than patients. Pathology and clinical laboratories, emergency rooms, dialysis and hepatitis wards, operating and recovery rooms, dentistry units, and blood banks are the most dangerous areas.

HBV is transmitted by needle injection of contaminated blood or serum, by blood transfusions or dialysis, or through cuts or raw skin surfaces. Technicians may inadvertently stick themselves with needles after drawing blood from the veins of patients or carriers of HBV. This virus is also present in the saliva, tears and semen. Studies in dialysis units have also shown that it can contaminate and be transmitted through needle clippers, gloved hands, and any equipment or instrument which has come into contact with blood from a patient or carrier. One newly admitted patient in 100 is a carrier, affording multiple risks of infection. But HBV is *not* transmitted through the stools, as is HAV. When hospital staff members suspect that they may have inoculated themselves, they are injected with hepatitis B immune globulin, which is extremely costly. It may cause pain or shock and is not guaranteed to prevent or reduce the severity of the hepatitis they may acquire after two to three months of anxious waiting. An effective HB vaccine has recently been approved by the FDA and should largely eliminate the carrier state.

The physician-carrier poses a dilemma. What is the risk of transmission of hepatitis to patients? Should clinical practice be prohibited: Dr. R. E. Sampliner of the University of Massachusetts Hospital has stated the concensus that ill physicians be excluded from patient contact until recovery and blood tests show that they are not carriers. If the doctor is a chronic carrier, containing the virus in his or her blood for over 6 months, spontaneous clearance is infrequent. Gloves must be worn for any procedure involving a break in the skin. Saliva and blood contact with patients must be avoided by sterilization of all exposed instruments. There must be no eating or drinking in patient care areas. Unfortunately, no method to remove the virus from the blood has yet been found.

Laboratory evidence of current or previous infection with HB was found to be more *than 3 times as common among physicians and dentists* surveyed at a convention in Arizona than in first-time blood donors. Fourteen percent of these professionals had a history of viral hepatitis; 3½% of dentists had hepatitis with jaundice during their training and professional careers. (It must be remembered that most hepatitis does not display jaundice.) The degree of risk of medical or dental personnel transmitting hepatitis to their patients has not been established, although it does exist. In 1976 and 1977, reports of an asymptomatic oral surgeon infecting 55 patients, a dentist with chronic HB, 13, a general practitioner, 12, a nurse, 11 and an inhalation therapist, 4, were published in various journals. In 1981, seven clusters, of nosocomial HB, totalling 137 cases, were reviewed. The greatest group was traced to two oral surgeons who operated without gloves. After they donned gloves, no additional HB infections occurred in their practice. Hospital employees carried HBV in their blood twice (0.8%) and dentists three times (0.9-1.7%) as often as the general population and are thus more likely to be asymptomatic carriers.

Hepatitis A is seldom contracted by hosital patients or staff, who have no more risk than the general population. It is not transmitted by blood and has only a short carrier state via the feces. It has an incubation period of two to six weeks, averaging one month. Epidemics occurred in January, 1982, when 12 persons in a Queens, N.Y. hospital, including four physicians, five nurses, one patient and two visitors, acquired nosocomial HA. In 1977, 11 of 55 staff members of a California hospital who cared for a child who had marked fecal soiling of her body and bedding were affected.

A 21-month-old girl was admitted to a Los Angeles hospital in 1978 because of dysentery. Approximately one month later, three physicians developed HA—the first laboratory confirmed instance of HA being transmitted from a patient *without jaundice* to hospital personnel.

NA/NBV now accounts for 80% of post-transfusion hepatitis, but is present in only 25% of patients admitted with hepatitis. It is becoming more prevalent after dialysis and has been transmitted to patient-care personnel after needle punctures. The stools may also carry the infection. Its incubation period is midway between that of HA and HB; approximately 45 days. It is frequently unsuspected because jaundice occurs less often than in HA or HB but may cause a concealed, chronic carrier state.

Despite the explosion of knowledge about viral hepatitis, post-transfusion and post-dialysis hepatitis remains a problem that just won't go away. Its magnitude is masked by the long incubation period, its frequent mild symptoms and the absence of jaundice in most cases. Laboratory tests, although helpful, are not sensitive enough to eliminate all the carriers from the pool of donors.

In June 1978, the Mayo Clinic reported that three to five of each thousand transfusion recipients became carriers of HBV or NA/NBV, 72% without having had jaundice. In that year, the American Medical News, an AMA publication, reported that if blood from paid donors was used, the risk of a recipient acquiring hepatitis is 3.5 times that of blood from volunteers. According to the AMN, the John Elliot Blood bank in Miami supplied 55 hospitals with blood, 80% from paid donors. These hospitals performed 144 heart or blood vessel operations in which large quantities of blood were used; 21% of these patients developed hepatitis.

Shingles (Herpes Zoster) is a painful eruption, generally involving one side of the chest. Because it is caused by the virus of chickenpox (varicella), many cases of this generally mild pediatric disease spin off from contact with zoster or other cases of varicella. In weakened patients or those awaiting surgery this complication can be serious. Young interns and nurses have contracted varicella from patients.

Other Viral Diseases: During my army duty I was surprised by the number of pediatric diseases such as varicella, German measles (rubella), and red measles (rubeola) among young soldiers who were hospitalized for other conditions. These occur in civilian hospitals as well and their complications in adults are more severe than those in young children. The cytomegalovirus (CMV) can cause a type of hepatitis and, like varicella, is particularly dangerous in pregnancy because it may cause fetal deformities. Herpes can also spread from patient or personnel sources. Cold sores or mouth blisters may be trivial, but genital herpes in females, which is not necessarily transmitted sexually, can be precancerous. Herpes may also cause life-threatening disease in the newborn, acquired during its passage through the birth canal.

An epidemic of nosocomial Influenza B virus infection occurred in a Huntington, W. Va. hospital recently when 29 patients and several staff members contracted the disease within four weeks. Only one had received influenza vaccine during the past year. The excess cost was estimated at $460 per patient, totalling $13,000. Although there were no fatalities in this series, in other clusters there were added deaths from pneumonia, influenza or both. Patients in nursing homes are particularly vulnerable. In one example reported by the CDC, during February and March of 1982, 38 of 116 elderly residents of a home in Georgia developed influenza, and for many, the disease was fatal.

Nosocomial Fungal Infections

Fungi include yeasts, molds, and mushrooms. With the advent of antibiotics which alter the bacteria normally present in our bodies, with chemotherapy for malignant disease, and with the use of drugs to prevent rejection of transplanted organs by suppressing immunity, fungi have been invading greater numbers of patients during the past several decades. The CDC believes that the trend will continue upward because the predisposing factors will also increase. The problem is compounded by the many adverse effects of antifungal drugs such as griseofulvin and amphotericin B, and by the fact that diagnosis is made definite only by biopsy or autopsy. There are no well-established X-ray or clinical laboratory criteria for many of the invasive fungal diseases.

Death from infection plagues many cancer patients. Although bacteria account for most of the fatal infections during therapy, fungal infection has been increasing in recent years. A study at Barnes Hospital in St. Louis could not find a single case in patients with leukemia and lymph node tumors from 1919 to 1941, but in 16,000 autopsies for all causes, fungal infections were found in one case in a thousand. After the introduction of antibiotics in 1941, the incidence rose to 11 cases in each thousand autopsies. And in 1962, it sextupled to 66 per thousand. At the Sloan-Kettering Cancer Center in New York there was a 15-fold increase from 1950 to 1959, and fungi complicating leukemia doubled between 1959 to 1964.

The Jefferson University Medical College in Philadelphia performed 1,200 autopsies on cancer patients during the ten years from 1966 to 1975. Over 7% of these had fungus infections, but during the first 5-year period the incidence was 5.1%, while during the second, it was 9.3%. (Under 3% of patients dying of non-malignant disease had fungal infections.) The enhancement of fungal invasion by radiation, antibiotics and chemotherapy, as well as the advanced age of many of the patients, accounts for this increased risk. Leukemia leads the list with 23%.

A 1979 report from the University of Cincinnati College of Medicine described 77 adults who had 85 episodes of nosocomial blood stream fungus infections (fungemia). Their risk factors included antibiotics, intravenous and urinary catheters, simultaneous bacterial infections, recent surgery, and intravenous feeding. Fungemia could be distinguished from bacteremia only by culture. Eleven (14%), developed severe eye inflammation, three became permanently blind, and 29% died as a result of the fungemia; 33, or 42%, recovered spontaneously when their catheters were removed or antibiotics stopped.

Fungal eye inflammation is a special risk during total parenteral nutrition (intravenous feeding), as demonstrated by the case of Sam Foster, who was shot in the abdomen during a robbery attempt. His spleen and left kidney were removed and the operative wounds became infected, requiring surgical drainage. He was placed on TPN. He suddenly became more acutely ill after seven months in the hospital, with shaking chills and fever up to 104 degrees. Candida, a yeastlike fungi, was recovered from the blood and the catheter tip. The total parenteral nutrition catheter was removed but two more blood cultures found candida. Subsequent blood cultures, however, were negative, and IV hyperalimentation was resumed. Three weeks later, Mr. Foster complained of blurred vision and severe pain in his right eye. An ophthalmologist found severe inflammation and amphotericin B was started. The inflammation subsided but impaired vision remained. He deteriorated and after four months, died of heart and kidney failure.

Another example of how serious the nosocomial complications of modern treatment can be is the case of a 22-year-old army corporal whom I shall call Martin Jones. Martin was tinkering with a gasoline field stove when it exploded, causing severe burns over two-thirds of his body surface. He was rushed to a nearby hospital where a catheter was inserted into a leg vein to permit administration of fluids and blood. Large doses of penicillin and steroid hormones were given and dressings were applied under pressure. A week later streptomycin and chloromycetin were added. At this time the dressings were removed, revealing that the burnt areas were foul-odored and heavily infested with maggots. These were cleaned out under anesthesia. Martin continued to have a high fever, sometimes rising to 106 degrees. Despite adequate fluids and antibiotics, he lost awareness of his surroundings and had visions of gun-battles. He became comatose and died 2½ weeks after the accident.

Autopsy revealed that Martin's death was caused by numerous abscesses due to candida in the brain, heart, lungs and kidneys. This fungus is almost universally present and harmless to the healthy, but its invasion of vital organs was promoted by antibiotics and steroid hormones, compounding his general weakness.

It is not always necessary for patients to have deadly disease or drastic therapy for nosocomial fungal infection to develop. Philadelphia's Temple University Hospital has reported several such cases. One, that of a 53-year-old, otherwise healthy man, began with his admission in 1977 for total left hip replacement by an artificial joint (prosthesis) because of disabling arthritis. The operation was uneventful, but when the dressings were removed five days later, blisters were noted at the site of the adhesive tape. By the 12th day these had developed into ulcers. Biopsy and culture revealed mucor, an unusual fungus. Local treatment resulted in complete healing within two months. However, when this organism infects leukemic or debilitated patients it is almost universally fatal, and its diagnosis is seldom made before death.

Nosocomial Parasitic Infestations

A single-celled animal parasite, a protozoan called *pneumocystis carinii*, can cause violent pneumonia in patients who lack immunity because of treatment or congenital deficiency. Although it is probably spread by direct contact, we are not certain of this, and there is little that can be done to control it. In a series of British patients pneumocystis carinii was a major cause of death after bone marrow transplants. A 1980 report in *Pediatrics* related that of 67 infants two to 12 weeks old with pneumonia, 10, or 14%, had pneumocystis in their lungs. None of these had deficient immunity or any underlying disorder. Although they had no fever, all had severe shortness of breath, cough, and x-ray film shadows. New tests and new antibiotics permitted early diagnosis and recovery in these otherwise healthy infants.

Strongyloidiasis is an infestation of the small intestine with an invasive parasitic worm, ⅛-inch long, which, with its eggs, is found in the stool. It occurs primarily in the rural South in areas having poor sanitation. Although the Center for Disease Control found the national average to be two cases in a thousand, it reported that New York City, with its many immigrants from the third world, and Kentucky had over one for each hundred people. About half have no symptoms, but abdominal cramping, bloody diarrhea, pneumonia-like invasion of the lungs and death occur.

New, severe infestations with these parasites, which usually cause few symptoms, occur in patients receiving treatment to prevent rejection of transplanted organs, primarily kidneys. The first fatal nosocomial cases of disease due to creatures visible to the naked eye were reported late in 1981 in the *American Journal of Clinical Pathology* by Dr. Lawrence H. Boram of the Jewish Hospital in Louisville. He described three patients receiving corticosteroids who were infested with strongyloides, none of whom lived under unsanitary conditions. One, a 22-year-old male, had been placed on dialysis for kidney failure in March of 1977. In February of 1978, a kidney transplant was performed and he was maintained on cortisone. A month later he developed signs of rejection, for which he was given other steroids and low-dose radiation. He failed to respond and his kidney wound became infected. He then developed severe intestinal inflammation with persistent diarrhea, and strongyloides parasites and their eggs were found in his stools. He rapidly deteriorated and died in June.

A previous study in 1974 reported 32 patients with strongyloidiasis, 24 of whom died, all having received treatment to suppress immunity. What will be the next animal parasite to be awakened to deadly invasion by medical intervention?

Special Pediatric Nosocomial Hazards

Most healthy babies enter the world with a clean slate. But if they require lengthened hospitalization, especially if premature and in intensive care, they are at significant risk. The Children's Hospital in Boston reported in 1981 that 15% of infants in its ICU contracted a nosocomial infection. The bacteria are transmitted by contact with the mother's genital tract during delivery or with the hands of personnel caring for the infants. Reports in the late 1950s and early 1960s described plagues of skin infections in nurseries due to staphylococcus. These frequently invaded, causing breast abscesses and bone inflammation, or osteomyelitis. This has fortunately not recurred and now we chiefly see an inflammation called the "Scalded Skin Syndrome." At one time this was wrongly thought to be preventable by bathing in a mild antiseptic called hexachlorophene, (PhisoHex) which has been discontinued because of its toxic effects.

Because intensive care and new antibiotics have increased the survival rate of newborn babies, the first 26 days, or neonatal period, remain a risk period for bacteremia and meningitis acquired from organisms resident in the nursery. Most of these, which originate in the intestinal tract, still make a significant contribution to infant illness and mortality and can only be eliminated by scrupulous attention to handwashing and sterilization of equipment and linens.

Although bacterial infections have been emphasized, the frequency and importance of viral nosocomial respiratory tract infections in pediatric patients have generally been underestimated. Recent studies have shown that these exceed all others in pediatric services. Colds and symptoms such as sore throats and cough are so common that they are thought to be trivial and their importance as forerunners of pneumonia may be overlooked.

Sometimes antibiotic treatment can weaken the bacteria that cause pneumonia in newborns, resulting in failure of the bacteria to grow on blood culture. The Children's Hospital of Columbus, Ohio studied 111 cases of fatal pneumonia in infants less than one week old occurring from 1974-1978. Although among other germs, 19 cases of streptococcus pneumonia were uncovered, 41 showed no indentifiable organism.

As advances in medicine have prolonged longevity of children with cancer, cystic fibrosis, chronic kidney disease and congenital immunity deficiency, the percentage of these children in hospital populations has increased. They are also frequent visitors to outpatient facilities. The infections they contract are analogous to those of the premature. New antibiotics and vaccines for chicken pox and hepatitis B have been developed. But this problem will not go away, and it is certain that the numbers of children at greater risk for nosocomial infection will increase in the foreseeable future.

Nosocomial Hazards to Hospital Workers

These dangers are commonly invisible but widespread. Many of those in greatest jeopardy know little about the risks they take. Hepatitis, staphylococcus and streptococcus infections, and typhoid have been discussed earlier in this chapter, as have been the work areas of greatest danger. There are many other, less frequently considered infections, which in their totality, make hospitals veritable combat zones!

Pregnant employees' fetuses are exposed to viruses which may cause severe deformities if the mother is exposed during the early months after conception. The risk from rubella is well known but the recently discovered cytomegalovirus (CMV) presents similar perils. Blood tests have been developed to identify this virus and contact with such patients must be avoided.

Diphtheria is decreasing, but 200 to 300 cases, one-third in adults, have been reported annually in the United States in the past decade. It has been found that no more than half of medical students or personnel have been immunized. This danger is only potential because during a recent outbreak all immunized personnel remained unaffected.

Although many cases of cold sores or fever blisters are unrecognized in the hospital, susceptible patients in the categories already discussed may have serious illnesses due to the herpes virus. Hospital staff who develop inflammation or blisters on their hands may not only spread the virus to patients but to their own mouths or genital tracts. Genital herpes is precancerous and may also affect the fetus. Scrupulous hand-washing, glove-wearing and avoidance of work in areas where such cases are hospitalized should be practiced as in all other infectious situations.

Measles now frequently occurs in young adults and may cause abortion and prematurity if contracted furing pregnancy. Because histories are unreliable, blood tests for immunity will determine which persons should be vaccinated.

Six percent of reported mumps occurs in adults over 19 years old. One adult male in five with mumps will develop inflammation of the testicles (orchitis), which can cause permanent sterility. Some may have nervous system inflammation. In 1971, several interns and medical students working in pediatrics developed this unpleasant complication.

During the influenza season, hospital personnel are exposed to a greater degree than those in other occupations. Because of the interaction between patients, personnel and visitors, it is difficult to document nosocomial spread. My experience as a pathologist and director of laboratories has taught me to expect an inordinate absenteeism during influenza outbreaks.

Although the incidence of tuberculosis in the United States has gradually declined, in 1980, 28,000 new active cases were reported. If the infection is unidentified in a patient, it constitutes a hazard for personnel as well as other patients. The tuberculin test, which indicates not active disease, but immunity due to past contact with the bacteria, is frequently negative in young student nurses, many from rural areas. However, almost all become positive by the termination of their training, although clinical disease seldom develops. Their risk is greatest, with that of medical students and residents following. As mentioned previously, tuberculosis is not extinct among pathologists.

Chickenpox (varicella-zoster) virus is highly communicable, but a few adults have escaped the disease and remain susceptible. Patient care personnel are more vulnerable than others and should be removed from duty until the skin lesions have subsided or the 21-day incubation period has passed without sign of the disease. If complications which are more common in adults like herpes zoster, pneumonia or brain inflammation (encephalitis) develop, the illness is no longer trivial.

Needle-stick injuries may also seem trivial, but a study of 316 reported cases from 1975 thru 1979 at the University of Wisconsin Hospital revealed that these accounted for one-third of all work-related accidents. Dr. Denis Maki and Rita McCormick, R.N., reported that housekeeping and laboratory staff suffered the highest percentage of needle accidents, but nurses experienced 60% of these injuries. The study was prompted by a severe case of hepatitis B originating from an accidental needle stick. The total cost to the hospital in a 27-month period was $6,331.

A comprehensive plan for management of hospital personnel exposed to communicable disease was presented by Dr. Jerome O. Klein of Boston City Hospital at the 2nd International Conference on Nosocomial Disease, held in 1980. Dr. Klein mentioned outbreaks of whooping cough (pertussis) and Legionnaires' Disease but gave no figures for employees. He reviewed the recommendations of the Study on the Efficacy of Nosocomial Infection Control that every hospital should have a plan including the following: directions for the management of each of the common infectious diseases, directives for employees at special risk, such as those who are pregnant and those who work in high-risk areas like newborn nurseries, clinical and pathology laboratories, blood banks, or hemodialysis units, assessment of the infectious disease experience of new employees by history, skin tests for tuberculosis and blood tests for rubella and hepatitis B and a plan for subsequent tests during employment, a continuous program of education for employees in infection control, and coordination of policies among administration, employee health service and infection control committee.

The first study of nosocomial infection was made shortly before the revelations and recommendations on sanitation made by Drs. Semmelweis and Holmes. A surgeon at the University of Edinburgh found that 2,000 amputees in hospitals had a much higher death rate from infection than a similar number whose limbs were removed in their homes. He called these infections a disease, "hospitalism." The strides made by Pasteur and Lister prevented millions of infectious deaths and many thought that the problem was solved. This illusion was dispelled during the 1914-1918 war but was revived in the antibiotic era. With the development of resistance by bacteria and new invasive varieties, our hopes have again been frustrated, even though on balance, benefits have exceeded harm.

At the first International Symposium on Nosocomial Infection, in 1971, Sir Robert Williams described the advances made since World War II and the methods of monitoring developed during the 1960s. In summation he said, "The one outstanding omission from almost all the studies of preventive measures is any attempt to measure *cost effectiveness*. We could devise any number of elaborate preventive measures, but even if money were unlimited, the ability of personnel to observe a plethora of precautions is limited, no matter how vigorous the admonitions of the hospital infection committee. It should be our aim to determine those procedures whose value is really established; we have so little documentation of the good achieved. One of the principal reasons we have failed to persuade our colleagues in hospitals to do the antiseptic things we think they ought to is that we have rarely provided them with convincing evidence that if they do, their patients will get better more quickly or survive in significantly greater numbers."

What progress have we made since Sir Robert's eloquent but dubious synopsis? We know more about the part the patient plays in the development of nosocomial infections. Immunity or lack of immunity are the most important factors. Resistance to invasion is reduced by chemotherapy, by lowered white cell counts in the blood, which occur in certain leukemias and anemias, especially those secondary to drugs depressing the bone marrow, and by medication given to patients receiving kidney or other transplants. We have no reliable tests to identify incompetence of immunity.

We understand more about the risk of bacteremia associated with the use of equipment or supplies which are supposedly sterile, especially those used in invasive procedures and for intravenous fluids and nutrition. This was demonstrated by the widespread outbreak of bacteremia caused by contaminated intravenous fluid from one manufacturer.

There is less concern with the general hospital environment but more emphasis on specific sites and procedures as well as new organisms which have emerged during the past decade, principally those causing Legionnaires' Disease, cytomegalovirus infections and their relatives, and parasites such as pneumocystis and strongyloides. We have also learned that short-term prevention of infection may be effective by chemical means, especially in high-risk patients prior to surgery for the insertion of foreign objects, such as heart valves or artificial joints. The risk of infection may not be great when these procedures are used, but the consequences of infection can be disastrous.

We have developed tests for the indentification of hepatitis A and B, for their differentiation from NA/NB, and for the recognition of carriers of these viruses. However, only Maryland requires that carriers be reported to the State Health Department, and the law is ineffective because carriers cannot be registered without their informed consent, which is seldom given for fear of job loss. Now that HB vaccine is available, the law is unnecessary.

With a few exceptions, the recommendations, so laboriously considered and recommended for each hospital department by overworked staff committees, have not resulted in success. Many meticulous sterile procedures involving catheters, isolation, and intravenous fluids have not resulted in lowering the infection rate.

We still have no precise data regarding the hazards of beards, flowers and the water in their vases, stethoscopes, wheelchairs or the relation of showerheads to Legionnaires' Disease. Sir Robert Williams' 1971 challenge has not been met. We just don't know about the effectiveness of our elaborate surveillance system. The SENIC and JCAH recommendations are based on insufficient hard evidence that they will be effective. To fulfill them, says Dr. Eickhoff, would require that a 400-bed hospital employ "at least two full-time nurse epidemiologists, a full-time secretary and a well stocked xerox machine, together with innumerable hours of work by the chairman and members of the infection committee and others of the professional and administrative staff of the hospital." This would add immensely to the already unbearable cost of medical care with no assurance that its outcome would be beneficial. As an example, Grady Hospital in Atlanta recently identified 91 nosocomial bacteremias. Thirty-two of these were related to various invasive or respiratory assist procedures, and in 25, all recommendations were followed. Only seven deviated from standards. Therefore at least 84, if not all, could not have been prevented.

The flip side is that if, as in another study by Dr. M. R. Britt of the University of Utah College of Medicine, all high-risk patients with fatal underlying diseases are identified on admission and antibiotics and invasive procedures *used minimally*, nosocomial infections can be reduced by half. Since the patients ultimately die of their disease the "benefits" may be questioned by many, except for those benefits relating to reduced cost.

It is time for the medical profession and the public to accept the inevitability of mortality. Medical intervention, too often prolongs, not life, but the process of dying without dignity, with added pain and emotional trauma to the patient and family.

In a previous chapter I discussed the fitness or "wellness" phenomenon that has become a nationwide movement. Although there is no solution to the human dilemma, we can avoid many of our sorrows and needless expense by adopting a measure of responsibility for our health in order to prevent illness requiring hospitalization. Except for obvious conditions requiring intervention, like severe traumatic injury, localized inflammations and tumors needing surgery and medical emergencies, people must be taught to care for themselves before they become patients, while they are patients, and after they have been patients. They, with their physicians, must carefully weigh the risks of hospitalization against its benefits. If, as in some respiratory viral diseases, a patient has one chance in a hundred of dying from hospital-acquired infection, how many indications for hospitalization are there that warrant this hazard?

The best way to avoid nosocomial infection is to *stay out of the hospital whenever possible.* If you are ambulatory or can be transported by family or friends, home, office, or outpatient care should suffice for most illness or injury. If you must be admitted, get out as soon as possible. The growing movement towards outpatient surgery and the construction of facilities in which the patient returns home after a few hours of observation will reduce not only costs, but infectious and other complications, with the saving of many lives.

Dr. Paul Gertman, chief of the Boston University School of Medicine health care research section, agrees that there is marked over-utilization of hospitals and ancillary services in the U.S., from 10-50% of admissions being unnecessary in Massachusetts. Once admitted, there is overuse of nursing personnel, of tests for routine procedures, and particularly in terminal cases. "Every oncology [cancer] patient gets a complete profile, even when there is no indication." This fruitless intervention increases the risk of infection (and other iatrogenic complications).

As the public becomes better informed of the risks, demand for hospitalization should slacken unless it is really necessary. Intelligent people do their best to reduce their own personal risk factors leading to illness by adopting a prudent lifestyle.

7.

HOSPITALITIS—THE INHUMAN ROUTINE

Mrs. Margaret Feldman was anxiously awaiting hysterectomy. Medication had not controlled her excessive uterine bleeding which was causing anemia. Her gynecologist ordered a transfusion of two units (about a liter) of blood the day preceding the operation. The nurse deftly inserted a needle attached to a plastic tube connected to a clearly labeled blood container. "Why are you giving me type B blood when I *know* I am an A?" Mrs. Feldman asked. "Oh, my God!" exclaimed the dismayed nurse as she instantly yanked out the needle. By chance, I was walking through the hospital corridor and overheard this exchange through the open door. We confirmed that the blood was intended for Mrs. Madge *Fieldman* who occupied the adjoining bed. Why weren't the patients' wrist bands checked? Human error again proved the truth of Murphy's Law. If this mistake had not been detected by the alert Mrs. Feldman she would have suffered a serious, perhaps fatal, transfusion reaction due to destruction of the incompatible blood cells entering her circulation.

Radiation damage and infections, discussed in earlier chapters, are among the most important injuries sustained by patients. They are only two of the many physical and emotional perils that lurk in the total hospital environment. Administrators and staff are greatly concerned with risk reduction, focusing on a common element—the occurrence of an event which causes an unfavorable outcome.

These events are termed "patient incidents" and require the completion of an incident report for subsequent review and action. Reducing incidents will result in fewer malpractice claims and consequently lower malpractice insurance premiums. These premiums have increased from $200 million in 1972 to $1.2 billion in 1977, and account for almost 3% of already unbearable hospital costs. It is estimated that if the present trend continues, insurance costs will surge to over $10 billion by 1989.

The report usually includes such information as the type of incident—errors in medication, tests and/or treatment, the type of injury: abrasions, bruises, sprains, fractures, head injuries, burns, infections, internal injuries, heart or breathing arrest or adverse medication effects, the extent of injury: minor, severe or fatal, the location of the incident, the personnel involved and the sequence of events leading to the incident, and contributing factors—staff training and communication, patient behavior, equipment that contributed to or caused the incident, and safety devices available at the time.

From February of 1978, through June of 1979, 5,500 incident reports were submitted by nine Iowa hospitals. Almost three-fourths resulted in no known injury, one-fourth were minor; 1% were severe and 0.1% fatal. Almost half were traumatic, with falls accounting for 36% of the total. Some thirty-six percent were medication errors, including omission of medication or wrong medication, dosage or timing. Treatments, tests, and "miscellaneous" comprised the remaining 15%. Three-fourths occurred in patients' rooms, with nurses the most frequent personnel involved. A 1980 report from the University of Florida recorded 432 incidents with a similar ratio—166 (38%) were falls and 137 (32%) were medication errors.

The data obtained from these reports can enable a hospital to take action to reduce the frequency of errors. For example, my hospital took great pride in its bright shining floors which were constantly being waxed and polished. When several patients slipped and fractured wrists and collarbones, the housekeeping department effectively shifted to a non-skid surface dressing. However, it has not been shown that less common accidents can be predicted, and no research has shown that the costly studies required of hospitals by state laws are effective. Each incident has its unique set of contributing factors.

A 1979 British study did not yield significantly different results from those performed in the United States. Accidents to patients peak slightly at ages one to 20 and rise again dramatically after 60, with incidents involving the very young and the very old predominating. The areas of most frenzied activity had the highest accident rates: for example, operating rooms, x-ray, outpatient, and emergency departments. Of approximately 2,200 incidents not involving medication or surgery, falls comprised 1,800. Cardiac patients and those under sedation are more likely to fall out of bed. Unattended patients, even fully conscious, may fall off narrow stretchers while awaiting transfer to other areas. If there are no guard rails, as in the case of a 56-year-old lady who broke her thigh, the hospital cannot deny liability.

Here is a typical case of negligence: An 80-year-old woman being treated in a Massachusetts hospital for a mild heart attack was given a sleeping drug by a nurse who raised the upper bedrails only. Shortly after midnight, Mrs. Moon awoke to go to the bathroom. She was able to slip out under the upper bedrails and staggered to the hallway, where she fell and broke her hip. An operation was deferred because of her poor general condition and she was not able to walk without pain or assistance afterwards. In a suit against the hospital, she was awarded $20,000 because the jury agreed that the nurse was negligent in not having raised the lower rails. She should have anticipated that the shaky patient would become confused.

The inventory of injuries due to defective, malfunctioning or misused equipment includes scalds and burns, cuts from equipment and shaving prior to operation, trauma from violence and miscellaneous accidents of every conceivable variety—doctors' eye burns because of sparking arcs from electrically illuminated equipment such as cystoscopes or the explosion of an infra-red lamp cutting the faces of patient and operator, x-ray equipment falling on the patient's head or causing electric shock due to a short circuit, burns from lights, cautery instruments, heating pads, smoking materials, incubators, thermal mattresses and fires, several of which in oxygen tents have been fatal, cuts from broken thermometers, needles, and guide-wires used in catheters, collapse of chairs or beds causing head injury, and strangling in restraining jackets. The list is endless.

Self-inflicted injuries after drug overdosages, incidents in which patients set themselves on fire while smoking, and suicides performed by jumping out of windows have all been reported. One such attempt, which caused paralysis from the waist down resulted in the hospital being sued for negligence on the ground of insufficient supervision.

A similar malpractice suit may involve all hospital personnel attending a patient: A resident in surgery was an innocent bystander as a member of the operating room staff of an esteemed teaching hospital in upstate New York. He was assisting his chief in a routine hernia operation. All was going well, when suddenly the middle-aged patient gasped, became blue and expired. The anesthesiologist had left his post at the head of the table and one of the attendants stepped on a loosened tube, causing a kink and depriving the patient of oxygen. This tragedy resulted in the resident being party to a multimillion dollar malpractice suit, since everyone in the operating room was included. The case was settled out of court for several hundred thousand dollars (but the resident suffered no financial loss since the hospital underwrote his malpractice insurance).

Despite all efforts aimed at quality control and orientation of personnel, the human factor inevitably frustrates "fail-safe" instructions. My laboratory included a blood bank with a special cylindrical refrigerator containing "lazy Susan" shelves on which approximately 100 containers of blood, many reserved for specific patients, were stored. The blood had to be maintained at a narrow temperature range of 1 to 6 degrees centigrade. The refrigerator had an automatic visible graphic temperature recording chart and was attached to an alarm system. If the temperature fell below or rose above these limits a red light would flash and a bell would ring. For additional safety in case the night technician were called away, a bell would ring in the central telephone operator's station. The emergency maintenance crew would at once be alerted to remedy loss of current or malfunction in the refrigerator. Numerous precautions were instituted to prevent the wrong bottle of blood from being removed. No one was allowed to open the door but the technician in charge, and the blood could be given only to a registered nurse or physician, who had to sign a book containing identification of patient and blood by name, age, sex, type, and number. Despite this care, several years ago at 4 A.M., the temperature rose above 6°C while the technician was not in the blood bank. The bell rang in the telephone operator's station. As a new employee, she had not yet been told of its purpose, and because she was nearsighted, she could not read the small sign indicating the bell's function. Annoyed, she placed a bit of folded paper under the clapper. When her replacement arrived at 7 A.M. she asked, "What is this damn bell for?" Commotion ensued—the maintenance and blood bank crew all rushed to the refrigerator and found that the last person to dispense blood had inadvertently left the door ajar. All 100 units were unfit for use at a loss of over $5,000, but more important, many patients who needed transfusions had to wait almost a whole day before the proper types of blood could be obtained from other sources. The major surgery scheduled that morning was cancelled at great loss of time and added expense because surgeons will not operate unless blood is readily available to replace blood lost from any unexpected bleeding that might occur.

A 60-year-old, apparently healthy teacher, noticed mild chest pain in 1976. This increased with exertion and progressed to unbearable angina. After an EKG and coronary angiography, a bypass of her left main coronary artery was deemed necessary. She was prepared by intravenous medication and firmly strapped to a litter with tubes and electronic equipment in place. For reasons not disclosed, surgery was delayed for two days. The patient was obliged to lie motionless on her back in an extremely uncomfortable, spread-eagle position, for 48 hours, anxiously awaiting a dangerous operation. An attending nurse admonished her, "If you move you will die." Despite this inhumane preparation, the operation went well. After several weeks, she was discharged. As she was being wheeled to the waiting car, she asked her escorting nurse, "Why are these wires sticking out of my chest?" Only then, did the surgical staff remember to remove the monitoring device which had been implanted during the operation.

The Overuse of Intensive and Coronary Care Units (ICUs and CCUs)

Although many people are now alive who would not have survived a disastrous head injury, heart attack, breathing difficulty, or drug overdose unless they were treated in an intensive care unit, the overuse of these costly, "hi-tech" facilities has concerned many thoughtful critics. Not only are many admitted to the ICU who don't need it, but its complexity generates iatrogenesis. Also, adverse results elsewhere may send a patient to the ICU.

ICUs originated as postoperative recovery rooms, but starting in the 1960s, they were also used as CCUs to detect rhythm irregularities after heart attacks. Later, their function was expanded to include monitoring heart failure not associated with coronary disease; breathing difficulties due to lung disease, coma, blood borne bacterial disease, and bleeding from the stomach or intestines.

In 1981, Dr. William A. Knaus of George Washington University Medical Center reported in the Journal of the American Medical Association that half of the critically ill patients admitted to the ICU did not require its electronic monitoring. Nursing care and close observation would have been sufficient. Over 80% of patients admitted for auditing breathing, blood pressure, and heart rhythm (vital signs) needed no active treatment. These conclusions were the same as those of similar studies at the Massachusetts General Hospital. The statement conflicts with the widely held belief that most ICU patients are near death but have a chance to survive with the aid of intricate, mysterious machinery and require continual treatment through catheters and needles inserted into their noses, mouths, urinary system, and blood vessels.

The advantage of the ICU is that the sickest patients are closely grouped in a small area in which trained personnel and complex equipment can help them immediately when the need arises, at any instance around the clock. The flip side is the eerie scene confronted by patients and visitors. The ceaseless activity under continuous artificial glare, the waltzing blips on the cardiac monitor screen, the disco-like light flashes, the frequent emergencies, and the ever-present threat of death, exacerbated by the seemingly sinister gadgetry, all provoke intense anxiety. The patient cannot move, reach for a glass of water, or turn on his side without either dislodging the wires attached to his chest by suction cups or shortcircuiting them against metal objects like safety pins or parts of the bed. The expense is two to three times that of ordinary bed care, without considering extras for medication and tests.

There are no controlled trials to substantiate reduction in death rates or length of illness compared to ordinary care. Unfortunately, many patients with heart failure or lung disease survive the ICU but die soon after discharge, negating its true objective, which is not merely to keep them alive while they are in the hospital but to improve their chances of survival and the quality of their lives *after release.*

Almost half the admissions to the ICU are patients with chest pain, but only 3% of these are actually proven to have coronary heart disease (192 patients in the Massachusetts General Hospital ICU who were suspected but not proven to have coronary heart disease were charged an average of $2000 a day while they endured this distressing experience. Their doctors, *to play safe,* sent them to the ICU.) If coronary disease is confirmed, it is impossible on the basis of tests to select those who will improve independently from those who will really require intensive treatment. Doctors fear that a wrong guess from a calculated risk might result in a malpractice suit. If heart muscle damage (myocardial infarction) is eliminated, the patient should be moved elsewhere after 24 hours' observation.

Despite the slowdown in hospital construction, there has recently been a 4% annual increase in ICU beds. Only 10% of hospitals with over 200 beds had ICUs in 1960, but by 1981 they were present in 99% of hospitals and are occupied by 42,000 patients each day. More selective admission to the ICU would help to reduce the medical care cost explosion to $287 billion in 1981, up from $12 billion in 1950.

In *The Metamorphosis,* Franz Kafka described a family's reaction when a young man was transformed into a giant bug. Initial sympathy and helpfulness changed to boredom, loathing and desire to end this repulsive intrusion into their lives. This is symbolic of the position of a patient, especially in the ICU, who is made to endure a few extra weeks or months of dying. Additional perils and emotional shocks assault the sufferer, who is metamorphosized into an inhuman chemical mechanism, deprived of dignity and confronted constantly by fear. What progress has been made to alleviate terminal terror since Leo Tolstoy wrote *The Death of Ivan Ilyich* in 1884? Martha Lear's 1980 anecdotal account, *Heartsounds,* is a sequel to *Ilyich.* She has dramatically demonstrated the over-valuation of technology and the tendency of the ICU to rob the patient of personality. Her husband, Dr. Harold Lear, 53, suffered three heart attacks (surely hastened by his 3-pack-a-day tobacco addiction). The second attack left him with agonizing angina. As a veteran physician, he found that young interns and residents overcompensate for their lack of experience by callous arrogance. The staff doctors resented any attempts he made to assert his feelings, preferring passivity and acceptance of their God-like eminence. Because of a scheduling error, coronary angiography was performed without the prescribed intravenous valium sedation. The anesthesiologist arrived later. This resulted in extreme tension and anxiety in addition to the burning pain. After a double bypass, he was sent to the ICU where he was expected to remain two days. Instead, he stayed nine days during which he sustained another MI and brain damage. The course of his illness was agonizingly erratic. During his seven hospitalizations, Murphy's Law again prevailed. Once, a neophyte nurse doubled the flow of oxygen required, causing inflammation of his nasal lining. The tube was replaced by a face mask, but later that night it was discovered that the line from his oxygen supply was disconnected. Other medication errors caused his lungs to fill with fluid (edema), almost ending his life by some years earlier than his disease did finally.

Once in the ICU, a patient is more likely to suffer iatrogenic mishaps than when undergoing routine bed care. In October of 1980, the Journal of the American Medical Association published a report by Dr. Norman S. Abramson which reviewed 4,700 admissions to the ICU of the Presbyterian-University Hospital in Pittsburgh during the 5-year period from 1974 through 1978: 21% of these patients died; 145 incident reports were made. Two-thirds (92) of the incidents were due to human error and half of these involved the misuse of equipment. The rest included *communication errors,* for example, written or verbal orders misunderstood or noted but not carried out, laboratory samples, charts or patients mislabled, and understaffing by nurses which resulted in deficient care.

To the one-third of incidents due to 53 equipment malfunctions must be added the 43 due to human error in their use. July and August, and the hour between midnight and 1 A.M. witnessed the peak of mishaps, suggesting that vacation periods, the summer influx of new "wet-around-the-ears" young physicians and nurses, and changing shifts contribute to iatrogenesis. (My own impression is that adverse occurrences in all hospital functions peak during holidays when the staff is depleted or temporarily replaced by inexperienced personnel). Patient harm resulted in half of the reported incidents, most (43%) with fatal results. If the patient was unattended, harm resulted in 75% of the incidents, indicating that *mechanical safety features cannot replace well-trained, experienced people.* Dr. Abramson and his colleagues believe that the occurrence of harm is underestimated because not all incidents are reported, although an incident is more likely to be disclosed if it results in patient harm. Unfortunately, trends indicating poor design, abuse, or poor maintenance of equipment, or factors contributing to human errors are difficult to detect from the data available in incident reports. Perhaps complexity itself is the culprit in compounding hazards.

When patients in the ICU are receiving mechanical respiratory support, most often for emphysema or pneumonia, over half die during or soon after support is discontinued. Drs. Driver and Lebrun of the University of Nebraska Medical Center found that 26 such patients received inadequate calories, proteins and vitamins. Their appetite was suppressed and they were unable to eat sufficient food. Their average daily intake was equivalent to six small chocolate bars with almonds. This reduced their ability to withstand nosocomial infection.

Not only does iatrogenesis increase in the ICU but iatrogenesis plays an important role in causing patients to be sent to this robotic life support system in the first place. Dr. Patrick Trunet of the Mondor Hospital, Crèteil, France found that mishaps in treatment accounted for 41, or 13%, of 325 patients admitted to its ICU from August, 1978 to August, 1979. Nineteen mishaps, or 46%, were preventable, 8 were fatal, 13 were life-threatening and 20 were moderate. Many were related to misuse or to the wrong dosage of drugs, and others were linked to various medical and surgical maneuvers. Cause and effect relationships were firmly established. Particularly important was the conclusion that *almost half of the incidents were avoidable.* Those that were unpreventable were due to the natural course of the illness. The attending physician gambles on the risk-benefit ratio, but the patient loses in this game of Russian roulette.

Medication Errors

Errors in medication given in hospitals average 12%, according to a recent study by the Health Care Financing Administration. Professor Neil Davis of the Temple University School of Pharmacy said, "In a hospital with a daily census of 300 patients, this could mean as many as 131,400 errors per year—an error rate of only 1% would mean 10,950 each year, or 30 errors each day." Although many are caught in time, others do cause serious iatrogenic damage. Davis and Professor Michael Cohen have gathered 150 examples in a book, *Medication Errors: Causes and Prevention,* published by George F. Stickley Co. in 1981. "It's one of the great hidden problems in medicine today and none of us can afford to hide it any longer," Cohen said. Physicians and hospital administrators have not been eager to reveal the extent of damage caused by these errors, now more serious because of the increased potency of drugs and their adverse effects. Although many humorous tales have been told about physicians' handwriting, deciphering instructions not only wastes valuable time but may result in wrong medication or dosage. Among the more important causes of error is the confusion of "U", a symbol for units, with the letter O. To avoid this problem, "U" should be spelled out as *units.* Like the authors, I have seen ten-fold overdosages, especially with insulin, which result in lowered blood sugar (hypoglycemia) and shock. I know of a 19-year-old schizophrenic patient undergoing insulin shock therapy who died of hypoglycemia because of such overdosing.

Medication orders, especially when telephonically blurred, are often misinterpreted by nurses or naive patients. The book lists 400 "sound-alike" drugs that have caused confusion. I have been told by a colleague that he directed a female patient to insert rectal suppositories for hemorrhoids twice daily. When, after several days, she returned to complain that her discomfort had increased, he examined her rectum and found that she had neglected to take the aluminum foil wrapping off as he had instructed! Neophyte nurses, taking orders by phone, have been known to mistake "per os" (by mouth) for per arse, with results begetting levity but no damage. Many communication errors result from voice distortation and extraneous noise when using electronic dictating and transcribing equipment. My pathology reports were all dictated on a recorder and then transcribed. New secretaries or typists frequently brightened my day by typing cerebral "kotex" for cortex, "eerie syphilis" for erysipelas, "very close veins" for varicose veins, and "mighty Jesus" for meningitis. Though communication errors may sometimes produce humorous results, the medication errors they may cause can often be fatal. For instance, mistaken prescriptions caused 12 deaths in two small hospitals in Riverside County, CA, during 1981 resulting in overdoses of lidocaine, a heart stimulant.

An Ohio pharmacist improperly substituted a generic diuretic, furosemide, not approved by the FDA in 1980, for the approved prescribed Lasix. He sold this drug to a 62-year-old woman three times. She died in April, 1981 of heart failure, allegedly because the furosemide did not perform properly. The pharmacist has been indicted for manslaughter. This case sets a new precedent and perhaps indicates that the unapproved substitution of less expensive drugs may be a wider problem than is realized.

The patient who is being treated for several conditions by one or multiple physicians presents a common problem. For example, a 60-year-old woman with hypertension, asthma, bladder infection, stomach ulcers and depression was treated with a new medication that blocked her other medications' effects and aggravated her depression. Other drugs, acting together, caused excess water and salt retention. An alert hospital pharmacist was able to advise her physician to correct these incompatibilities.

Hexachlorophene (HCP-pHisoHex) had been used from the 1950s to 1972 for preoperative surgical scrubbing, bathing of babies to prevent infection, postoperative wound care, and as a general disinfectant. It was present in many handwashing preparations on hospital sinks and in scores of over-the-counter items. Human poisoning through apparently healthy skin was first reported in 1959. Dr. John B. Wear of the University of Michigan Hospital collected 10 cases in 1962 in which patients had been mistakenly given a liquid containing HCP instead of milk of magnesia which it resembled. Most of the dosages were dispensed in paper cups. All patients quickly developed nausea, vomiting, cramps and diarrhea of varying severity. Some went into dehydration and shock. All recovered, though some required intravenous fluid administration. In other incidents, two adults died of mistaken ingestion of HCP, and there were four infant fatalities after treatment for burns or skin disease which resulted in severe brain destruction.

But it was not until January, 1982, that a report of a 1972 epidemic of hexachlorophene poisoning affecting 204 French children, 36 of whom died, was published. A talcum baby powder that hexachlorophene had been mistakenly added to in twice the concentration used for disinfection (6%) was used on these children. They developed skin ulcers and brain damage manifested by drowsiness, fever, convulsions, coma, and death. This tragedy was covered up for nine years because French law prohibited publication until the conclusion of litigation. However, the FDA of the U.S. issued a regulation requiring that all over-the-counter products containing HCP could be sold only by prescription.

Seven elderly patients died because of a construction blunder. The air and oxygen lines were crossed when hospital rooms were remodeled in 1980, but the rooms were not used until November. The mistake was not discovered until February 1981, when a doctor asked for a check of the system because his patient's condition was incompatible with the results of a blood test. Ten other patients' conditions worsened, but they survived.

Emergency Errors

"I'm Sorry Mrs. Jones, but You Don't Have Hypertension," was the heading of a JAMA editorial in 1978. Many patients who seek help from the emergency room rather than their own familiar physician are found to have high blood pressure (BP), but subsequent re-evaluation finds their BP normal. Visits to "emergency" are usually under stressful circumstances which can raise the blood pressure 20mm or more above the norm. Only 56% of persons with high blood pressure in a community screening program were verified as hypertensives on a second examination. Many readers will remember that, during insurance examinations, their repeat blood pressure was lower than the first. This overdiagnosis can cause unwarranted anxiety and apprehension among patients. Physicians are not certain of the importance of this short-lived hypertension. Since *sustained* hypertension is an important cause of coronary disease, heart attack and stroke, recheck is necessary, with added expense and apprehension.

When patients are so ill that they must be taken to the emergency room by ambulance, Murphy's Law is again invoked. A 1981 survey by Illinois state investigators showed that private ambulances were in violation of safety regulations over five times as often as public ambulances. But more than vehicle safety is involved. Shortages of medical supplies, rough and callous treatment of patients, fraud, and theft were uncovered.

When a patient is brought to the emergency room or is found anywhere in or out of the hospital without breath or pulse, there is no choice but to administer cardiopulmonary resuscitation immediately—mouth-to-mouth aeration by forced breathing and closed chest cardiac massage by pressing on the lower breast bone 60 times a minute. The flip side is that CPR can result in transmittal of infectious viral disease. Autopsies on unsuccessful cases have demonstrated, among other injuries, fractured ribs, especially in the elderly and in children, fat particles from bone marrow in the brain and lungs, laceration of the liver and/or spleen, bleeding into the chest or heart, tears of blood vessels with hemorrhage, and even rupture of the heart. This damage, which is not necessarily fatal, can be prevented by strict adherence to the prescribed techniques which are taught in many schools, YMCAs and other facilities.

Damage has also been documented among CPR trainees. Many develop muscle sprains in their lower backs and necks. The danger of infection with herpes, mononucleosis and hepatitis is present when training manikins are improperly cleaned. Acute inflammation of the joint between the jawbone and the lower skull causing painful chewing has occurred after prolonged mouth-to-mouth respiration practice. Less common, but more serious are the heart attacks among sedentary volunteers. Therefore, it would be prudent to be physically fit when such training is started.

Faulty Physicians

Despite licensing requirements, the public has difficulty in detecting incompetent and/or unethical physicians. A review by the Georgia Board of Medical Examiners in September of 1981 stated that "41% of the physicians surveyed indicated that the board is not being made aware of most of the cases involving questionable behavior or incompetence." The situation is aggravated by the prevalence of Medicare and Medicaid mills, in which many low-caliber doctors make up in volume for their lower fees. The best hospitals and doctors not only admit iatrogenesis but are subjected to criticism and audit. We have no figures regarding incompetent doctors since they usually work in inferior hospitals and clinics where such records, if compiled, are not published.

Patients often complain about arrogant, unfeeling young interns and residents. But sometimes their work schedules approach 100 hours weekly; I recall certain periods of my own training when I endured 48-72 hours of continuous duty. Sleep deprivation can cause lack of concentration, difficulties in problem-solving, depression, irritability, loss of memory and extreme sensitivity to criticism. This can lead to bad temper and impairment of relations with patients. Many psychological problems arise which later lead to alcoholism, drug addiction and even suicide. I vividly remember the poor physical condition of most of the young doctors I examined when they entered military service compared to officer candidates from other occupations. The caveat, "Physician, heal thyself," is too often disregarded.

Several anesthesiologists became worried after they arrived at Wilford

Hall (Air Force) Medical Center in San Antonio, Texas in 1975. They refused to work with one surgeon because seven children died during or shortly after his surgery for inborn heart defects. More than half of the children he operated on died. The mortality rate for all his heart surgery was 43%, although the average for the other surgeons was 6%. A review by the hospital Commanding Officer excused this discrepancy by noting that he operated on only poor-risk patients. In 1978, the surgeon was then sent to the Milwaukee Lutheran Hospital on "temporary duty." There he became party to a $20 million malpractice suit alleging that he hooked up a heart-lung machine backward during a coronary bypass operation, depriving the patient's brain of oxygen. She was left a speechless quadriplegic, according to TIME (Feb. 1982) and was awarded almost $2,500,000. The surgeon returned to Wilford Hall as Chief of Heart Surgery. Cardiologists who observed his technique and the judge who rendered his opinion agreed that he was rough and careless and that it was a "shame that one surgeon's mortality was six times that of the others." Despite this record, he received an excellent recommendation by his commanding officer, retired from the Air Force and entered private practice in 1980. This is an example of the all-too-frequent bureaucratic cover-up of incompetency which victimizes unknowing patients in government and private hospitals, even in those of high repute.

Hospitals share qualitative differences with industries and colleges. New community hospitals and older ones in decaying inner-city neighborhoods do not recruit the best-trained residents or senior staff physicians of maximum ability. They will hire almost any warm body. Established centers, especially those connected with medical schools, are more selective. They will accept only doctors with superior credentials and promise. If on entering a hospital you observe a predominance of foreign, non-English-speaking personnel, it is evident that the best trained and capable physicians want to work elsewhere.

In emergencies like severe heart attacks or major traffic accidents, it is important that you know which hospitals are staffed around the clock by able, supervised medical personnel. Such are generally indicated on major highways by signs pointing to Trauma Centers. The recent growth of groups of competent primary care physicians who contract to staff emergency rooms is a development which should bring better care in sudden catastrophic illnesses or accidents.

Many medical societies have committees for helping "impaired physicians," a euphemism for doctors whose careers are being blighted by alcoholism or drug addiction. The unusual stresses, the irregular hours, and the easy availability of drugs cause doctors to be more vulnerable than most. Dr. W. S. Halstead of Johns Hopkins Medical School, a pioneer surgeon, was addicted to morphine, and Sigmund Freud experimented with cocaine. Many addicted doctors have managed to continue their work with the help of their society's committee, which uses techniques resembling a more sophisticated version of Alcoholics Anonymous.

To all outward appearances, Dr. Edgar Morton was a happy and successful dermatologist with a pretty wife and two teenaged children. Only after he was found dead at 41 in his sealed garage with his car motor running did his hospital colleagues discover that he had been under psychiatric care for alcoholism and barbiturate addiction. His marriage was foundering. Doctors and patients who phoned him at night reported that he was often incoherent. Some recalled that he frequently could not be found and had missed many appointments and committee meetings. Many of his patients sought other doctors because they had recently found him brusque and discourteous. One would not care to be in the hands of a surgeon with a similar impairment.

Hazards to Hospital Staff

Another important concern is the protection of personnel from toxic chemicals. Although these are present in many areas, they are most likely to affect personnel in the laboratory, where surgical and autopsy specimens are prepared, examined, diagnosed and stored, and tests are performed on blood, urine, body fluids, excrement, and miscellaneous material unpleasant to the uninitiated. The Occupational Safety and Health Administration (OSHA) has issued regulations regarding the exposure of technicians. In keeping with the Reagan Administration's deregulation policy and because of the variability of reagents and time of exposure, individual laboratories are allowed more latitude than are industries.

Almost everyone is familiar with the unique acrid odor of formaldehyde, a gas which is dissolved in water to make *formalin,* the most common preservative for tissues removed at surgery or autopsy. It is also, when combined with various perfumes, the principal ingredient of embalming fluid. Cough, running noses, itchy eyes and wrinkled, roughened fingers have been the expected occupational hazards of pathologists and their assistants. Every doctor remembers student days of fume-filled anatomy rooms and pathology demonstrations with pickled organs. When I was an instructor, my chief had a skin allergy to formaldehyde and had to wear special gloves. There is no evidence that non-smoking medical personnel have excess cancer of the respiratory tract, but cancer of the lung is increased among workers in plastic, printing, insulation and other industries which use large amounts of formaldehyde. Tobacco smoke contains a high concentration of formaldehyde. Animal studies show that this chemical causes severe inflammation of the kidneys and bladder.

One of the most toxic chemicals to which anesthesiologists and their assistants are exposed is nitrous oxide ("laughing gas") which inevitably leaks from their equipment. This has caused impaired performance, loss of dexterity and slowing of thought processes. There have been numerous recent studies revealing that pregnant anesthesiologists and nurse-anesthetists have an increased risk of stillbirths and congenitally deformed offspring. Even the wives of male anesthesiologists share this risk. There are so many different toxic chemicals to which anesthesiologists are exposed that it is difficult to pinpoint the precise compound or combination of agents responsible for the damage.

Not only are female personnel exposed to anesthetics at risk, but hexachlorophene in soap also has recently been incriminated. An extensive Swedish study showed that all women medical and paramedical hospital staff have an increase in malformed infants and newborn deaths. In 460 births of children of nurses and other hospital workers who frequently washed their hands with soap or used hand cream containing HCP, there were 25 severe malformations of the esophagus, anus, central nervous system and heart. There were 46 "minor" birth defects, such as cleft lip, extra fingers, slight heart defects and bony dislocations. This incidence of 15% is five times higher than the 3% found in the general population and the 3.4% in nurses who did not use HCP.

An *unpublished study* originally done by Sterling/Winthrop, manufacturers of HCP, showed that there was a four-fold increase of abnormal fetuses in rats tested with oral HCP—an obvious cover-up. It has also been found in the blood of women after washing and in the cord blood of fetuses whose mothers had a single pre-delivery bath using HCP containing soap. HCP-containing detergents are belatedly no longer used in U.S. hospitals, except by prescription and for surgical scrubs.

Many of the waste chemicals and plastic disposable equipment used in hospitals are disposed of through the usual sewer outlets. Even if not radioactive, they can have a serious environmental impact. As the use of disposable equipment increases because of the high labor cost of cleaning and sterilizing reusable material, this worldwide problem is expected to become more serious and will require government intervention. In the long term, only a reduction in the use of the disposable equipment, and recycling will be the solution.

Nursing Homes Are No Place Like Home

Although their function is to separate the chronic, terminally ill from society rather than cure or palliation, nursing homes share the problems of hospitals. Perhaps the least agreeable aspect of our fragmented family structure is that there is often no place for incapacitated elderly parents. Their last years are hopelessly endured in warehouses for the dying containing a total of 1,300,000 inmates at an average charge of $15,000 to $18,000 per annum. There are few good nursing homes, mostly non-profit, many mediocre and some disgraceful. Old age, which should be a triumph, has become a disaster for many. A proverb laments, "One mother can take care of ten children, but ten children can't take care of one mother."

The infirm inhabitants of nursing homes cannot assert their rights. They are often forgotten by friends and family whose visits are often not frequent enough to induce operators to make showcase displays of tender care. Many corners are cut by unscrupulous owners or managers seeking profits, resulting in a chronic shortage of maintenance staff, doctors and nurses, and a personnel turnover of 200% each year. Inspectors have found monstrous mismanagement such as patients with bedsores lying in sheets soaked with urine and agitated elders tied to chairs.

Federal and state regulations are frequently violated and instances of fraud and mistreatment are rampant. Since half of the payments are made by Medicare and Medicaid, there are governmental critera of acceptability. However, enforcement lags. The JCAH has recently instituted voluntary inspections and will accredit nursing homes, as it does hospitals, if they meet strict standards.

Even if nursing homes were models of comfort and care, they would not provide surcease from the sense of anguish and loss caused by separation from accustomed surroundings, home, friends, and family. The two-edged sword of prolonged life because of better sanitation, immunization, lifestyle and medical care has created this macabre, pre-mortem industry.

Mrs. Betty Woodson is 94. She has been unaware of her surroundings and has not recognized her family for two years. Since then she has been confined in a superior nursing home. At 89, she was still alert and responsive, but her left leg was amputated because of diabetic gangrene. Progressive deterioration followed. Her loving and concerned children, nieces, and nephews, now senior citizens with their own medical problems, had no way of caring for her in her own or their homes. At 93, after a year of vegetation in the nursing home, gangrene of her right leg developed. Her doctor insisted on amputation again. The family was divided. Some felt enough was enough and that Mrs. Woodson should be permitted to die without further futile and expensive surgery. Others prevailed that she eke out her last breaths, no matter what the economic or emotional cost. So her remaining leg was amputated and she remains a barely living relic.

The ethical questions raised by Mrs. Woodson's case are inescapable human dilemmas. How long do we prolong vegetative life? While the aged are still responsive, would not the provision of home nursing care be less taxing to everyone's emotions and finances than these dismal depositories?

Can We Reduce These Hazards?

A study by the University of Tennessee's Center for the Health Sciences in Memphis, concluded that preventable factors may be involved in over three-fourths of hospital admissions. Of 136 admissions, the investigators found that destructive personal habits and lifestyle, failure to comply with instructions for controlling illness, and lack of community resources played the largest role. The illness itself was preventable in 44% of the cases, which were mostly due to excess use of tobacco and alcohol. Patients' failure to comply with professional health care by stopping effective treatment, or delaying office care when symptoms were obvious, caused 21% of the admissions studied.

The rapid increase in free-standing ambulatory surgery and emergency centers (not connected to hospitals), from 55 in 1978 to over 500 in 1982, has reduced many of these risks. If the condition is not life-threatening and overnight stay can be avoided, infections and costs can be halved.

I am skeptical that the real, underlying issues have been faced by administrative or medical authorities. The problems of self-induced illness requiring hospitalization will not be solved even partially, until governmental and private insurance agencies, supported by all of us, sternly decide to stop paying or to impose sanctions for the consequences of willful destructive behavior. If this approach is thought too harsh, those whose lifestyle enhances health should be rewarded by tax and insurance allowances, encouraging others to profit by their example.

8.

THE DIAGNOSTIC DILEMMA—ITS EFFECT ON OUTCOME

Medicine is a science of uncertainty, and an art of probability.
Sir William Osler, Regius Professor of Medicine, Oxford University
1905-1919

"In the distant past, symptoms were often confused with diseases. Fever was a disease as well as a symptom, and so were the colic, 'yellow jaundice' and edema," editorialized Dr. Samuel Vaisrub, in 1979. Modern practice emphasizes the changes in bodily structure and chemistry which underlie the symptoms. Jaundice, for example, can be caused by many different types of liver disease or by blood destruction, and can even be simulated by overeating carrots. All of these basic causes have different outcomes and require different treatment.

"Diagnostic overkill," resulting in the "Ulysses Syndrome" which can be carried to extremes if redundant, repeated, elaborate and costly tests are performed when simpler ones would suffice, has been discussed in previous chapters. But even simple, inexpensive tests are less important than careful histories and physical examinations and information, understood by the patient, of the risks and self-perceivable signs of complications that occur after medication or surgery. If the patient becomes aware of adverse effects, treatment may be stopped, or new measures instituted in time to prevent disaster.

How often are diagnostic errors made? Dr. Richard Cabot of Massachusetts General Hospital reported the first analysis of these errors in the JAMA in 1912. He compared the diagnoses in 3,000 autopsies with evaluations made before death. Many of the pitfalls he found still exist today. "Rheumatism" turned out to be a complex of bone disease from syphilis to cancer. Dr. Cabot cautioned, "Rheumatism is one of the most dangerous of all diagnoses to the conscientious physician." "Malaria" was often tuberculosis, syphilis or abscess of the liver. "Hemorrhoids" often hid cancer of the rectum. Dr. Mark W. Sheehan reviewed many reports, totalling 32,200 autopsies, in 1978. The incidence of misdiagnoses varied from 6% to 68%, averaging 25% in clear-cut cases and up to 45% when the diagnosis was given as probable. Although laboratory tests and x-rays are frequently necessary to support an unsure diagnosis based on clinical findings, they have been excessively relied upon. The disease may not be seen, it may not be noticed or it may be misinterpreted. In one study, five radiologists interpreted 100 chest films and 25% of important abnormalities were overlooked by one or more of the specialists who read them.

The literature is replete with articles regarding the risks of surgery. Although there has been a plethora of advice on the cost and misinformation brought about by diagnostic testing by internists, few reports of the *degree* of danger have been published. As techniques, equipment, and type of patients change, new adverse effects are not adequately monitored despite the need for physicians to have precise knowledge of the risks involved in order to arrive at a sound decision for management. The *Index Medicus,* a guide to medical journals, has no subject heading for hazards. Without this knowledge, a doctor cannot always determine whether a new symptom in a patient is a result of the illness—or iatrogenic.

This is the first book to reveal to the consumer the risks of medical and surgical diagnostic maneuvers, although many volumes have been written about the hazards of drugs. Alerted patients will be able to grant or deny truly informed consent to procedures suggested by their physicians, and to participate fully in the decision-making process.

"One of the troubles of our age is that thought habits cannot change as quickly as techniques—with the result that as skill increases, wisdom fades."—Bertrand Russell

A 1981 survey in the *Scottish Medical Journal,* showed that in 1152 hospital autopsies, 39% of the main clinical diagnoses and 68% of the diagnoses contributing to death were not confirmed. Accuracy of diagnosis did not improve with a longer hospital stay but did correlate with the clinician's confidence in his main diagnosis. But 25% of "fairly certain" diagnoses were wrong. The number of laboratory tests was not related to either the diagnostic accuracy or the outcome of the illness.

There is more to be said about Frances Hartman, whose story was begun in Chapter 6 (Nosocomial Infections). Her penicillamine-induced aplastic anemia included pallor and weakness due to shortage of red blood cells and infections due to loss of the protective function of the white cells. Platelet deficiency resulted in easy bruising, excess bleeding under the skin and from the gums and rectum and over-abundant menstruation. Mrs. Hartman was neither warned of these risks nor of the signs she might notice if an adverse reaction occurred. She was given a typed information sheet that mentioned that penicillamine might possibly cause blood formation problems. This meant little or nothing to her as she was not informed of specific symptoms to be watched for. She was, however, instructed to have blood counts and urinalysis every two weeks.

The penicillamine supressed her joint pain and was continued in increasing dosage. Her blood counts and urinalyses remained within normal limits. On July 1, 1977, she went on vacation with her doctor's consent. During the last week of July, after she skipped two blood counts, a friend noticed that she had "black and blue" marks on her body. Later, she noted additional small bruises, a "pink tooth brush," and heavy menstruation. These caused her no alarm, but on August 22, she suddenly developed weakness, bleeding from the gums, nose, rectum and vagina and large bruises all over her body. Alarmed, she called her doctor who sent her to a hospital, where it was found that her bone marrow was not functioning and her blood cells and platelets were decreased to "panic" levels (aplastic anemia). Because this disease has a fatality rate of 25% and only 10% experience complete recovery, even with bone marrow transplants, Mrs. Hartman was in serious trouble. If she had been aware of the nature of the adverse effects and if penicillamine was stopped late in July, when bruising was first noted, it is probable that her anemia would not have been as severe and she would not have had to endure the next two years of multiple hospitalizations, transfusions and urinary infection. In September she was sent to the hospital for a marrow transplant. This hospital had promised that matching marrow donors were available and waiting. When she arrived there, however, it was found that they were unsuitable and therefore the transplant was not performed. Because of her infection she was subjected to the additional iatrogenic risks of antibiotics and intravenous catheterization. It was not until the spring of 1979 that she began to recover. She is still "borderline" anemic and there is no way of forecasting her outcome, whether complete recovery, chronic low grade anemia or recurrence. A simple, humane explanation of the possible bleeding tendency in terms understood by a layperson could have avoided this expensive and harrowing ordeal.

Although Mrs. Hartman's tests were among the simplest available,they illustrate the greatest modern medical mistake—the *over-valuing of technology.* Normal x-ray studies do not exclude the possibility of cancer of the lung, stomach or bone. Normal EKGs do not exclude the possibility of heart disease. The converse is that abnormal tests do not necessarily point to the patient's symptoms and may occur in the absence of symptoms! Even biopsies which show malignancy may be fallible because: the symptoms may be due to some other cause; the tissue removed may not be representative and may have missed the diseased area; there are some conditions that are difficult to diagnose; and three different pathologists may offer three different opinions.

I have already illustrated how it is not only possible to overvalue but to mislead by technology. This is deplorable but there are also circumstances in which it is absurd to do any investigations. How can an aged person, paralyzed by a stroke, unable to speak and incontinent, be benefited by multiple tests? Medicare, Medicaid and private insurance funds are being depleted by this fruitless quest for causes. People must pay more out-of-pocket now than before this insurance was available. Rates for doctors' services rose 12.5% in 1981 and additional insurance is necessary to cover deductibles and excess costs. But who determines how much of this expenditure improves the outcome for the patient? We are constantly bombarded by cries of alarm in the media over the care of the poor and the elderly. I have never heard any commentator or journalist discuss the waste of public and private insurance funds in futile testing which has become routine merely because equipment and payment are available. And does anyone cite the iatrogenesis engendered? We like to think that even if the patient dies we have done all that was possible to help and that the more that was done, the better. But in many cases the patient's condition is *worsened* by all this activity. Except in severe injuries, despite all spectacular remedies, the recovery of most patients is due more to nature than to anything that doctors do!

The New York Times of December 27, 1978 reported the claim of a Congressional subcommittee that there were 2 million unnecessary surgical operations that year, with 10,000 fatalities. The degree of unnecessary surgery has been well publicized, but other excessive diagnostic procedures have received little attention from the media. Despite criticism by many medical leaders, the number of diagnostic procedures continues to increase and probably will continue to do so until insurance funds become more selective and pay only for processes which improve outcome and the quality of life. While it is true that innovations like the CAT scan have replaced many dangerous and painful invasive procedures, the same can not be said for most new techniques. In addition, it may require years of observation to determine the value of an innovation for improving outcome and increasing survival, and by the time a judgment is reached, the procedure may be obsolete.

Syphilis, for instance, was assumed to cause devastating effects on the heart, blood vessels and brain if not treated. In 1955, a Swedish study showed that 85% of untreated syphilitics had normal life spans, and over 70% showed no evidence of the disease at autopsy. This does not mean that syphilis should not be treated. It does indicate that until the early 1940s, the risk/benefit ratio of treatment with highly toxic arsphenamine was greater than thought. Penicillin, which is much safer, has reduced this risk.

Another example is that of radioactive scanning for brain tumors. At Johns Hopkins Hospital, these procedures increased 1,000% from 1962 to 1972, and earlier diagnosis could be made. The wait from awareness of symptoms to operation dropped from four years to one year, but survival after operation did not improve, since less than half of the patients were alive two years later. There are as many brain surgeons in Massachusetts, with a population of 5 million, as in England, with a population of 50,000,000. The ten-fold ratio in Massachusetts' favor has not given the unfortunate neurosurgical patients there improved survival. It merely means that more procedures useless to the patient are being performed.

But even with common, easily diagnosed illnesses like hypertension and diabetes, diagnosis is often faulty and the disease undetected. Physicians, like airplane pilots and flight controllers, are human and sometimes labor under stress, boredom and fatigue, which causes them to make errors of judgment and omit essential procedures. One of the most productive and easiest tests is blood pressure measurement. A study at Baylor University College of Medicine has shown that 20% of patients entering the emergency room did not have their blood pressures recorded and 66% of those with elevated blood pressures were not treated for hypertension. I have often seen otherwise careful examinations for varied complaints in which the blood pressure was not checked or was overlooked. Laboratory reports, adhering like shingles to a page in the patient's chart, are often not noticed, causing physicians to miss signs of high or low blood sugar.

Many simple tests are important, but many others are unnecessary unless the patient's symptoms and other findings point towards a disease which tests can confirm.

The JCAH requires that hospitals have utilization committees whose purpose is to determine the necessity for hospitalization and its duration in the hope that it can eliminate the wastage of beds. But once a patient is admitted these committees ignore the amount of services provided. When my 240-bed hospital was filled with patients in 1961, my laboratory performed 100,000 tests annually. By the early 1970s with the same number of patients, our building program had almost tripled our laboratory working space and we were performing over 600,000 tests. The radiology department's expansion was even greater. There was no discernible benefit to mortality rates or length of hospital stay, while work and costs sextupled. Between 1975 and 1978, laboratory tests, many unnecessary, increased 27% and now account for over $10 billion, or 25% of hospital charges in the U.S. Because physicians are responsible for ordering hospital admissions and tests, they generate 70% of hospital care costs.

In 1981, the Hospital of the University of Pennsylvania inaugurated a program to detect and correct over-utilization of diagnostic services. Charts of patients who have had three or more of the same tests in a week are audited. A panel of twelve physicians established criteria to justify these multiple procedures. If these criteria are not met, the attending physician is notified. An extensive educational program regarding the value and cost to the patient of each investigative procedure has been instituted and physicians can compare their over-utilization with that of their peers. Only time will tell if all this watchdog activity will justify the time and expense involved.

MISDIAGNOSIS—CAUSE AND EFFECT

Ultra-technical equipment solves fewer problems than careful history-taking, physical examinations, and communication, not only with the patient but with the clinical laboratory and x-ray departments. This is not just to select the best and smallest number of tests necessary for patient benefit, but to prevent overlooking important data in the maze of paper documents and stressful situations. Most diagnostic delusions are not due to lack of knowledge but to failure to do simple things well. Human error, promoted by haste, overwork, and loss of sleep, can undo the most careful planning by the best trained and most conscientious physicians.

History and Physical Examination Blunders

Will Rogers said, "The best doctor in the world is the veterinarian. He can't ask his patients what is the matter—he's got to just know." Rogers' remark was superficially sage but actually specious. Obtaining a revealing history is a fine art based on knowledge not only of medicine but also of the patient's background and environment. Anyone who has watched or listened to skilled interviewers like Oriana Fallaci, Studs Turkel, Phil Donahue or Barbara Walters will understand that many people must be carefully coaxed to reveal past experiences.

Because of withholding information regarding a skipped menstrual period, pregnancies have been missed. They have been misdiagnosed as fibroids, resulting in miscarriage or the surgical removal of a pregnant uterus. This was often deliberate and accepted by both doctor and patient before abortion was made legal. Abdominal pain due to tubal pregnancy may still be diagnosed as appendicitis if a history of missed menstrual periods is not elicited, if it is deliberately withheld or if the pregnancy test is either not awaited or false-negative.

Appendicitis is one of the most common complaints requiring operation, but it is frequently misdiagnosed, especially in children, pregnant women and in old age, when its signs and symptoms may be atypical. Conversely, overdiagnosis has resulted in many unjustified appendectomies; surgical surveillance has reduced this rip-off. Approximately 200,000 cases occur in the U.S. each year, with over 2,000 deaths, a high rate for a disease considered innocuous. There were 339,000 appendectomies with many of the removed appendices showing no disease in 1973.

One 68-year-old man who had pain in the right lower abdomen told his family physician he thought he had appendicitis. The doctor disagreed and told him he had colitis, for which he prescribed medication. No tests were performed. Mr. Casper felt worse the next day and the doctor told him to take an enema. This increased his pain and his wife called a surgeon who operated immediately and found the appendix had ruptured due to the delay, with peritonitis resulting. Mr. Casper recovered after a stormy convalescence. Many whose surgeries are delayed through misdiagnosis are not so fortunate.

When, because of lack of beds, a patient with suspected appendicitis was transferred to a county hospital, failure to read records permitted an enema to be given, resulting in rupture of the appendix with fatal peritonitis.

While on a beach picnic on Long Island several years ago, a young physician badly cut his foot on a partially buried broken bottle. He went to a first aid station and allowed the nurse to administer tetanus antitoxin, forgetting that he had had severe skin itching after a similar injection while in the army, indicating that he was allergic to the serum. Almost two weeks later, while making hospital rounds with his Chief and other junior staff members, Bob was surprised to find everyone staring at him. "You're swelling up," exclaimed one colleague. Then Bob became conscious of generalized itching, puffiness of his face and hands, heat, asthma-like difficulty in breathing and dizziness, a typical example of delayed serum sickness. He was immediately taken to the emergency room, where adrenalin was injected, providing immediate relief. For several weeks he had a gradually subsiding mild fever and swollen glands in his armpits and groin.

Allergies or hypersensitivities, common with tetanus toxoid or antitoxin, penicillin, or narcotics, but possible with almost any drug, may be overlooked. Reactions such as those due to previously administered agents may have been noted in old records which are not available in emergency situations. Many allergic reactions have been fatal. I know a primary care physician who was shocked when a middle-aged woman died in his office, almost immediately after a varicose vein in her leg was injected with a solution intended to cause it to close. A trial skin injection with a small amount of the solution had been negative.

Diabetics are in particular peril because miscalculation of insulin dosage and deficient diet may result in lowered blood sugar, also known as hypoglycemia, with insulin shock instead of high blood sugar. If carbohydrates are not given immediately brain damage or death will occur. If, conversely, the patients face impending coma because of high blood sugar and acidification of the blood (ketosis), they may be mistaken for alcoholics and placed in police lockups. This happened to a respected Pennsylvania clergyman who was found staggering down the street. He was discovered dead in the morning.

If diabetes is undiagnosed in a pregnant woman, her baby will generally be abnormally large, causing difficult delivery and, frequently, stillbirth.

A false diagnosis of diabetes will result in unnecessary treatment and emotional problems.

When matadors are gored by bulls, the injury is obvious. But when a 62-year-old dairy farmer was escorting a truckload of cows to market, one tossed her head and the flat side of her horn struck his neck under the right jaw. He barely felt this minor blow but felt dizzy that afternoon and was admitted to the local hospital. Two physicians could find no evidence of injury. Two days later, his left side became paralyzed (hemiplegia), he lapsed into coma and died on the 4th hospital day. An autopsy revealed that his right carotid artery, the main vessel supplying the brain, was completely filled with blood clot and that the right half of his brain had suffered destruction from lack of blood supply. If this blockage had been suspected on the first day and confirmed by arteriography, the blood clot could have been surgically removed through endarterectomy with at least partial recovery.

Invisible neck injuries are becoming increasingly common. They are often unrecognized when other major injuries are present. Restraining harnesses in roller coasters may slip from the shoulders; wrestling, judo, automobile accidents, chiropractic manipulations and compression by certain eye tests like ocular plethysmography have resulted in fatal clotting in the carotid artery. If the neck bones are injured, careless handling of the patient may cause damage to the spinal cord, resulting in paralysis.

Physical examinations can be faulty because of errors of omission, detection, and interpretation, rather than deficient technique. Goethe said, "One sees what one knows." The doctor's hands and eyes will be effective only when there is a background of information and reasoning. During my pre-war retreat from pathology, I examined the mayor of a nearby small Appalachian town who was suffering from severe abdominal distress. I felt that he had gallbladder disease but noted that his voice was very hoarse. He whispered that this speech difficulty had been increasing for almost a year. His family doctor, then on vacation, had been prescribing various gargles, but had never used a mirror to visualize his vocal cords. I found the mayor had an ulceration of his right vocal cord, presumably malignant. In the hospital, x-ray examination of the chest revealed a large cancer of his right upper lung which compressed the nerve supply of his vocal cord, causing it to be paralyzed and consequently ulcerated. The mayor received radiation therapy but died several months later.

Despite all the lessons learned in training, the rectal examination is frequently not done because it is tedious or unpleasant. Due to this dereliction, patients with intestinal obstruction from tumors, adhesions or twisting have had this condition misdiagnosed as "intestinal flu." I have seen a certified internist, examining a patient with generalized joint pains, carelessly omit not only the rectal, but also the blood pressure exam, although these are the two easiest, safest, least expensive and most valuable procedures in terms of detecting treatable disease. Dr. Rosalind Krasnoff, a brilliant young pathologist, was co-author of a monograph on tumors of the bowel. Despite her insight, she neglected to have a rectal examination when she noticed a trace of blood in her stool, assuming it was due to a recurrence of her hemorrhoids. Later, cancer was discovered, which ultimately proved fatal. Clarence DeMar, who ran in the Boston Marathon for 46 years, had extensive studies of his cardiovascular fitness, but suffered a similar fate at the age of 70. His early investigation had not included a rectal examination.

Many deaths from head injury have resulted from failure to take x-ray pictures of the skull or CAT scans after falls or blows, especially in the case of alcoholics, children and the elderly. But the CAT scan, estimated to be performed one million times annually in this country, should not become the neurologist's "chest x-ray." Its expense precludes its use in minor trauma, simple headache (even if periodic), or fainting or dizziness, without abnormal neurologic signs. There are no data on the overuse of the CAT scan, but many hospitals refuse to omit it, fearing future malpractice litigation should brain damage manifest later. Some 40% of CAT scans will be positive if abnormal neurologic signs are present, compared to 1% of ordinary skull x-ray films. The risk is small because the dosage of radiation is not increased. If intravenous contrast agents are used to enhance the picture, the risk of death is one in ten thousand and is increased by advanced age, diabetes, heart disease or overly large doses of the compound. The cost of the scan is offset by the lessened necessity for later invasive procedures and greater safety and comfort to the patient.

Foreign bodies in the eye have been overlooked through failure to do x-ray studies after minor injuries, sometimes resulting in blindness. Tuberculosis, even with its present reduced incidence, may progress to cavitation and hemorrhage if undiagnosed radiologically.

In June, 1981, the *Western Journal of Medicine* discussed the documentation of radiologic errors in 20 to 50% of lung cancers. The University of California in San Diego collected 79 consecutive cases of confirmed lung cancer. Eight of these had erroneous x-rays before cancer was proven. During the next two years, 143 cancers were diagnosed, but 19 x-ray errors were found. These 27 errors included 22 cases in which the diagnosis had been missed, 4 in which abnormalities were found but misinterpreted, and 1 in which there were errors of detection and misinterpretation at different times. The diagnosis of lung cancer had been delayed months or years after the first x-ray abnormalities had been unrecognized, which adversely affected what little chance of surgical cure existed in almost half of the 27 cases.

Why these mistakes? Busy or rushed radiologists, failure to compare previous films and study old reports, and scars from previous inflammatory disease which obscure new shadows all played varying roles. One mass was thought to be an aneurysm; three, chronic pneumonia; and another, an enlarged artery. An error rate of about 30% seems unavoidable under present circumstances, and many malpractice suits are instituted for these blunders, although the substantial rate of error in common practice reduces the justification and the chances for success in a liability action. Communication errors compound the mismanagement. The reviewers found several cases in which the correct diagnosis was ignored or not read by the referring physician and others in which patients missed or refused further evaluation or follow-up.

Diagnosis of Non-Existent Disease

Sophie Higgins had visual difficulty and multiple tests were performed. One of her blood proteins was found to be slightly abnormal. Although a later bone marrow biopsy was within normal limits, she developed headaches and further visual impairment. A specialist treated for a fatal bone marrow cancer called multiple myeloma "because of the progressive nature of symptomatology." So shocked was she by the diagnosis of cancer that she suffered severe depression, quit her job, separated from her fiancé, and made arrangements for her funeral. She was treated with chemotherapeutic agents for five weeks. After four months she had no signs of cancer. She was reexamined at the Memorial Sloan-Kettering Cancer Center in New York, where it was concluded that she did not have multiple myeloma.

Many people are wrongly diagnosed as being diabetic because of an inadequate blood glucose (sugar) test. They flunk this test because their bodies cannot utilize insulin, which regulates the concentration of glucose. This occurs most often in the obese, which explains why so many overweight persons are "cured" of non-existent diabetes when they lose weight. Drs. Roger W. Turkington and Howard K. Weindling of the Milwaukee Diabetes Center observed 334 diabetics for 18 years. They found that serious complications such as blood vessel and kidney disease, neuritis, and blindness occurred only in patients lacking insulin and were not predicted by the glucose test. It is for this reason that many are opposed to publicity advocating the use of diabetes detection tests frequently offered by hospitals. Newer tests of insulin utilization are more reliable.

More serious is the misdiagnosis of leukemia. There are several diseases which, in their early stages, resemble this dread blood cancer. Most have a more favorable outcome; but, if treated with potent chemotherapeutic agents, the patient may experience severe adverse reactions. Mongolism, or Down's syndrome, may have blood changes resembling leukemia, but these spontaneously disappear in early childhood while the mental deficiency remains.

39-year-old Joe Scavelli became pale and weak in 1976. He was found to have enlargement of his spleen and the lymph nodes in his armpits and groin. A blood count revealed severe anemia and an increased percentage of white blood cells called lymphocytes. Joe was hospitalized and a hematologist performed a bone marrow biopsy. Abnormal lymphocytes predominated, suggesting a diagnosis of chronic lymphocytic leukemia. Chemotherapy was started, causing severe nausea and vomiting. Most of Joe's hair fell out. There was no improvement and after several weeks of drug treatment most of the joints of his hands and feet became swollen and painful. Other tests and a review of his blood elements were performed. A rheumatologist was consulted and, after several months of observation, it was decided that Joe did not have leukemia but a rare type of arthritis called Felty's syndrome. Leukemia has no relation to the non-fatal, Felty's syndrome but both may present atypical, confusing signs and symptoms in their early stages.

Why Sandford Baum, a popular, public-spirited businessman in an Appalachian college town was told by his urologist that he had cancer of the prostate before a biopsy was performed is not known. When Mr. Baum consulted this specialist, because of urinary discomfort, the urologist felt a stony mass through the rectum. Two pathologists who reviewed the belated biopsy agreed that cancer was not present. Mr. Baum had an inflammation called granulomatous prostatitis which feels like cancer to the probing finger. Since the urologist was a medical school professor, it seems unpardonable that he made his taken-for-granted diagnosis known to patient and family with unnecessarily severe alarm before it could be confirmed microscopically.

Psychiatric Iatrogenic Disorders

As in Mr. Baum's case, anxiety and depression will result from an incorrect diagnosis of a catastrophic disease and often persists after the threat to life has been disproven. If a pre-malignant condition such as herpes or an x-ray burn is present, cancer phobia may destroy the victim's peace of mind. It may occur after the removal of a benign, malignant or misdiagnosed tumor, especially of the breast. Wrong diagnoses may cause extensive exploratory operations in a fruitless search for cancer. This has occurred in chronic bowel inflammations like diverticulitis or when a discrete shadow (coin lesion) in a lung are disclosed on x-ray films. The latter case poses an inescapable dilemma for doctor and patient. The lesion is probably benign and harmless but—can they take the risk of not being sure? The operation itself is not without danger, but the risk of not removing a potentially curable cancer is greater.

Misdiagnosis in Elderly Patients

Mr. Baum's father, David, was a hearty and vigorous 77, but had been complaining of pain in his legs on walking moderate distances for several years. He had been seen by a certified internist who ascribed his pain to narrowing of the leg arteries due to arteriosclerosis but did not bother to palpate his abdomen. One morning the senior Mr. Baum developed severe abdominal pain and collapsed while attempting to get out of bed. He was taken to the local hospital where he was found to be in shock with a rapid, feeble pulse and loss of blood. Because facilities were insufficient, he was transferred to a larger hospital in Pittsburgh, where the diagnosis of a ruptured ballooning (aneurysm) of the main abdominal artery (aorta) was confirmed. If Mr. Baum's abdomen had been palpated previously, the pulsating, clot-filled mass should not have been overlooked. It could have been surgically removed and a dacron tube implanted with only slight risk, and his circulation would have been restored. Once ruptured, however, there was insufficient intact blood vessel wall for the prosthesis to be successfully inserted. Mr. Baum died of internal hemorrhage after a futile attempt by a vascular surgeon to complete this operation.

In 1979, *Geriatrics* published a report from the University of Leuven, Belgium, where 276 emergency, non-surgical admissions of elderly patients were investigated. In 103 cases the referring physician did not suggest a diagnosis but in 63 of these, the disease should have been accurately identified. Tuberculosis, low blood sugar, thyroid disease, anemia, kidney failure, and low blood pressure, resulting in many later fatalities, were unrecognized, often because the patient was over-sedated. The final diagnoses after hospital study and/or autopsy agreed in distribution with those of a previous report from England of 1,500 elderly patients. Acute stomach and intestinal diseases were surprisingly more frequent than heart attacks or strokes. Liver and gallbladder disease followed. Physicians may feel very helpless when faced with multiple symptoms in the elderly, but the number of correct diagnoses was higher in patients who were referred by their own doctor than in those referred by a physician they had not seen before. Whether or not the remaining years of desirable quality of life would have been improved by more accurate pre-hospital diagnosis was not determined by these studies.

Errors Due To Record Mix-ups or Communication Failures

These non-medical mistakes have resulted in operation on, or medical treatment for, the wrong patient or wrong organ. Last year an unlucky bridegroom-to-be had a castration instead of the circumcision for which he was admitted. Another patient, whose name bracelet was ignored, had a thyroidectomy instead of a cervical biopsy. Other unfortunates have had operations on the wrong leg, mistaken amputations, and transfusions with the wrong blood type. Hospitalized patients—be alert!

Misdiagnosis Due to Pathology Errors

Most non-professionals do not understand the function and scope of pathology. *Pathologic anatomy* is concerned with the diagnosis of cancer and other diseases by biopsies and the gross and microscopic examination of tissues removed by surgery or from autopsies. *Clinical pathology* includes hematology (blood counting and clotting), immunohematology (typing and cross-matching of blood for transfusions and parentage exclusion), chemistry, microbiology (bacteriology, mycology or fungus study, virology and parasitology), and clinical microscopy, a potpourri of urinalysis, and the examination of biologic fluids (spinal fluid, sputum, amniotic fluid, joint fluid, semen, pus, etc.). *Cytology* ("pap" smears) occupies an intermediate position, although it is generally included in pathologic anatomy. There is much overlapping of functions and variation of administration. In some large teaching hospitals and other countries, clinical pathology or some of its subdivisions are controlled by the Department of Medicine or are autonomous. This has led to intramural conflict and "executive suite" rivalries because considerable funds and positions of power are involved. The hospital pathologist is usually called the "Director of Laboratories." Although with one or more associate or assistant pathologists he or she is responsible for overall supervision, quality control, budget planning and training of residents and other personnel the pathologist personally performs pathologic anatomy functions but except in special cases, is seldom involved in the actual execution of the myriads of clinical pathology tests.

Biopsies, generally considered the most accurate tests for cancer, are not infallible. There is no absolute margin between benign and malignant in many cases and when a slide is sent to many experts for their opinion, multiple diagnoses may be returned. This leaves the local pathologist in a dilemma. Some surgeons and patients expect a definitive answer but sometimes only time and the autopsy will tell. I'm sure that Harry Truman was not thinking of pathologists when he said, "The buck stops here," but it is often applicable when there is difference of opinion regarding the presence of cancer.

Jimmie Greenfield, the 12-year-old son of a successful Florida physician, complained of severe local pain in his left shin bone after a basketball game. As the pain persisted, Dr. Greenfield ordered an x-ray study which revealed a small tumor. The anxiously awaited biopsy report revealed a malignancy, osteogenic sarcoma. The pathologist was so certain of his diagnosis that he did not think a second opinion necessary and, with the surgeon, recommended amputation of the leg. Dr. Greenfield, however, flew to New York with the slides and showed them to the bone cancer experts at the Sloan-Kettering Memorial Cancer Center. After study and consultation, they pronounced the tumor benign and recommended merely local excision. Ten years after this operation, Jimmie is in perfect health with no sign of recurrence.

Enlarged lymph nodes are particularly troublesome since the differentiation between Hodgkin's disease, other lymphoid tumors and benign enlargements due to inflammation is often extremely difficult.

Biopsies frequently are not done when necessary for diagnosis, especially in lesions of the mouth, skin, lymph nodes and breasts, resulting in failure to diagnose cancer in time to prevent spread. When an attempt is made to tie or cut the fallopian tubes for sterilization through a small incision or by a tubular instrument called a laparoscope the failure to send tubal tissue to the laboratory for confirmation may result in an unwanted conception.

Quick-frozen sections are the source of considerable anxiety. Although their accuracy has improved with new equipment, there are serious emotional as well as organic illness problems when the waiting surgeon receives a report of malignancy and removes an organ or limb, usually a breast, only to be told, 20 minutes later, that the tumor is actually benign. I have long recommended that no major surgery be performed on the basis of a frozen section report in certain situations calling for difficult pathologic decisions. Sections should not be done to satisfy the curiosity of the surgeon. Studies have shown that a 24 to 48-hour delay does not increase the mortality rate of breast cancers and allows time for the permanent section to be carefully reviewed before a final pathologic diagnosis is made. The patient is then not horrified when she awakens from anesthesia and finds that a mutilating operation has been performed. The wait allows time for consideration of the risks and, if the operation must be performed, the patient knows what to expect.

Pathologists have more difficulty providing clinically useful information since fine needle biopsies and flexible fiberoptic instruments became popular. Although these techniques penetrate further and reach areas previously inaccessible without open surgery, which is needed less often, they provide smaller samples, which are often more difficult to interpret. It has been found that, in *complex* cases, pathologists specializing in a single organ system like the kidney, skin or brain, had correct diagnoses in 75%, while general pathologists averaged 62% accuracy and trainees, 55%.

The average hospital pathologist examines and reports 5,000 cases annually, mostly the routine gallbladder, uterus, appendix, curetting, etc. Few of the less usual bone, brain or borderline cases among the common specimens are received. Therefore, problems in identifying unusual abnormalities frequently arise. When in doubt, the slide is shown to a colleague, or sent to a pathologist who has established a reputation in the study of the tissue in question. These second opinions eliminate many misinterpretations and save the pathologist sleepless nights spent worrying over the possible unnecessary removal of a breast, limb or other organ.

Even in clear-cut cases, the pathologist, being mortal and subject to human frailties, may err, especially in stressful situations or when faced with heavy workloads. The specimen submitted may be improperly prepared or preserved, especially when obtained by a non-specialist. Pressed for an answer, the pathologist may give an opinion even if the slide does not satisfy his requirements. This attempt to save time and help a colleague may, in fortunately few cases, lead to disaster for the patient.

Rosalind Tower, 32, had a dark mole removed from her left ankle in May of 1974 by a dermatologist. The specimen was sent to a pathologist who reported that it was benign. During the next 2½ years, Ms. Tower visited the dermatologist on eight occasions for other minor skin problems. During the last few visits she pointed out dusky discoloration around the side of the incision. The doctor reminded her of the benign report. In May of 1977, she consulted another doctor who also told her that the old incision site was benign. However, in 1978, she noticed a small lump in her left groin. It was removed by a surgeon and the hospital pathologist pronounced it malignant. A short time later the same surgeon removed the discolored scar of the ankle wound. The pathologist reported a "black cancer" (malignant melanoma). A wide excision of the mole site was performed with skin grafting to cover the defect. Although there is no evidence of recurrence at this writing, Ms. Tower will live with the "sword of Damocles" for many years and will require additional plastic surgery. I can recall many similar cases, most soon fatal.

Unlike Dr. Quincy, pathologists may make mistakes. The differentiation between an active mole and early malignant melanoma, like that between a benign or malignant lymph node tumor, can be very difficult and has caused many a pathologist prematurely graying hair.

Early in 1981, the Justice Department investigated a large laboratory, Automated Medical Services of Ohio (AMSO), which had analyzed almost 640,000 "Pap" smears of women employees and their dependents at 76 U.S. and 18 foreign air bases under a government contract in effect from 1972 through 1977. In 1978, several AMSO employees charged that the slides were being carelessly processed and many were incorrectly diagnosed. Air Force pathologists who reexamined a group of slides turned up a significant amount of misclassification. These women were advised to have the test repeated. Information regarding the number of cancers missed or falsely diagnosed was not available. The firm went out of business shortly after the investigation, and a number of lawsuits are pending by women who sued either the Air Force or the firm and its director, charging negligence.

Shortly after her marriage, Flora Miller, a lovely 22-year-old girl, had a routine "Pap" smear. It was pronounced positive for cancer but a follow-up biopsy showed only suspicious changes. Without waiting for confirmation, a hysterectomy was performed. No cancer could be found in the uterus. Since the young husband desired children, marital discord followed, leading to divorce.

Although the American Cancer Society no longer advocates annual "Pap" smears for women at *low* risk, those at *high* risk may not find yearly smears sufficient to prevent death from cervical cancer. If the malignancy is extremely aggressive, fortunately uncommon, it may spread from its onset; screening, no matter how frequent, will then be insufficient for detection in time to prevent invasion and metastatic spread. At the gynecologic department of Yale Medical School, ten cases of invasive cancer of the cervix, seven fatal, were discovered in women who had had negative "Pap" smears less than a year previously. Their ages ranged from 20 to 29, all were sexually active, and they had an average of 3.2 pregnancies. There were also five errors, with original false-negatives showing cancerous or precancerous changes when repeated.

The diagnosis of lung cancer by "Pap" smears of the sputum is beset with even more pitfalls than cervical cancer. Bronchitis, fungus infections and previous radiation may all cause changes in the cells which resemble cancer. Of course, no further treatment should be instituted until the disease is localized by x-ray examination and proven by biopsy.

Clinical Laboratory Errors and Iatrogenesis

Most patients complain that blood is withdrawn from their veins too often. Physician-patients protest that subdivisions of a single specimen could be sent to the various laboratories needing samples. Until the last century, blood-letting was a panacea for almost every disease. Monks were bled to counter the accumulation of semen due to celibacy. This therapeutic vampirism has now become diagnostic vampirism, and can result in iatrogenic anemia. Regardless of the reason for admission, many routine tests are required by the hospital, anesthesiologist or surgeon, and residents add their quota. An example is that of a patient who was hospitalized for 3½ months, during which time 121 blood counts and 111 chemical examinations were performed. It was estimated that a total of three liters of blood were removed. In one study of 64 hospitalized patients, 26 became anemic and one required blood transfusion.

In big teaching hospitals especially, students practice their jabs on patients, their ineptness frequently destroying veins and requiring different vessels for future specimens. Patients develop sore arms, inflamed, clotted veins, pain and fever, and may faint, causing falls and injury. Stacks of data accumulate, which add handsomely to hospital revenues, but are of questionable value to the patients' recovery.

The CDC estimates that there are approximately 15,000 clinical laboratories in the United States. Half are in hospitals and most of the remainder are private commercial facilities which serve physicians' offices, small hospitals and nursing homes. There are 30,000 to 80,000 small laboratories in physicians' offices. Over 5 billion tests are done annually, averaging 24 for each person in this country. Around one-hundred forty independent laboratories are located in Chicago. Some are large interstate operations with a central facility and branch offices where specimens are obtained and forwarded to the central laboratory. Smaller facilities are located in medical office buildings, shopping centers and converted stores. Some are corporations, owned by groups of certified pathologists, others by doctors, chemists or technicians. Pathologists must nominally serve as directors if tests involving tissues or cytology are performed. These enterprises may be extremely lucrative and the media have frequently exploited horror stories of "kick-backs," "sink tests" and other unethical practices by marginal operators.

State laws and standards vary, but the CDC monitors the performance of on-site inspections conducted by state examiners. It checks laboratories paid by Medicare or Medicaid or engaged in interstate commerce under terms of the 1976 Clinical Laboratory Improvement Act. It mails samples to the laboratories for analysis and notes the accuracy of the returned reports. This method has been criticized by the U.S. Department of Health and Human Services, which says that the 1,000 laboratories engaged in interstate commerce that are checked by the CDC identify the test samples and give them special treatment for best results.

If a local laboratory cannot do the infrequent or esoteric tests, it is possible for a specimen to be collected in the early afternoon and flown to California or New Jersey, where the largest laboratories, equipped to perform the most unusual tests, are located. An electronic print-out is then received by the referring physician or smaller laboratory the next morning.

Is this burgeoning industry, estimated to consume 8% of medical cost dollars or almost $20 billion annually, beneficial to the consumer? Some tests, particularly biopsies, are crucial to diagnosis and treatment, others substantiate diagnoses already made, but most are of little direct value. The key questions are—did the attending doctor do anything different as a result of the finding? And, did the different treatment favorably affect the outcome? During my training, a wise professor taught: "Before ordering a test, decide what you will do if it is (a) positive or (b) negative. If both answers are the same, don't do the test."

The fallacy of multiphasic screening of well persons by multiple automated blood chemistries was discussed in Chapter 2. But even with sick, hospitalized patients, simple tests are often best, according to an JAMA editorial in 1981. Ultratechnical procedures should complement clinical judgment but not replace it. A common myocardial infarction requires $500-worth of chemical studies, and an abdominal tumor cannot be operated on without expensive CAT scans and other imaging procedures, because of the tendency to regard lack of extensive technical documentation as poor practice of medicine. Perhaps the decrease in federal and state contributions to health care will have a salutory effect in restoring clinical judgment to maximum importance. The journal *Medicine* has recommended "proceeding immediately to the diagnostic test most likely to provide a diagnosis," rather than wasting time on a routine and expensive sequence of examinations. "The application of the doctor's five senses often exceeds the best that technology can offer," the report continues.

Since most clinical laboratory tests are now performed by electrochemical, automated machines with abundant controls, technical mistakes are less common than in the past. No longer do technicians have to skillfully manipulate Bunsen burners, test-tubes and slides for most routine work. Samples of blood are placed in small containers in turntables which rotate automatically after a button is pushed. Unseen by the eye and untouched by human hands, they are mixed with the appropriate reagents, whirring or clicking sounds are heard and, in a few minutes, a numerical report is printed in several copies, ready for distribution to the requesting physician, the hospital chart and of course, the billing office. Asterisks indicate abnormal results. Each JCAH-approved laboratory must maintain a chart indicating "panic" values, which are those that must be brought to the physician's attention immediately because they indicate a result at variance with that expected or which requires immediate treatment. The College of American Pathologists maintains a voluntary quality assurance program (QAS). Therefore, significant unreliable results are now rare and mistakes occur mainly through clerical and distribution errors and the ever-present human factors. A few tests are still done in emergencies, singly and manually with insufficient controls, or the result may be overlooked, as in the case of Fred, whose low blood sugar report was completely disregarded.

Despite the technical wizardry of automated equipment, spurious results can occur due to unexpected factors. Many have relevance to patient management. Platelets, small particles concerned with blood clotting, may be included with minute debris, abnormally small cells and fragments of cells, thus giving falsely elevated counts. This occurred in the case of an elderly woman who was severely burned. The mechanical counter gave a result almost three times higher than a precise manual method.

A commercial artist, Selma Jones, complained of loss of weight and vigor, excessive thirst and appetite, and poor healing of a minor cut on her foot. Suspecting diabetes, her doctor ordered a blood sugar test and sent the specimen to a commercial laboratory. The report was normal. With these symptoms the blood sugar test should have been repeated, but the doctor looked for other causes. Several weeks later, Selma became comatose and only heroic measures saved her life. The control chart on the automatic analyzer showed no discrepancies so it must be assumed that this report was intended for another person. Because of inept clerical personnel it was never determined who received the report intended for Selma. This case illustrates the fallacy of relying on a single laboratory report which contradicts clinical judgment.

Over 20,000 American infants were born with congenital deformities in 1964 due to an epidemic of German measles (rubella) which involved many expectant mothers. Vaccines, tests for rubella, and abortions of fetuses borne by women who contracted rubella during pregnancy have reduced these calamities to less than 25 known cases annually. However, a CDC survey, reported in *Laboratory Medicine* in February of 1982 showed that 11% of participating laboratories were unable to correctly perform a test showing that a mother-to-be was immune to rubella and that therefore her baby would not be at risk. Half of the laboratories could not correctly assay the degree of immunity.

What appears to be an abnormally high or abnormally low result of a laboratory analysis may be the effect of drugs, particularly narcotics, diuretics ("water pills") or intravenous or intramuscular injections. Tests for overactive or underactive thyroid glands are among the most important supplements to clinical judgment, but are also commonly subject to interference by a host of compounds which cause false results. It would be impossible to learn all the different agents and combinations, but charts have been prepared showing the effects of medications on the results of blood and urine tests. Unless this is known, the attending physician may receive a misleading report. Alcohol and smoking may also interfere with results. Strenuous physical exercise will cause a release of enzymes suggesting muscle disease and if the patient has chest pain, this may cause the physician to suspect myocardial infarction. Even the psychological stress of the anxiety preceding blood withdrawal will increase the white blood count. If the constricting tourniquet is kept on the arm for three minutes, the blood protein will increase. Blood taken after meals will show increased sugar and fats.

Tests sometimes tell too much. A 60-year-old man with an enlarged prostate had four tests for an enzyme called acid phosphatase, all of which were elevated, indicating the possibility of cancer. But it has been found that one in ten people has these elevations for no discernible reason. Several doctors who palpated the prostate, found it to be soft, with no indication of cancer. In this case, the doctors' clinical judgment must prevail.

"Pap" smears are big business, estimated at $500 million annually for over 60 million procedures. Many commercial laboratories, some processing hundreds of thousands of smears annually, attest to the profitability of this enterprise. Well women have been indoctrinated that this is a painless and beneficial health measure that should be repeated at regular intervals.

New tests are continually being introduced in the hope that they will improve diagnosis and outcome in established illnesses. Many are used without clear evidence of their benefit. Very often the precision obtained in practice does not equal that of the originators of the method. But they may have psychotherapeutic value for the physician. Some patients are so ill that there is little that can be done for them, but it is always possible to order more tests to create the illusion that something is being done to help. If the patient is terminally ill, the doctor can order daily blood counts and chemistries. This psychotherapy is also for the patient's benefit. The doctor can say, "I have done these tests and you do not have diabetes, you have no kidney disease and your liver is fine." This reassurance helps to quell fears and anxieties.

"Supply-side" economics has long been true in medicine. Doctors who attend a seminar or read of a new method are quick to jump on the bandwagon. Hospital administrators love any expansion of activity that increases their cash flow. But the criterion for acceptability must be a more precise diagnosis that will improve treatment and outcome. Reduction of discomfort, risk, cost and time lost from work, as well as saving the physician's consultation time, must also be considered. Hypotheses on the effectiveness of tests can never be tested sufficiently in experimental trials. Only in widespread, long-term clinical use will the validity of a new procedure stand or fall.

9.

PREVENTING AND TERMINATING PREGNANCY

". . . some political and social activities and practices . . . are detrimental and even dangerous for the community as a whole, here and everywhere. I mention here only the fight against birth control at a time when overpopulation in various countries has become a serious threat to the health of people and a grave obstacle to organizing peace on this planet."

Albert Einstein—1954

The most important political, religious, moral and medical event of recent history has been the explosive expansion of the human race. We must add the population proliferation to our list of iatrogenic evils. Good intentions—urban hygiene, medical care and universal immunization of children—not balanced by birth control, have raised the birth/death ratio. Infant mortality has decreased even in impoverished countries, permitting survival to maturity in misery. Destruction and depletion of natural resources, soil erosion, desertification, deforestation, urban sprawl, and pollution of air and water all result from the inability of the environment to absorb the additional wastes and to fulfill the additional needs of too many people. This is the global evil that plagues us today. But birth control, indispensable for the survival of civilization, has risks for the individual.

Oral Contraceptives—Perils of the Pill

When Sarah Dalton was a 19-year-old sophomore at a Midwest college in 1975, she joined the ranks of her liberated classmates and starting using the Pill. Six months later, she experienced severe cramps in both legs which progressed to painful spasms, and sharp abdominal pain developed. Then both legs became completely paralyzed. She was taken to a renowned hospital where diagnostic study indicated that the paralysis was caused by a blood clot in a large artery supplying the nerves to her lower extremities. Treatment was of no avail. She sued Ortho Pharmaceutical Corporation, manufacturer of her oral contraceptive. In 1980 she was awarded $3.8 million. She has since become a consumer advocate, speaking about the problems of the Pill from her wheelchair.

The Pill, which has been available since the early 1960s, has liberated women from primary dependency upon their male partners for contraception. By 1981, 40% of U.S. females aged 15 through 44 were regularly taking oral contraceptives (OC) and 54 million were estimated to be using them worldwide.

The first reported instance of OC-related blood clotting in a pulmonary (lung) artery occurred in Suffolk, England in 1961. By the end of that decade, it was discerned that women on OC were at increased risk for thrombo-embolic (blood-clotting) disease in many systemic sites. Since 1961, studies in the U.S., England and Scandinavia have demonstrated an increased risk for heart attack (myocardial infarction or MI), stroke and thromboembolism. OC users over 35 years of age triple their risks from one in 1,000 to three in 1,000 if they smoke cigarettes. Unapparent blood clotting, which is more common than overt disease, also occurs three times as frequently in smokers who use OC. The clots usually dissolve spontaneously.

This increased risk, which is due to the clot-enhancing estrogenic component of the pill, is of long duration. A 1981 study at the Boston University Medical School reviewed 556 women who were admitted to 155 hospitals. The longer the women took the pill, the greater was their risk of MI. If OC were used for more than nine years, the risk was increased two to three times and persisted up to nine years after discontinuance. After menopause, the risk declined to normal expectations.

Those of blood types A, B and AB are genetically predisposed to have three times the risk of those of type O (12/10,000, compared to 4/10,000 per year). Half of the MIs have been fatal but only 5-10% of the stroke victims have died. Deaths of OC users from stroke and MI combined total 22-24 per 100,000 per year and are concentrated in smokers over 35 years old.

Dr. Bruce Stadel in the *New England Journal of Medicine* recently summarized the risks of OC compounded by other dangers. For MI, the greatest additional risk (40%) is caused by smoking over 15 cigarettes daily. Hypertension increases the risk 13%, diabetes, 2%, and high blood fats, 4%. Dr. Stadel also concluded that the increased danger was centralized in smokers and those over 35. For non-smokers, the annual risk increased from one in 100,000 at age 15 to 19 to 18 in 100,000 at age 40-44. However, to place the hazards in perspective, their total for non-smoking OC users is only *25% of the expected complications of normal pregnancy* occuring with OC for women below age 35, and equal to the risk of pregnancy after age 35—21 deaths per 100,000 per year.

MI, stroke and blood-clotting in other large arteries are the principal complications of OC, but other undesired effects occur. Although gynecologists prescribe OC, other specialists see most of the iatrogenic aftermaths. But if pregnancy occurs within a month after discontinuing OC, there is a substantially greater risk of tubal pregnancy, the birth of twins, cesarean delivery, stillbirth or a premature infant. There may be a decrease in the quality and quantity of breast milk. A delay in conception after discontinuance of OC was reported in the *JAMA* in 1982. Dr. Shai Linn of the Harvard School of Public Health showed that 25% of 3,000 such women did not conceive for 13 months or more, compared to 10% of those who had used other methods such as the diaphragm, spermicides or intrauterine devices (IUDs). A smaller percentage took three years or more to attain desired conception.

Greater promiscuity increases genital herpes, and the risk of cervical cancer. (A study of 17,000 women by the Kaiser-Permanente Medical Center showed no increased risk for breast cancer, and other studies have shown no additional cancer of the uterine lining.) There have been reports of loss of vision, double-vision and discomfort with the use of the new extended-wear contact lenses due to excess fluid in the eyeball. Gallbladder disease, high blood pressure, irregularities and cessation of menstruation are occasional effects.

The "morning after pill" (DES) is reasonably potent in preventing pregnancy if given in sufficient dosage after a single unprotected intercourse. But large amounts of DES must be given twice daily for five days after exposure. Because it increases the risk of cancer of the uterus and damage to possible offspring, it is no longer recommended as a post-coital contraceptive.

Vaginal Creams, Foams and Jellies (Spermicides), and Diaphragms

A total of seven hundred sixty-three infants of mothers who used only vaginal spermicides within 10 months of conception were recently reported on by Dr. Hershel Jick of the Boston University Medical Center. The rate of congenital defects in these infants was 2.2%, almost twice the expected rate. Ten exhibited loss or deformities of limbs, rare types of cancer, penile deformities or Down's syndrome (mongolism). These *serious* flaws occurred at five times the expected rate and confirmed previous studies which had postulated that the process of fertilization of the ovum was harmfully affected. Spontaneous abortions were almost twice as common as in a comparison group. Even more recent studies show that the risk is present, although at lower levels.

Vaginal inserts (suppositories) are handy, but seldom used. They must be implanted 15 minutes before intercourse to allow melting and must not be washed out for an hour afterwards. They are not as effective as most other methods, with 8 pregnancies for each 100 users per year.

Before the development of OCs, the diaphragm plus spermicides for maximum protection was the technique most used in the developed world. No deleterious effects had been reported for the various models except for their ineffectiveness when incorrectly inserted or displaced during intercourse, and their unesthetic, messy interference with coitus. In October, 1981, however, the *NEMJ* carried a report by Dr. E. E. Horowitz of toxic shock syndrome associated with the use of a diaphragm and later that year, several other cases were reported. Drs. Lucy Loomis and Henry Feder of the University of Connecticut Health Center wrote of a 23-year-old who inserted a diaphragm which she was unable to remove. Two days later, she developed fever, vomiting and diarrhea. She went to a hospital emergency room where the diaphragm was easily extracted. However, after 36 hours she returned with fever, joint and muscle pain and sore throat. She had low blood presssure, a red rash, "strawberry tongue" and a pink cervical discharge from which staphylococci were cultured. Antibiotics were administered and she appeared well, but 11 days after the onset flakes of skin peeled from her palms and soles.

Intrauterine Devices (IUDs)

In 1970, 22-year-old Sally Greco was delivered of a 7-pound boy with no unusual events. Six months later she had a polyethylene IUD (Lippe's loop) inserted. She experienced considerable pain and bleeding and the loop was removed after two months. For the following two years she took an OC, but it was discontinued because she developed high blood pressure. In 1973, a polyethylene Dalkon Shield was inserted which also caused pain and bleeding. She tolerated it for a year but then discontinued all contraception. She became pregnant in October, 1974. In her 15th week she developed severe vomiting, abdominal pain, diarrhea and pallor. She was markedly anemic and had low blood pressure and a rapid pulse. Blood was transfused while an operation found the uterus ruptured and a fetus, 10 inches long, floating free in a pool of blood. The uterus was repaired after removal of the fetus and afterbirth (placenta). Several other uterine ruptures after or during IUD insertions have been reported, but many are believed not to have been disclosed.

IUDs were first used in 1909 and were made of such diverse material as wire, silver and silkworm gut. The present generation are composed of copper, plastic or stainless steel. Their advantage over other contraceptives is that they require little or no follow-up care and minimal motivation. But they fail to prevent pregnancy in 3% to 5% of users each year. Pregnancy may occur in a fallopian tube, which can rupture and hemorrhage into the abdominal cavity. There may be excessive bleeding and uterine infection with or without abortion. Fatal bacteremia can result. Perforation of the uterus may require operative removal. Spontaneous expulsion of the Lippe's loop occurs in 18% to 24% of all cases, but the loops may remain in place for as long as five to ten years before encrustations irritate the uterus. Dalkon Shields were removed from the market in 1975 because they caused more complications than other devices and were difficult to insert. The Cu 7 is slender, easier to insert and causes less bleeding and cramping. But it has a high rate of spontaneous expulsion and must be changed every two years because of corrosion of its copper component.

An English report in 1981 showed that most women with IUDs were very sexually active and 24% had contracted gonorrhea. Some of these developed inflammation of the fallopian tubes and often sterility. Fungus infections occur in up to 5% of IUD wearers, as discovered in a study of 70,000 women.

Male Contraceptives

Despite its dangers, the pill has emancipated women from conventional sexual codes and is partly responsible for the recent disturbing increase in venereal disease, often due to organisms which resist antibiotics. Hence, public health authorities advocate a return to the condom. These familiar protective sheaths were first used in the 1700s and were originally made of sheep intestines, later replaced by rubber and plastics. Failures in contraception caused by condoms may result from defects in manufacture, tearing, or leakage after culmination if the flaccid penis is not promptly removed from the vagina. Some find that they are messy and reduce stimulation. If used properly, only 4% will fail annually, but studies have shown that two-thirds of users discontinue use after the first year.

And what of the male contraceptive? An editorial in the *NEMJ*, in September of 1981 described research now in progress on a synthetic gonadotropin-releasing hormone which decreases sperm production. Eight volunteers at Vanderbilt University were taught to give themselves injections of the hormone, which can also be taken as a nasal spray or in nose drops. The same substance is being tested on women, raising the possibility of developing a unisex contraception. After six to ten weeks, the sperm counts dropped precipitously, and in two they almost disappeared. At present it would be unacceptable because it also results in hot flashes and decreased libido and potency.

SURGICAL CONTRACEPTION—Cutting the Cords and Tying the Tubes

Vasectomy

This simple procedure—the removal of a short segment of each spermatic duct (vas deferens) which can be done under local anesthetic in a few minutes in a doctor's office—is becoming increasingly popular. It has been estimated that 35 million men, 6 million in the U.S., have had vasectomies. Serious political unrest occurred in India a few years ago when the government tried to induce pious Hindus to undergo vasectomy (with gifts as incentives).

Vasectomy leaves sexual performance unimpaired but causes permanent sterility, although experiments with removable plugs and reconstructive plastic surgery have been conducted with dubious success. Its possible relation to the development of hardening of the arteries (atherosclerosis-arteriosclerosis) was reviewed at a 1981 American Heart Association meeting. Experiments with vasectomized monkeys on high-fat, high-cholesterol diets showed more atherosclerosis than in non-vasectomized primates fed similar food. In 1981, a collaborative American study, of almost 5,000 vasectomized men showed that they had no increase in heart attacks compared with 24,000 men whose spermatic cords were intact. However, according to researcher Nancy Alexander, "the survey involved mostly men who had had relatively recent vasectomies and atherosclerosis may take ten years or more to develop." A larger scale study of the relationship of vasectomies to atherosclerosis, MI and strokes is now underway.

An editorial in the JAMA in June of 1981 reviewed the literature on complications of vasectomy. The late Dr. Harold Lear wrote "A Note of Concern" in the *JAMA* in 1972. He related the results of a survey of 6,100 men who were observed for an average of four years. A slight increase of enlarged prostates, narrowing of foreskin (phimosis) and inflammation of the testes was noted. But the risk was low enough to make the procedure acceptable. Dr. J. W. Squires' article in *Surgery, Gynecology and Obstetrics* in 1976 discussed 242 vasectomies, of which six developed serious complications: gangrene of the scrotum, local blood accumulations (hematomas) and persistent pain. In six cases there was spontaneous regeneration of a spermatic duct. Only a few men among over 10,000 vasectomized at the Chicago Midwest Population Center developed decreased libido and impotence, according to a letter from Don C. Shaw, its Director. There was only one instance of epididymitis—a superb record.

Closing the Fallopian Tubes—Sexual Tubal Sterilization (STS)

Until recently, when a couple desired to dispense with temporary contraceptive methods, the husband usually prevailed upon his wife to have her fallopian tubes ligated or sectioned instead of submitting himself to a vasectomy. Women's consciousness-raising and the ease of the procedure increased the number of vasectomies. Formerly, closure of the tubes required a vaginal or abdominal operation and was frequently performed after cesarean section. The insertion of a lighted tube (laparoscope) through the umbilicus, leaving no visible scar, has now made this procedure more acceptable and its frequency is rising. A segment of each tube can be removed, or closure can be performed by cautery (fulguration).

When tubes were sectioned and a short segment removed, a pathologist could examine the fragments and certify that tubal continuity was interrupted. The newer methods of fulguration, tying, or use of a plastic clip may mistakenly be performed on the nearby, similar, round ligament and there is no way to prove that the tube was closed. The risk of failure is slightly less than 1%, which is comparable to that of vasectomy.

Most American women receive general anesthesia, since air injected through the slender laparoscope for better visualization of the tubes causes discomfort. Dr. Herbert Brown wrote in a 1981 *JAMA*, that the length of stay need not exceed 4-6 hours postoperatively. He described free-standing clinics, set up in camps in India, where thousands of STS's were performed with only local anesthesia and minimal postoperative supervision. The Association for Voluntary Sterilization estimates that 4 million STS's were performed in the U.S. from 1976 through 1979 and that the elimination of overnight hospitalization could save $360 million each year.

Besides intestinal burning and failure to close the tubes, serious complications, although few, have occurred. The procedure is impossible or dangerous if adhesions from old operations or inflammations such as tuberculosis are present. The aorta, bowel and stomach have been perforated, requiring immediate operative intervention. A fatal hemorrhage from disruption of a liver tumor was recorded several years ago. Although STS is conveniently performed after cesarean or vaginal births, complications are more likely at this time and it should be deferred for several months.

As divorce and remarriage increase in the U.S., more women are seeking surgery for reversal of STS, according to Dr. Arthur F. Haney of Duke University. Because STS has been enhanced by the adverse effects of OCs and IUDs, more reversals are desired when remarried women wish to have children by their new husbands. The reversal surgery has about a 50% success rate.

A new method—squirting a few drops of liquid silicone rubber into the tubes through a thin instrument inserted through the vagina and uterus, thus forming flexible rubber plugs—is safe and perhaps reversible. "The results are extremely encouraging," said Dr. A. J. Kresch of Stanford University in November of 1981. There have been no failures (pregnancies) with normally formed plugs among the most recent 500 volunteers. The procedure, which is being tested on carefully selected women in 10 cities, takes about half an hour, can be done in a doctor's office with local anesthetic and costs about half as much as other types of sterilization. A satisfactory plug, however, is not attained in 10 to 15% of the cases. Early in the study, nine pregnancies occurred in 125 women whose plugs were considered inadequate. Over 600 women have undergone tubal plugging since 1978 with no important iatrogenic incidents. The FDA will soon decide if the procedure can be licensed for general use.

ABORTION—THE EMOTIONAL ISSUE

Sally Sue Culp, a 24-year-old West Virginia schoolteacher, found little in common with the semi-literate young mountain men of her generation. She met a local businessman at a school board meeting. Mutual attraction developed into clandestine intimacy and soon Sally was pregnant. But it was 1959 and Sally's only recourse was to visit an ex-nurse who lived on a small farm near town. This lady was reputed to have come to the aid of distressed young women and older women who already had more children than they desired. An abortion was performed in a spare bedroom with the most sterile precautions possible under the circumstances. Several days later, Sally's bloody discharge became foul and she developed high fever, abdominal pain and myriads of tender blue spots over her trunk, arms and legs. She was taken to a small rural hospital, 12 miles down the valley and given antibiotics and intravenous fluids, but her general condition deteriorated. She went into shock and died on the 12th day after the abortion. Blood cultures were positive for streptococci.

Sally's abortion was performed in unsanitary conditions like those of home delivery. Others have been attempted with lye or permanganate uterine douches, slippery elm twigs, coat hangers, knitting needles or stiff catheters. It is no wonder that not only infection, but perforation of the uterus with damage to the intestines and peritonitis occurred so often during the period of illegality. Even when performed by doctors, the secretive circumstances and their often less-than-optimum standards and character caused a high incidence of infections and fatalities. I was once informed by a state's attorney that these doctors would not be prosecuted unless their illegal abortions were known to cause complications. "Dr. Sunshine" operated openly in a palatial mansion on Gramercy Park in New York for years. His good results, police connections and prompt 50-50 fee-splitting with the referring doctor guaranteed his unhindered services. Chicago also had a "society" abortionist on posh Michigan Avenue, well known to most middle and upper-class women.

Despite the fulminations of the so-called "moral majority" and "right-to-lifers," nobody favors abortion as a primary means of contraception. It should be resorted to only when other means have failed, or if prenatal examination indicates that a congenitally deficient infant will be born. Women will have abortions, legal or not. Iatrogenesis will increase with illegality, as it has in the past.

Dr. George Ryan, president of the American College of Obstetricians and

Gynecologists, affirmed recently on TV that abortion during the first trimester is "twenty times safer than normal pregnancy." Four months earlier he had condemned the "human life" bills now pending in Congress and warned that such legislation "would be a return to the documented hazards of illegal abortion." Before abortion was legalized in 1973, "an estimated 200,000 to 1.2 million illegal abortions occurred each year in the U.S. Until 1970, over 100 women died each year as a result of abortion complications and thousands of others were hospitalized with serious or critical illnesses."

An abortion ban would have very serious societal consequences. There are currently 1 million teenaged pregnancies every year, 400,000 terminated by abortion. If these went on to delivery, the cost to taxpayers for additional welfare would be $40 billion. A cut in funding for abortions is paradoxical when the government is trying to reduce expenditures. Violent crime and unemployment would also increase as these predominantly disadvantaged children reached maturity.

Iatrogenic Effects of Abortion

Most women choosing abortion are white, unmarried and childless, one-third teenagers and another third aged 20 to 24. This is a departure from the past generation when the average woman having an abortion was middle-class, married, and had two or more children. The CDC determined that there were 1,239,000 legally induced abortions in 1979, 7% more than in 1978—over one abortion for every three live births. There were 20 deaths from legal and, for the first time, no deaths recorded from illegal abortions, indicating that the latter have markedly decreased. Nine additional deaths were due to spontaneous abortions, approximately half the usual toll. The death rate decreased from 4.1% in 1972 to 1.5% in 1979. It is believed that the actual number of abortions is 20% higher than the CDC calculation, or 1,540,000. Despite these figures, an estimated 736,000 women in 1978 and 641,000 in 1979, had unwanted births because they were unable to obtain abortion services within a reasonable distance, according to *Family Planning Perspectives.*

There were ten deaths reported since 1972 from ruptured tubal, and one from abdominal, pregnancies following attempted abortion and two after spontaneous abortions, indicating mistaken diagnoses of uterine pregnancy. Most of these abortions were performed by suction and a minority by sharp scraping (curettage). Risks increase with advancing age, black race, low socioeconomic status and multiple previous pregnancies.

As in the U.S. before 1973, when abortions are performed for conditions threatening the health or life of the mother, iatrogenesis increases. A report from Winnepeg, Manitoba analyzed the complications of 2,100 therapeutic abortions during a 5-year period. There were no deaths, but tearing (laceration) of the cervix serious enough to require suturing occurred in 25 cases or 3% of those done by suction curettage. There were four (0.5%) uterine perforations, nine (1.1%) hemorrhages, three of which required transfusions, and 19 anesthetic complications, such as severe vomiting or irregular heart beats. Over 1,000 were performed by injection of medication (prostaglandin) into the amniotic sac (amnioinfusion), mainly after the third month. Major complications included sensitivity reactions to the medication, incomplete abortion requiring curettage for completion, and urinary and other infections. Delayed bleeding and pelvic inflammation were also noted. Abdominal operation including opening or removal of the uterus was done in 290 cases with 17.7% having major complications, urinary and wound infections predominating.

These complications exceed most U.S. reports, because many more (35%) were performed after the third month by amnioinfusion and open surgery and because facilities were limited.

The Rhythm Method—Family Planning Without Intervention

Critics warn of the failures of abstinence from sexual relations during mid-cycle as a means of birth control because of its poor success rate. Impregnation can occur during the beginning or end of abstinence. The fertilization of overaged ova by overaged sperm increases the risk of having miscarriages or children with birth defects. Women's cycles do not occur with mathematical regularity, and one mistake each year means a baby each year. But the adverse effects of the Pill, IUDs, spermicides and abortion have revived interest in the rhythm method. New methods employing better detection of temperature change at time of ovulation (the Sympto-thermal method) and changes in the cervical lining (the Billings method), developed in Australia, are becoming more popular, especially with observing Catholics. However, these require complicated charting of menstrual and ovulatory cycles and dedicated motivation by intelligent participants. The variability of menstrual cycles does not permit prediction of widespread success.

IATROGENIC EFFECTS OF SUCCESSFUL CONTRACEPTION AND ABORTION

The increase in teenage pregnancy is now accompanied by a parallel opposing phenomenon—an over 15% rise in the birth rate in mature women. Now aged 30-44, many of the daughters of the baby boom of the 1940s and 1950s are having their first child. The U.S. birth rate dropped to 14.5 babies per 1,000 population in the 1970s, but has been rising and is expected to exceed 17.5 in 1982. Many of these have had successful careers in the arts, business and professions. They marry later than their mothers and are reluctant to interrupt their professional progress to have offspring until they feel secure in their upward mobility.

Advances in management and improvement in physical fitness have raised the age of increased risk to 35. But as age increases, the hazard is that diabetes, high blood pressure, arthritis, respiratory ailments and kidney disease are more likely to develop and cause problems during pregnancy and delivery.

Defective infants are more than twice as likely to be born to 40-year-old mothers than those at 25, and defective births quintuple after age 45. Eggs (ova) and sperm not only age naturally, but have had more time to be attacked by pollution, pesticides, drugs, viruses and radiation. Mongolism (Down's syndrome) and dwarfism due to retarded bone growth (achondroplasia), are the greatest congenital risks. Many fetal defects can be detected by amniocentesis, the insertion of a long thin needle into the cushioning "bag of waters" (amniotic sac) and the withdrawal of fluid-floating cells which can be studied for genetic flaws. It can also be tested for abnormal chemicals, which signal the presence of Tay-Sachs disease or spinal cord and brain defects. But faulty hearts and intestines, cleft lip and palate, and clubfoot cannot be predicted by amniocentesis. The procedure carries a slight danger of infection, induced miscarriage and damage to the fetus. However, the opportunity to detect and abort an abnormal fetus is worth the risk to most women of any age.

The U.S. is not proud of its maternal mortality rate. Although fewer than one in 10,000 women die in delivery, 16 countries do better. Women over 35 have five times the mortality and twice the miscarriage rate of women in their early 20s. Getting pregnant has problems. Not all of the older women's menstrual cycles produce ova and their aging husbands' sperm cells are more likely to be defective.

Years of successful contraception now take their toll. After the discontinuance of OC, it may take 13 to 15 months for conception to occur. Infertility and miscarriage are two to three times more likely after two or more abortions. Gynecologic disorders such as uterine and tubal infection, sexually transmitted or exacerbated by IUDs, and benign fibroid tumors and particles of misplaced uterine lining in the pelvic cavity (endometriosis) can all prevent successful nesting of a fertilized ovum in the uterus.

These handicaps were demonstrated by a study of 2,000 women who had artificial insemination, reported in the *NEMJ* in February of 1982: 73% of those under 25 became pregnant in the first year; 74% of those 26-30; 61% of those 30-35 and 54% of those over 35 became pregnant.

Because so many women use contraceptives, are sterilized and/or have abortions, the term reproductive mortality—a measure of the hazards of fertility and fertility control—is more appropriate than maternal mortality. Reproductive mortality (RM) may be (1) *pregnancy related:* ectopic pregnancy or abortion, spontaneous or induced, or (2) *contraception related:* due to OCs, IUDs, or barriers such as diaphragms and spermicides or sterilization.

Since 1955, there has been a 73% decline in RM, down from 7.8 to 2.1 per 100,000—a total of 2,703 to 999. The CDC has shown that, in 1975, almost half of the remaining deaths—472 women—died from complications of contraception and sterilization. The decline in RM has been less dramatic in the age group 35-44 (41%) than in the group 15-19 (81%), and, in the older group, the contraceptive-related mortality has actually increased, especially in cigarette smokers. OCs alone accounted for 350 deaths.

Deaths from abortion have declined phenomenally from 1955 to 1975, while those from IUDs and sterilization have shown no significant change. Since 1975, it has been estimated that RM has decreased due to an awareness of the hazards of OCs and a decline in their use, but OCs still account for 45% of RM.

In summary, the overall risk of RM has shown a sharp decline since 1955, but there is still an increase in deaths due to OCs in women over 35. Any further decrease in contraceptive risks will have as great an impact on public health as improvement in pregnancy mortality rates.

The most important, but usually overlooked, risk of deferred pregnancy is that of breast cancer, which will strike one in 11 American women in their lifetimes. As I have explained in Chapter 2, women who are "elderly primiparas" or childless have a significantly greater chance of developing breast cancer than do those who have had several pregnancies before the age of 25. Research concerning the anti-breast cancer effect of pregnancy terminated by abortion has not yet produced conclusive results. From the biomedical point of view, it would be better to have babies first and careers later.

10.

PROCEDURES—INVADING THE SKIN, CIRCULATORY SYSTEM AND OTHER OPENINGS

Surgeons' income and prestige traditionally exceeded that of other doctors. So-called health insurance (actually illness insurance), originally developed to protect patients from the high cost of surgery. As private and governmental insurance gradually grew to cover almost our entire population, benefits were expanded to include diagnostic tests and x-ray examinations. "Procedures" are lucrative equivalents of minor surgery but use no knives. With new devices to penetrate the circulatory system, cardiologists became invasive. Radiologists perform arteriograms, venograms, arthrograms, encephalograms and lymphangiograms. Other specialists probe all orifices, organs and hollow spaces.

During the past generation, improvements in long, slender, illuminated fiberoptic instruments have enabled specialists to inspect and treat disorders of organs formerly accessible only by open surgery. These snake-like devices can be wormed through natural openings or through the skin, umbilicus or scars of old operations, leaving imperceptible evidence of their passage. A little skin anesthesia is required and most procedures can be done on an outpatient basis. As expected, they are overused, but for the most part they have eliminated the need for more costly and dangerous surgery. Gastroenterologists advanced from their primitive proctoscopes and sigmoidoscopes and learned to insert new fiberoptic instruments further up and down the digestive system and its ramifications. Pediatricians give exchange transfusions and kidney specialists devised dialysis. The closest that pathologists get to a living patient is when they do needle biopsies of the bone marrow in small hospitals which do not have hematologists on their staffs.

Surgical specialists, too, have departed from the scalpel for many maneuvers. The cystoscope, for examining, biopsying and operating on the urinary tract and prostate, was the first in importance. Bronchoscopes and esophagoscopes followed. Now, general surgeons and gynecologists use laparoscopes which can be used to observe the interior organs and perform small biopsies and cauterization procedures. Obstetricians do amniocentesis for diagnosing and operating on the fetus and orthopedists look at joint cavities through arthroscopes.

Most non-surgeons also perform procedures which pay more than thinking and decision-making services. This creates an incentive to increase the volume of instrumental maneuvers, since insurance will reimburse a patient $50 for a 10-15 minute instrumental examination of the lower bowel (sigmoidoscopy) and more for an examination of the stomach (gastroscopy) or lower bowel (colonoscopy), but will not pay the same for a half-hour or longer office visit. Needles and catheters are inserted into veins and arteries and left in place for feeding, monitoring, transfusing and dialysing by everyone from nurses and residents-in-training to their chiefs. Spinal, abdominal and chest taps are routine in all branches. Even the simplest of these techniques, which do not require actual cutting through the skin and leaving a wound large enough to require suturing, have their hazards.

Spinal Taps (Lumbar Punctures)

One summer morning in 1980, 13-year-old Sarah Constanza woke up complaining of severe headache. This did not disturb her mother very much because Sarah had been having headaches for six months and her doctor had reassured her that headaches were common in early adolescence. But the headaches grew worse and by the late afternoon convulsions developed with intermittent loss of consciousness. Sarah was driven to a nearby hospital where a doctor performed a spinal tap by inserting a long slender needle between segments of the spinal column in the lower back and into the space around the spinal cord to get a sample of protective fluid. The spinal fluid pressure was found to be higher than normal. In less than an hour, Sarah became comatose and her breathing and heart beat stopped. She was put on a life support system but was soon declared dead.

Although spinal taps are among the most common procedures performed in hospitals, these taps can be very dangerous if the fluid pressure is elevated. If the fluid is removed too rapidly, the brain stem, which contains the respiratory center, will be pushed down into the canal containing the spinal cord with frequently fatal results. There are other hazards. Between 1972 and 1981 at the Boston University Medical School, 271 children with bacteremia, mostly secondary to ear infections (otitis media), pneumonia or acute pharyngitis, had lumbar punctures. Nine of these, all less than a year old, developed meningitis, fortunately responding to antibiotics, with no fatalities.

Headaches occur in one of four patients after spinal taps, are mostly deep and throbbing, frequently cause neck muscle spasms, and are accentuated by movement.

Ten-year-old David Manners had surgical removal of a benign brain tumor when he was four years old. During this hospitalization he had nine spinal taps. He remained well for 6½ years, when he developed pain his left calf, aggravated by sneezing and coughing, and began walking with a shuffling gait. Spinal x-ray films with contrast media showed complete blocking of his lower spinal canal by a tumor which was removed and found to be composed of skin elements. Three cases of such epidermoid tumors found in the spines of children following spinal taps were reported in 1977. These benign but troublesome tumors were first demonstrated to be related to single or multiple spinal taps in 1956, when six cases were reported in children who had been given intraspinal antibiotics for tuberculous meningitis. Many other instances were found in a search of the literature. In most cases, the stylet filling the canal of the needle was not used, resulting in the implantation of skin fragments which then grew and formed tumor-like masses.

Spinal taps in alcoholics can be dangerous because these patients frequently have bleeding problems. Their blood platelets, which assist in clotting, are often decreased in numbers due to the toxic substances present in "moonshine whiskey." The resultant blood clot around the spinal cord can cause nerve damage and paralysis. Similar dangers are present in patients with bleeding tendencies from other causes such as leukemia and purpura.

Sometimes spinal taps are not possible because of severe arthritis, infection of the skin of the lower back, or obstruction by spinal tumors. The needle may then be inserted with great care by an experienced physician just below the skull (cisternal puncture). The complications are the same as in a lumbar puncture except that injury to the brain stem is possible if the needle is advanced too deeply.

I have begun my discussion of procedures with spinal taps because they are so commonly performed for diagnosis and the instillation of medication, anesthetics and dyes for x-ray visualization. They comprise 15% of invasive procedures, second to cardiac catheterization at 20%, which has been discussed in Chapter 3. In a study of 303 patients at the University of California in 1978, 47% had at least one invasive procedure, but many patients had multiple maneuvers for a total of 231. Thirty-five other procedures were performed, with bone marrow needle biopsies, chest taps (thoracentesis), endoscopy (gastroscopy, colonoscopy, bronchoscopy, cystoscopy, etc.), abdominal taps (paracentesis), needle liver biopsies, nerve blocks, and skin biopsies leading, in descending order. Twenty-nine complications occurred in 22 patients, of whom 5 required additional treatment and 12 had prolonged hospital stays.

Here I might remind readers that Dr. Steele's 1981 report of almost 500 iatrogenic events, discussed in Chapter 1, included more than 120 from invasive procedures, although drugs led with 208.

Needle Biopsies

Biopsies of internal organs done by inserting a long needle through the skin and removing a thin cylinder of tissue are increasing in frequency. Their purpose is to establish a diagnosis, evaluate the results of treatment, determine the underlying cause of the illness and, if possible, predict the outcome. They have the advantage over scalpel biopsy in that they can be done at the bedside with local anesthesia to the skin by a non-surgical specialist, and can replace an open surgical procedure. Biopsies of different organs vary in usefulness and many more are done than are warranted for patient benefit.

Liver needle biopsies are the most frequent and are useful in distinguishing jaundice caused by blockage of bile ducts (which requires surgery), from "medical" jaundice such as hepatitis or cirrhosis. In over 20,000 procedures, hemorrhage and peritonitis from leakage of bile were the most common complications, causing fatalities in one or two per thousand biopsies. Almost 10% were inadequate and had to be repeated because the needle missed a localized tumor. One-third of all patients developed transient pain in the abdomen, chest or shoulder.

Kidney needle biopsies are done less frequently. Although they are valuable to the doctor as the most accurate diagnostic tool, it is difficult to understand, from the patient's point of view, how a more exact microscopic diagnosis of chronic kidney disease, almost always incurable, can beneficially alter the outcome of the individual case. Rarely, culture of the tissue may grow bacteria not found by repeated urine cultures and help in the selection of the appropriate antibiotic. Five percent develop complications like bleeding over the kidney capsule, blood in the urine (hematuria), severe flank pain (renal colic), collapse of a lung (pneumothorax) paralysis of intestines (ileus), or laceration of the spleen with hemorrhage or low blood pressure. From 20 to 30% of the samples are unsatisfactory and require repetition to satisfy scientific curiosity.

Needle biopsies of the lung covering (pleura) may result in hemorrhage, fluid or air in the pleural cavity, with difficulty in breathing, collapse of the lung with possible death, or air under the skin. Since the vast majority of tumors that could be diagnosed would be inoperable and incurable, mostly secondary to a primary site elsewhere, the value to the patient may not be worth the slight risk, although the doctor's curiosity would be appeased. Benign tumors require excision on the basis of x-ray findings alone, without added discomfort and expense.

Needle biopsy of breast lumps should only be done in large centers where practiced expertise is attainable. A study of fine needle aspiration of 2,000 benign breast lumps in 1979 revealed that almost 2% were false-positives for malignancy. It is thus prudent to confirm all malignant diagnoses by standard microscopic sections. A negative needle biopsy does not mean that cancer is not present unless fluid is obtained and the lump—a benign cyst—disappears. In this case an operation may be avoided. But if the lump is still present, a surgical biopsy will be necessary to rule out cancer. The riddle of whether a minute cancer, in another breast area, has been missed by the needle may not be solved by mammography. This can delay curative treatment and reduce chances of survival by 20%. Surgical exploration is less likely to overlook a cancer.

Prostatic tissue can be obtained with a hollow needle inserted through the skin between the scrotum and rectum (perineum) or through the lower rectum with less chance of missing a cancer than needle biopsy of the breast. It is easier than cystoscopic biopsy. But in 1981, complications were reported, including blood in the urine, infection and fever, bacteremia, hemorrhage into the lower back tissues and clots carried by the blood to the lungs (emboli), with occasional fatalities. After 48 hours, one man developed fever and bacteremia from a very aggressive bacillus that causes gas gangrene. Treatment with massive doses of penicillin was successful. Another patient, biopsied through the rectum and infected by this organism, died.

While a patient may avoid hospitalization by going to a physician's office or an outpatient clinic and having a small specimen removed from a breast, prostate, lymph node or thyroid, this places pathologists in a difficult position. It is difficult in borderline cases to make an accurate diagnosis with the minute fragments they receive. It is to be expected that in smaller hospitals where the procedure is performed infrequently, more mistakes will be made. Pathologists are generally cautious enough in doubtful cases to wait for an open biopsy and to consult with a colleague before rendering a final diagnosis.

PUNCTURING THE SKIN INTO CAVITIES (PARACENTESIS)

Entering the Chest

After operations on the lungs or its coverings or after penetrating wounds, air, blood, pus or other fluid may accumulate and compress the lungs. Wide tubes are inserted through the gap for drainage, usually without difficulty, but the blood vessels between the ribs may be damaged, causing troublesome bleeding. The lung may be lacerated if it is not completely collapsed, and sometimes the tube may be unwittingly inserted below an elevated diaphragm with damage to the spleen or stomach, or to the liver, causing leakage of bile. Pain from pressure against nerves along the ribs is usually severe. Leakage of air under the skin may fill the underlying tissues causing a crackling sound and sensation. But most important is the ineffectiveness of the procedure, which requires frequent repositioning, additional tubes and sometimes open operation for success.

Chest taps (Thoracentesis): In April of 1980, 30-year-old Robert Burton suddenly developed stabbing pains in his left chest. X-ray films revealed that his pleural cavity was more than half-filled with fluid. A needle was inserted, but no fluid was obtained and two repeated taps were unsuccessful. He then went into semi-shock, with pallor, low blood pressure and falling blood count, while the pain continued. An abdominal operation revealed that his spleen, which was enlarged, had numerous bleeding lacerations, and two liters of blood were in the abdominal cavity. The thoracentesis needle had penetrated the diaphragm, causing this damage. Numerous recent reports have discussed similar cases. All required removal of the spleen, which has its own dangers, discussed in the chapter on surgery.

Although thoracentesis is one of the most common and safest of procedures, a lung may collapse from inadvertent puncture. Air will fill the remaining chest (pleural) cavity. Infection may cause accumulation of pus. Pleural shock is a dreaded and unanticipated complication, occasionally fatal and probably due to air that enters the blood vessels of the chest and is transported to the heart or brain.

Abdominal taps are usually performed to relieve distention by fluid which accumulates in cases of cirrhosis of the liver. The dangers are perforation of a large vein which can cause fatal hemorrhage, oozing of blood caused by a coagulation deficiency, loss of sodium and potassium leading to coma and death, the sudden lowering of abdominal tension, causing the blood pressure to drop and fainting and collapse, and ubiquitous infections which may occur in these generally debilitated patients.

After an abdominal operation becomes infected, an abscess may remain. The pus may be drained through a catheter inserted into the abscess rather than by performing open surgery. This procedure is less dangerous than surgery but still has risks of disrupting the underlying organs. There were 11 complications in 61 patients, with six deaths from spread of the infection, in one series.

A helmet did not help 22-year old Russell Meadows who sustained an abdominal injury in a motorcycle accident. At the hospital, he was found to have a fast pulse and tenderness over his umbilicus. His doctors thought that he might have mild internal bleeding and decided to insert a needle containing a catheter into his abdominal cavity to determine whether or not blood was present. None was found, but a liter of dilute salt solution was administered. He immediately developed a firm penile erection and his bladder filled with fluid because the catheter had penetrated it. He voided 70% of the fluid and the remaining 30% was withdrawn by suction through the catheter. The unrewarding rigidity immediately subsided and the perforation of his bladder healed.

Pericardial taps are occasionally performed when fluid accumulates in the sac surrounding the heart in cases of kidney failure. Steroid hormones are instilled for temporary relief. Abnormal communication between an artery and vein, resulting in heart enlargement and strain, has been reported. Although this is a rare occurrence, it is an example of the unanticipated consequences which may occur with any invasive procedure.

Draining the Brain

Children with water-on-the brain (hydrocephalus) may have fluid diverted from the hollow spaces in the brain (ventricles) to the peritoneal cavity via a long thin tube. This can cause swelling of the abdomen, with hernia and even cysts between partitions formed by adhesions. As with all tubes used for any purpose, perforation and peritonitis add perils.

INVADING THE VESSELS: VEINS AND ARTERIES

The first physician who dared to administer fluids by vein was Thomas Latta of Leith, Scotland who saved the lives of many victims of Europe's devastating cholera epidemic in 1832. Several patients, however, died of large air bubbles obstructing the blood flow through the heart. In 1982, a niagara of over 100 million intravenous infusions will be performed in the U.S. "Water can save you, but it can also drown you," wrote Dr. Richard Duma of the Medical College of Virginia in 1976. "So it is with large volume parenterals. They can rescue your patient or they can injure or kill him."

In Chapter 6 (Iatrogenic Infections) I discussed the recall of 43 million containers because of product contamination, although "only" 54 deaths and 410 non-fatal illnesses were reported from this cause. The actual number of unsuspected fatalities and injuries must have been much greater. Although manufacturers take samples of each batch of fluid and the hospital pharmacy rechecks its stocks, it is obviously impossible to test the contents of each glass container or plastic bag and there is no way to guarantee that all are free of bacteria or fever-causing chemicals. Almost invisible hairline cracks or punctures which permit the entrance of bacteria or fungi have been found by careful inspection. Small, dust-like particles of material may cause damage to the small blood vessels (capillaries) of the lung, for instance, which results in breathing difficulties.

Most fluids contain drug products to which others may be added through connecting tubing by 3-way stopcocks or injection into the tube. It has been documented by the American Society of Hospital Pharmacists that many of these interfere with each other or cause increased toxicity. A veritable Pandora's box of thousands of different combinations is possible.

Inserting a needle or catheter into an artery requires more expertise than venipuncture. Fluids can be injected for monitoring the rate of blood flow. Over 80,000 patients annually are so tested each year in the U.S. At the University of Wisconsin Hospital, 56 high-risk patients had 102 arterial infusions, with eight bacteremias resulting from contamination of solutions or ice for chilling syringes used for needle insertion. Ninety-seven epidemics of nosocomial bacteremia have been reported from global sources since 1965; eleven of these (13%), were secondary to arterial infusions.

Damage due to angiography or cardiac catheterization has been discussed in Chapter 3. But procedures more advanced than x-ray examination are now routine. Invasive monitoring is performed via arteries, central veins, or the right side of the heart and its pulmonary artery. Blood samples can be withdrawn to determine oxygen content, blood pressure and rate of blood flow, and internal EKGs recorded. Dr. Ronald Vliestra of the Mayo Clinic has created a new term *catherapy* for treatments that can be performed with blood vessel catheterization. Arteries, even the coronaries, clogged by clots or arteriosclerosis can be opened, local treatment such as medication or freezing can be applied to specific areas, pacemakers can be installed in cases of disturbed heart rhythm, veins can be closed to prevent clots from becoming detached and fatally entering the lung circulation.

Since 1970, Swan-Ganz catheters have been used to monitor the pressure and flow rate of blood in seriously ill cardiac patients. Thought to be a safe procedure, the assumption is that the benefits outweigh the risks.

> Mrs. Joanna Cortran, 62, had severe, increasing chest pain or angina for several weeks in 1981. After angiograms she was found to have narrowing of three coronary arteries. Prior to bypass, a catheter was inserted through the right jugular vein in her neck, downwards to the right side of the heart from which the pulmonary artery carries blood to the lungs for oxygenation. In a few minutes, she coughed up a large amount of blood. Her chest was opened and the right pulmonary artery was clamped shut. But Mrs. Cortran continued to bleed and died. At autopsy, a puncture was found in a branch of the pulmonary artery, with hemorrhage into the lung.

Between 1975 and 1981, 1,500 Swan-Ganz catheters have been inserted prior to heart operations at the Columbia-Presbyterian Medical Center in New York. There were three punctures of a pulmonary artery (0.2%) with hemorrhage into the lungs and coughing up of blood, one fatal. Six perforations at the Yale-New Haven Hospital caused three deaths.

Relatively more frequent is clotting, which occurred in two-thirds of 33 patients at the Hopital Bichet in Paris who had venograms. Over half of these patients died, some from clots breaking loose to enter the lung circulation and others from infection. Almost 2% of 122 autopsied cases had lung involvement from clot fragments which floated from the catheter site. Reports of heart block and irregular rhythms, rupture of the pulmonary artery with hemorrhage requiring removal of a lung, lung collapse (pneumothorax), damage to heart valves, bacteremia, and knotting of the catheter in the heart further add to the Swan-Ganz hazards.

Minute electrodes have been inserted through veins in the upper neck for over a decade. Attached to a thin catheter, they are threaded through, reaching the heart muscle to serve as artificial pacemakers. However, they are frequently dislodged or misplaced, requiring repetition of the procedure or manipulative restoration. Fatal perforation is rare, but has been reported by various "catherapists" since 1971. The number of new complications has not yet been determined but awaits the test of time.

Catheters have been used to open clogged leg arteries since 1964 by means of a small inflatable balloon attached to their tips. Many a leg has been spared amputation by this non-surgical procedure (including that of Johnny Carson in 1980). The first coronary opening was done in Zurich, Switzerland in 1977 on a patient with severe angina, who walked out of the hospital in a few days; 266 of 410 subsequent attempts in various centers were successful by late 1980. However, in 36 cases (9%) the dilated arteries closed again and two deaths, both in the U.S., resulted in 1978. Seventeen acute MIs occurred and 20 patients required emergency bypass surgery after attempted opening by balloon-tipped catheters. The procedure—percutaneous transluminal angioplasty (PTA)—has been found suitable for only 10% of bypass candidates.

Professor E. Zeitler, a radiologist of Nuremberg, Germany has performed over 1,000 PTAs as of June 1982,* primarily opening the arm and leg arteries. His patients have suffered three perforations, none fatal, plus three deaths due to pulmonary emboli and heart failure. Other complications have been bleeding at the site of the catheter's entrance to the artery, and later, blood clotting, with a shutting-off of the circulation. He told me that in selected cases of coronary artery closure, PTA has been successful in Germany and Switzerland in 70% of attempts for at least two years. The procedure has not been done often enough elsewhere for precise evaluation of its risks.

Although leg arteries are now the most common site, the arteries to the kidneys are the most appropriate for PTA. Some 23 million Americans have hypertension, including more than a million from narrowing of a kidney artery. Over 1,000 PTAs have been done with a success rate of 90-95% at several centers in this country. There has been reclosure in 10-20%.

In children, arterial catheterization is usually performed for improving the accuracy of diagnosis of heart murmurs, congenital heart disease or brain damage but although it improves chances of survival, serious complications may occur. Cutting off or reducing circulation in a large leg artery, can cause shortening or even loss of a leg.

---

*Personal communication, June 19, 1982.

> One 9-pound newborn had a catheter placed in her umbilical artery, which branches from the aorta, for fluid administration. It was removed on the third day of life, but within 48 hours both legs became pulseless, blue and paralyzed. On the ninth day, via an abdominal operation, blood clots in the aorta and both main leg arteries were removed. During the next few days, both legs lost their circulation, the left foot became gangrenous and the infant died on the 15th day after birth. Autopsy revealed that the same arteries were completely blocked by recurrent clots.

Arterial damage in children is rarely as severe as in this case. Its risk is the same as in adults, with the frequent additional complication of defective growth and shortening of a limb. These have been found in a survey of several hundred cases from many hospitals. This iatrogenesis is most common under the age of eight years. Several children under 2 years lost most of their toes.

GETTING UNDER THE SKIN—LOCAL INJECTIONS

Almost every adult has had one or more local injections of a steroid hormone to relieve the pain of tennis elbow, bursitis, arthritis and a wide variety of distressing afflictions near a joint. Scores of such products are manufactured by the major pharmaceutical companies. Unfortunately, the pain is exacerbated for one to three days before relief that may last for weeks or months occurs. The danger of infection is always present. If given too frequently, there is the risk of tendon rupture, which recently happened to a neophyte runner whose heel area was injected, with subsequent rupture of his achilles tendon. The natural hormones of the adrenal gland will be suppressed, which will delay recovery after operations or other trauma.

Intramuscular (IM) Injections

Although IM injection has been used for over 100 years for the administration of drugs or fluids, it has many disadvantages and a few complications. Of 26,300 Boston patients, 46% received at least one IM injection, mostly for the administration of antibiotics, sedatives and iron preparations which cause excess irritation if injected directly under the skin. But absorption of the medication may be delayed, fitful or incomplete. Only 48 (0.4%) had important local adverse effects; the most frequent, abscess formation, occurred in 15 patients. Local swelling, hardening of the tissues, pain, redness and hive-like eruptions were more common with certain drugs than others. A relatively new antibiotic, cephalothin, was more often the cause of these troublesome complications than other preparations.

ENDOSCOPY AND INTUBATION—THE INSIDE STORY

When Dr. George Chapell, a British internist, and Robert Benchley wrote *Through the Alimentary Canal with Gun and Camera* in 1930, they did not realize how prophetic they were. We now insert weapons such as snares, forceps, electrocautery equipment and cameras. During the past generation, the development of fiberoptic instruments—long, slender and flexible sheaves of wispy glass fibers—has revolutionized the examination and treatment of almost all hollow spaces and organs of the body which were formerly accessible only by open surgery. One bundle brings light to the area to be examined and the other carries a color image back to the doctor's eye. Attachments permit photography or projection on a TV monitor for viewing and comment by colleagues and students. Side channels accommodate miniature tools: brushes, snares, forceps and cauteries. Blocked bladders or windpipes can be opened, biopsies taken and small benign tumors (polyps) or even cancers and gallstones removed. But pitfalls abound.

The blind insertion of tubes has been improved by the development of pliable plastic materials. They can be aided by x-ray procedures to reach the desired location, where food or fluid may be administered, secretions or excess accumulations removed, and tests performed. Despite their blunt tips, complications occur and many believe that confidence in their safety is not fully justified.

Through the Alimentary Canal with Light and Camera—Going Up

Because it is included in routine physical "check-ups," sigmoidoscopy is the most common invasion of the body through a natural opening. The question of its usefulness as a screening procedure for rectal and lower bowel cancer has been the subject of much debate. The insertion of a 10-inch, rigid, lighted tube into the anus, rectum and lower bowel is safe in the healthy examinee, but there are rare risks which resemble those of the more complicated colonoscopy. Cancers of the large bowel, for unknown reasons, have moved upwards and to the right, during the past two decades and most cannot now be detected by the probing finger or the sigmoidoscope.

Jonathan Kastor, a 62-year-old mechanical engineer, had no serious medical problems until March 1982, when he noticed dark blood in his stools. A barium enema was performed, enabling x-ray films to outline a small irregularity in the wall of his ascending colon, above the appendix. A gastroenterologist explained to Mr. Kastor that his bowel could be examined in the outpatient clinic with a flexible fiberoptic colonoscope which enables visualization of the entire large intestine and can remove small tumors by cautery under direct observation. "The most frequent complication," he warned, "is hemorrhage which occurs in less than 2% of all cases. Less likely, but more serious, is puncture, most often at the bowel's bends, especially if its wall is weakened by inflammation or if an outpouching (diverticulum) is entered. If a polyp is cauterized, the heat may cause weakening of the bowel wall, encouraging perforation. This will cause pain, and air will enter the abdominal (peritoneal) cavity outside of the bowel, which can be confirmed by x-ray examination. You must call Dr. Jones immediately if pain or swelling should happen." These risks were acceptable to Mr. Kastor since the procedure, if successful, would replace an open abdominal operatioin.

The snake-like instrument was inserted through the anus with little discomfort. It was deftly wormed around the right-angle bends at the spleen and liver and down the ascending colon to the site of the defect. A small tangle of coiled capillaries (angioma) was seen, from which a slow trickle of blood oozed. The bleeding spot was cauterized by an electric wire and the colonoscope was drawn out. The next day there was marked tenderness and distention of the abdomen. Mr. Kastor phoned Dr. Jones, who admitted him to the hospital. X-ray studies demonstrated air in the peritoneal cavity. An abdominal operation revealed a small bubble of liquid feces mixed with air, exuding from a minute opening in the colon. The perforation was sutured and an opening was made from the bowel to the outside of the skin (colostomy). Antibiotics were administered, but fever and pain persisted for a week. Several months after healing the colostomy would be closed.

Less common complications include distention of the small intestine with gas when air is injected to ease the passage of the colonoscope, partial perforation of the intestinal wall leaving a small abscess, collapse of one or both lungs, rupture of the spleen from pressure at the left 90-degree bend of the bowel, tears, with or without bleeding, in the covering (peritoneum) or support (mesentery) of the intestine, or hepatitis from contamination. More dramatic is the fatal explosion of methane gas in the bowel if unprepared by enema, during sigmoidoscopy (or colonic surgery). Colonoscopy can also cause deadly explosions when hydrogen is released by colonic bacteria, due to a chemical reaction with the solution used for preparing the bowel.

Through the Alimentary Canal—Looking Down the Mouth

It would seem logical that the replacement of rigid instruments by flexible fiberoptic endoscopes would have caused a decrease in the number of iatrogenic events. Paradoxically, there has instead been an increase in perforations and in the deaths resulting from them. The bullet-shaped head penetrates all layers, while the old rigid model generally merely scratched the lining. The American Society for Gastrointestinal Endoscopy has reported a complication rate of 1.32 per 1,000 procedures. There has also been hemorrhage from biopsy, inhalation of fluid or other material into the lungs, MI and cardiac and respiratory arrest.

Perforation of the gullet (esophagus) can happen during esophagoscopy or gastroscopy. Opening the channel of the esophagus, narrowed by old scars generally caused by swallowing caustic material, is done by different instruments called dilators and presents greater danger, with a complication rate of 4%-18%. Fiberesophagoscopy causes perforations in one case in a thousand. If the esophagus is inflamed or contains a tumor the risk of perforation is greater, especially if biopsy is performed. This catastrophe has a mortality rate of 9%-31%, exceeding that of all other alimentary tract punctures, and requires immediate surgical repair. It can result in abscess formation, air in the chest, fluid in the pleural cavities or abnormal juncture with the windpipe (trachea).

Because of its flexibility, the endoscope may curve back upon itself and become stuck in the esophagus or stomach. Sometimes manipulation, observed by the fluoroscope, can release the instrument but an abdominal operation (laparotomy) may be required.

Injuries to the stomach range from rupture to bleeding within the wall or vomiting of blood. The tear, which may be self-sealing unless located at the site of a tumor or performed after biopsy, can be up to ¾-inch long. If stomach contents or air is present in the peritoneal sac, an emergency operation is mandatory to prevent peritonitis.

> In May of 1980, Fred Corwin, a 59-year-old carpenter, developed pain in the pit of his stomach. Ten years previously, he had had open heart surgery for the repair of a narrowed mitral valve due to old rheumatic fever. Gastroscopy was performed with biopsy of a benign ulcer. A month later he became confused and drowsy, and lapsed into semi-coma with heart failure. A diagnosis of bacterial infection of his heart valve was made. An emergency operation to replace the damaged valve with an artificial one was performed and streptococci were found on the infected, removed valve. It was the opinion of his consultants that the bacteria gained entrance to the valve at the time of endoscopy. Mr. Corwin has been well since this ordeal. Similar cardiac patients may experience heart rhythm disturbances and even complete arrest of beating, with a mortality rate of 50%.

Because of their intricate lens and electrical systems, it is impossible to completely sterilize endoscopes. Infections following upper gastrointestinal endoscopy are uncommon, but must be foreseen. Pneumonia is infrequent, but has a mortality rate of 10%. It can result from the inhalation of fluid in the mouth because of mild trauma and the local anesthesia used in the pharynx to facilitate insertion of the instrument. Cases of other infections, such as bacteremia, inflammation of the bile ducts and of the pancreas, and infectious diarrhea with chills, fever, abdominal pain, nausea and vomiting, have been described.

A symposium in Germany reviewed 349 iatrogenic events during endoscopic operations using wire loops or cautery and found 88%

successful, but many caused perforation and/or serious hemorrhage. An intricate technique, the removal of gallstones through the bile ducts, which enter the intestine below the stomach, was tried 1,400 times. Acute inflammation of the bile ducts occurred in 21, or 0.7% of all cases. Six of these patients died. One series of 42 adverse events when benign tumors of the stomach (polyps) were removed included 37 hemorrhages, four perforations and one death.

Newer gastroscopes have a powered air supply and may cause expansion of the small intestine, with pain, tenderness and swelling which simulates the symptoms of perforation.

The Japanese have been leaders in devising more elongated endoscopes for the examination and penetration of the bile channel in the spot where it enters the upper small intestine (duodenum). Radio-opaque dyes may be injected or the opening widened by an electrical cutting current, and the gallstones removed. Over 3,000 such procedures have been done in Europe, and American endoscopists have been making pilgrimages to perfect their techniques. However, complications such as bleeding, inflammation of the pancreas and/or bile ducts and perforation occur in 6% to 8% of patients, with a mortality rate of over 1%. However, this is better than that expected with open surgical operations and requires shorter hospitalization.

Through the Alimentary Canal with Tubes and Catheters

When soft catheters are inserted through the nose into the stomach, discomfort is minimal but if they remain in place, inflammation of the nasal lining (rhinitis), nosebleed, sinusitis and ear infections have been reported. In cases of skull fracture the tube has been known to enter the cranial cavity, sinuses or the space behind the eyeball (orbit). If the patient is comatose it may enter the larynx, trachea or bronchus. This can result in food or medication being inserted into the lungs, with consequent pneumonia. There may be ulceration of the back of the mouth or larynx with scarring which, when healing, closes the airway.

The esophagus is most vulnerable. Some 60 percent of terminal patients in one study developed ulcerations, hemorrhages or perforation. Sometimes an abnormal protrusion or pseudodiverticulum is created. Newborns are similarly susceptible. Few of these injuries are recognized by the attending doctors. When these occur, there will be an increase in salivation, difficulty swallowing and/or air in the pleural cavities, under the skin, or about the heart. A special tube with a balloon tip, used to compress bleeding varicose veins in the esophagus secondary to cirrhosis of the liver is particularly culpable in these complications, with a 22% fatality rate. Other special tubes used to open a channel for feeding in cases of obstruction by inoperable cancer of the esophagus cause similar problems. They may also extend into, and perforate, the stomach.

Paramedics frequently insert a tube into the esophagus, blow it up and divert the air into the lungs. This causes perforation of the esophagus in up to 2% of the cases and, when air is introduced to dilate spastic narrowing (achalasia), perforation occurs in 4% to 6%. The presence of any tube at the junction between the stomach and the esophagus promotes inflammation due to entrance of acidic stomach juice, further leading to narrowing and obstruction.

Tubes seldom injure or perforate the stomach unless there has been a previous inflammation, ulcer, tumor or distortion, but if retained for longer than three days, pressure may cause ulceration and penetration. The action of the acidic gastric juice can cause hardening of the plastic tube, and its rigid end may injure the stomach wall. Commonly, the tube will coil and form knots within the stomach. This can cause it to become obstructed, and when it is removed it may injure the lining of the esophagus or nose. Sometimes it cannot be removed without open surgery.

Following operations on the stomach, tubes are often inserted for feeding. Hemorrhage, leakage or obstruction causing vomiting and dehydration have occurred in 1% to 5% of these cases, with rapid death unless the tube has been quickly repositioned. When the esophagus is closed by inoperable cancer, tubes are frequently inserted for temporary palliation by allowing the passage of liquid food. These may become displaced above the cancer and so fail in their purpose. Impaction of food and perforation occur, but less frequently.

Tubes may be inserted through the nose, past the stomach, or into the upper intestine for feeding, especially in children. This is considered safer than intravenous total parenteral nutrition. The plastic becomes semirigid after several days, converting it from sustaining to spear-like. Perforation can result from pressure and manipulation. In adults, the small intestine can fold about the tube in an accordion fashion with pain and vomiting and inversion into itself causing obstruction, with a 20% fatality rate. Complex knots requiring operative removal can also occur. A new development is suction biopsy of the intestinal lining. Five percent of these patients develop intestinal bleeding and some, pain and fever.

Tubes may be inserted through the anus into a twisted lower bowel to release entrapped gas and fluid and allow the intestine to straighten itself. This has caused severe inflammation and even perforation (which has also resulted from enemas in diseased bowels). After operations on the gallbladder and bile ducts, tubes may be inserted to promote drainage, with hemorrhage resulting from irritation of their linings.

THE BREATHING APPARATUS

Intubation

To facilitate respiration in severe pneumonias, during resuscitation, or in the administration of inhalation anesthesia, tubes are often inserted through the mouth and into the windpipe (trachea). Some are flexible and others are rigid. Although this is considered a routine procedure, it requires experience and skill. A group at the Hôpital Fernand Widal in Paris reported 12 perforations, six with each type of tubing. All were surgically repaired immediately and recovered. Ten of the 18 other cases, which were not diagnosed early and were repaired after a 12-hour delay, died, most with infection of the structures above the heart. Other instances of the tube penetrating the throat structures and entering the esophagus have been reported, with a mortality of 50% if not recognized and 14% if repair is attempted immediately.

A 50-year-old unnamed man was admitted to the ICU in semicoma after an overdose of heroin. His respiration was depressed and he was intermittently agitated. Intubation was attempted several times without success. Two days later, he developed pain in his throat, as well as fever and cough, and became blue (cyanotic). X-ray films revealed fluid in his pleural cavities. He was treated with antibiotics without benefit. On the 17th day an operation revealed a perforating tear, almost an inch long, above his vocal cords. This was sutured, but he went into shock and died the next day.

Bronchoscopy

The straight, rigid bronchoscope (RB) has performed wonders of diagnosis and extraction of foreign bodies from air passages since its virtuoso, Dr. Chevalier Jackson of Philadelphia, achieved international recognition for his mastery of this instrument. But in 1968, it was superseded by the flexible fiberoptic bronchoscope (FFB). Most authorities believe that the FFB is more versatile and safer, but the number of complications varies in different reports. If biopsy is performed through either type, lung collapse and hemorrhage, fever, pneumonia and bacteremia have been reported. When local anesthesia is used, reactions such as convulsions, fainting and cardiac arrhythmias have occurred due to hypersensitivity to the drug. Sometimes bacteremia localizes as meningitis.

A heavy smoker, 49-year-old Tom Perier had severe cough for several weeks. A chest x-ray exam revealed densities in both lower lobes. "Pap" smears of his sputum were suspicious, but did not confirm the presence of cancer. To confirm and localize this possible malignancy, an FFB was inserted under local anesthesia. An irregular elevation, a half-inch in diameter, was found in a right lower bronchus. A biopsy was performed which proved that the lesion was cancer. The next day Tom developed fever, chills and generalized weakness. Examination revealed a stiff neck. A spinal tap removed cloudy fluid containing pus cells and bacteria, showing that meningitis had resulted. Large doses of antibiotics were administered and the meningitis cleared up in four days. A month later, his cancerous right lung was removed.

Fatalities associated with the use of the FFB are rare. A recent U.S. survey of 17,000 procedures found only 12 deaths (0.1%) and 45 life-threatening complications (0.3%). Two of the deaths were caused by hemorrhage from tumors that were traumatized, and the others from heart arrest secondary to the medication used rather than the instrumentation. It was the opinion of the authors that the ease of the FFB procedure encouraged its use in cases where the information gleaned would not have been of benefit, especially to extremely ill, elderly patients.

It is difficult to assess accurately the iatrogenic rate of different hospitals because the type of patient and the severity of the underlying illness varies. In some, the FFB is passed primarily through the nose and in others, through the mouth. In teaching hospitals, in which residents or fellows in training perform most of the procedures, the complication rate will be higher. Dr. Donald Zavala, Professor of Medicine at the University of Iowa and a renowned bronchoscopist, has editorialized, "The 'good news' is that when performed in experienced hands, fiberoptic bronchoscopic procedures are safe, well tolerated by the patient and have a high diagnostic yield. The 'bad news' is that there is a tendency for physicians to overlook the inherent risks involved, mainly because the procedure is so readily performed."

Laparoscopy—Viewing the Viscera (Peritoneoscopy)

In 1982, Christine Fallows, 28, a physical therapist, was pregnant for the second time. She had severe uterine bleeding in the first month. Since an abortion seemed inevitable, a dilatation and curettage (D and C) was performed, but there was no evidence of pregnancy in the material obtained. To rule out a tubal pregnancy, laparoscopy was performed. Unfortunately, the manipulation of the long, slender instrument caused an artery to rupture and severe internal abdominal bleeding occurred, which caused semi-shock. At an emergency operation, the torn blood vessel was found and closed, but Christine required several blood transfusions and remained in the hospital for almost a month. A repeated D and C located products of conception in a corner of the uterus.

Laparoscopy originated in 1929 in Germany. Most of its complications have been discussed in Chapter 9 (Preventing and Terminating Pregnancy). It has become the second most common gynecologic procedure, with D and C still leading. But its use in the investigation and treatment of other conditions is increasing, particularly in the study of chronic liver disease. Almost all abdominal organs can be inspected and treated without overnight hospitalization. But many experienced operators believe that because of unanticipated accidents, laparoscopy should only be done in an operating room where immediate open surgery can be done if necessary to repair inadvertent damage.

Marjorie Faulkner, 32, had an uneventful dilatation and curettage for protracted uterine bleeding in May of 1980. The next day, however, she developed pain and generalized swelling in her abdomen. Before diagnostic laparoscopy which was to be done through the umbilicus to avoid scarring, a needle was inserted to allow the introduction of carbon dioxide gas for expansion of the peritoneal cavity. While the gas was blown in under slight pressure, she suddenly became pulseless and comatose. She was placed on artificial respiration but failed to respond and died a week after the aborted laparoscopy. Autopsy revealed that a large intra-abdominal vein had been punctured, which was bleeding profusely into the soft tissues of the lower back. The heart was filled with large air bubbles.

This tragic case, which resembles several others found in recent reports, illustrates that iatrogenesis can occur with accessory procedures as well as with the laparoscopy itself. A British report of 50,000 laparoscopies in a single year showed less than one death per thousand, but the intestine was perforated almost three times in each thousand, requiring open operation for repair.

Tuberculous peritonitis has rarely been seen in the West during the past generation. But with the influx of immigrants from the third world, it has made a reappearance. Indira Narotamdas, a 30-year-old recent arrival from India whose husband had pulmonary tuberculosis, complained of generalized weakness, painful and prolonged menses, and pallor. Her abdomen had a "doughy" consistency. Laparoscopy found myriads of minute tubercles studding her intestinal covering (peritoneum) and many dense adhesions. Because of its immobility, her small intestine was perforated by the laparoscope, requiring immediate surgical opening of the abdomen, removal of the injured loop of intestine, and rejoining the severed ends. In 600 cases of pelvic tuberculosis, it was believed by British surgeons that laparoscopy was used far too often and that perforations due to adhesions presented a great danger.

Visualization and/or biopsy of localized tumors of the bowel, peritoneum, pancreas, gallbladder and liver is much safer and more reliable when done under direct sight than when blindly performed with a needle alone, because injury to other organs and bleeding can be avoided or controlled in most cases. The confirmation of advanced disease by inspection and guided biopsy can avoid an unnecessary operation.

Other unusual complications are fungus infections, rupture of the spleen, peritonitis due to gonorrhea bacteria spreading from infected fallopian tubes, perforation of the uterus and gas entering the space surrounding the heart (pericardial sac). Burns from laparoscopy may not only damage the viscera but the abdominal wall; the operator, too, may suffer electric shock and burns of the hands and face due to malfunctioning electrical systems. Recently several cases of cardiac arrest or gas bubbles entering the brain following laparoscopy have been reported, with loss or blockage of circulation causing memory impairment and incoordination. One young woman has remained in a vegetative state for several years.

The instrument and its accessories are expensive, costing about $5,000, which is probably salutory since it would not be cost-effective unless it were used often enough after training to ensure familiarity with its iatrogenic consequences and achieve experienced manipulative technique.

A new and safer procedure, mini-laparotomy, is a true operation, but requires an incision only about an inch long above the pubic hairline. It causes far fewer complications than laparoscopy, significantly fewer burns, or perforations of the intestines or uterus, and its low death rate of 5 per 100,000 is even less than that of laparoscopy, which approaches 8 per 100,000.

The Urinary Tract

The common catheter has been used since antiquity to relieve obstruction at the bladder neck and permit urine to flow. Benign prostatic enlargement (hypertrophy or BPH) which occurs in many men past 60, cancer and failure of the bladder to contract due to loss of muscle tone after strokes, spinal cord injuries or operations are the most common causes. Meticulous attention to sterile technique must be observed to prevent infection, which may ascend to the kidneys. Continuous drainage before or after operative repair or in cases of nerve injury may be necessary. In males this drainage predisposes to inflammation of the urethra and abscess formation. The procedure is not always simple, since forcible insertion over an obstruction may cause pain and bleeding. In cases of complete obstruction, catheterization may fail and painful pressure must be relieved by surgical opening above the pubic bone (cystostomy). If catheterization is self-performed, as in previous years, infection will eventually result. There are tales of men who carried catheters coiled in their hat bands for emergency use, rather than submit to operation.

When the urethra is narrowed, most often due to previous bouts with gonorrhea, smooth, stainless steel rods called sounds curved at one end and well-lubricated, are inserted in graduated sizes to dilate the channel. The procedure is painful and has the same risks of infection as catheterization.

Cystoscopes, illuminated to visualize the interior of the bladder, carry the same risks as catheters and sounds. When used in infants, generally to diagnose congenital deformities, they have an additional danger. The cold irrigating fluid can cause extreme lowering of body temperature (hypothermia) if the procedure is prolonged and can contribute to increased mortality.

Although the cystoscope is inserted through the urethra without an incision unless the opening needs slight widening, trans-urethral resection (TUR) for removing the prostate is a major operation, probably the most formidable of invasive procedures. The prostate is chiseled out by an electrical wire loop and is removed in curved chips. Considerable bleeding occurs during the operation, which usually takes under an hour and may require transfusion if the procedure is prolonged. Because there is a continuous flow of fluid to wash out fragments and debris, water overload may occur with loss of salt, causing mental confusion, low blood pressure, heart failure, possible kidney damage and slow pulse. The fibrous capsule surrounding the prostate may be perforated, with leakage of diluted urine into the surrounding tissues causing intense inflammation and infection. Less common are inflammations around the testicles (epididymitis) and after healing, contraction of the bladder neck, causing secondary obstruction and requiring further surgery. As with all other urethral invasions, infection may lead to bacteremia and inflammation of the heart valves (endocarditis), especially in debilitated patients.

Of varying annoyance is sterility, since ejaculation no longer spurts from the penis but squirts backward into the bladder. This will cause impotence in a minority of still potent men. Much of this failure is psychogenic and is relieved by reassurance. If the muscle or nerves of the bladder neck are injured there may be failure to retain urine (incontinence), but this is usually transient. The patient seeking relief from the original urinary discomfort, urgency, frequency and dribbling may be disappointed that improvement is not complete. If the urinary opening is too narrow to admit the operating cystoscope it will have to be widened. After healing, urine may emerge as spray or in several streams.

The urologist is not exempt from injury. There have been a small but significant number of reports of electrical burns of the hands, face and scrotum of the surgeon due to defective grounding. This unexpected sudden shock can cause disruption of the procedure, with damage to the patient.

Amniocentesis

The fluid cushioning the fetus, amniotic fluid, was first withdrawn in 1956 to determine the presence and severity of blood destruction in the unborn children of Rh negative mothers. Since then great strides have been made and techniques have been refined so that it has become a routine procedure for many other purposes. In families known to have members with sex-linked genetic disorders such as hemophilia and a variety of muscular dystrophy in which only boys are affected, sex can be determined. High-risk genetic disorders such as Downs's syndrome (mongolism), Tay-Sach's disease (idiocy and blindness) and a host of other less well known abnormalities can be detected by a study of cells in the amniotic fluid. However, genetic counseling aimed toward preventing the transmissicn of defective genes and, in the cases of individuals who live to reproductive ages, halting the further production of dependent defectives, has only one weapon—therapeutic abortion, which is now under attack.

Amniocentesis, properly performed by inserting a long needle in the lower abdomen between the 14th and 16th week after conception and withdrawing 10 to 20 ml. of fluid, has a few pitfalls. There is a rare possibility of injuring a fetal limb or of entering a major uterine blood vessel. If fetal blood from the placenta or umbilical cord leaks into the amniotic fluid, the fetus will be imperiled. If the fetus' blood type is different from the mother she may be immunized and suffer reactions if future transfusions are required.

A new test for alpha-fetoprotein (AFP) can be performed on the amniotic fluid after the blood serum has been first tested and found positive. This will detect brain and spinal defects which make life impossible or unbearable for the infant and family. The AFP test is 90% to 98% positive, which means that 2% to 10% of defects will be missed. If a previous child has been defective, the chance that the fetus will be similarly afflicted is 1 in 20. The parents can then decide on the basis of the risk whether or not to terminate the pregnancy by abortion.

The possibility of fetal loss due to amniocentesis lies somewhere between 0.5 and 1.5%, although higher rates may occur in smaller centers where the procedure is done less often. If all pregnant women in the U.S. were screened for fetal brain and spinal defects by AFP testing each year, amniocentesis would be recommended in 51,000 cases with the possible detection of 2,300 defective fetuses. At a loss rate of 1%, approximately 500 normal fetuses would be unintentionally aborted. Ultrasonography to determine the degree of fetal damage can be performed before or after amniocentesis, but its value has not yet been accurately determined, nor is it available in all regions.

11.

THE UNCERTAIN SCALPEL— DRAMA IN THE OPERATING ROOM

The surgeon retains first place in prestige among doctors. In the popular imagination he is the epitome of dedication, resourcefulness, and courage in emergencies. The British aptly call the setting of his performance the operating theatre, with a cast of masked and costumed characters, ritualistic preparations, suspense, often unpredictable endings, and seats for spectators. Anxious well-wishers and families cluster in rooms or alcoves, in or near surgical suites, waiting to learn the outcome of an operation.

Some 24 million operations on 2½ million people are performed annually in the U.S. followed by 250,000 postoperative deaths; and the number increases 15% each year. Although the growth in population from 1971 to 1977 was 5%, the number of surgical procedures jumped 34% during that 5-year period. The greatest growth has been in cardiac, gynecologic (mostly tubal ligations and cesarean sections), prostatic and cataract surgery. Only appendectomies and tonsillectomies declined, the latter over 50%.

Hospital care accounted for 40% of our $287 billion medical care expenditure in 1981 and is increasing at an annual rate of 15%. Operating room costs comprise the largest percentage of this increase. There are more operations performed and more surgeons per capita in the United States than in any other country. Over one person in every 15 in the United States enters a hospital each year for one or more operations. The rate of increase in surgery is proportional to age. Those over 65 had more than 3½ times as many operations as did those under 16. The reasons for the increase are advances in technology which permit operations formerly considered too risky and increases in the availability of funds, facilities and surgeons in areas where they formerly did not exist. Medicare and Medicaid largely account for the vast increase in surgical utilization among the aged, the poor and non-Caucasians in urban areas. But the most important factor is that there are too many surgeons seeking operations.

From 1971 to 1975, the number of board-certified surgeons grew by 18%, seven times the growth of the population. The lure of increased income and prestige greatly increased the number of residents in training, resulting in a surplus of 30,000–40,000 physicians performing surgery. In some urban areas, the work load of young, well-trained surgeons is low, making it difficult to maintain skills. Only a small fraction of surgery is performed in life-or-death crises. Most operations are undertaken to relieve physical or emotional discomfort or disability. The benefit to the individual will eventually have to be carefully weighed against the cost and benefit to society as a whole.

All wounds inflicted by surgeons with scalpels or amputation knives have complications in common. Pain may last for weeks or months. Infections, usually occurring after the fifth day, accompanied by swelling, redness, tenderness and fever, occur in 2% to 4% of all surgical cases. Internal pressure may cause the wounds to burst open or the inner organs, still covered by their membranes, may protrude (herniate) from the gap, especially in incisions in the abdomen or flank in obese patients. There may be slow oozing of blood or serum, or rapid bleeding into or out of the incision. If the wound is originally clean, these mishaps raise the iatrogenic complication rate to 5%. But if wounds are infected at the onset or after the trauma leaving roughened edges, the complication rate may rise to 60%. Many of these iatrogenic complications could have been prevented by foresighted treatment.

After healing, especially in movable areas or following infection, ugly, giant scars (keloids) may occur, more commonly in non-Caucasians. They are most likely located in the zone between the ears and the chest. Conversely, the scars may contract, causing puckering and limitation of motion.

Shock, manifested by weakness, pallor, low temperature and blood pressure, sweating, decreased urine output, and rapid breathing and pulse may occur in extensive operations accompanied by bleeding and fluid loss. The patient will be thirsty, apprehensive, then irresponsive, and finally comatose. Shock is more likely to occur and to have a higher mortality rate (up to 60%) in cardiac patients and in those with bacteremia (bacteria in the blood) from wound infection, contamination of intravenous fluids, artificial respiration, or the insertion of artificial joints, blood vessels or heart valves (prostheses).

In 1979, a Congressional subcommittee estimated that 2.4 million operations were unnecessary, with a loss of over 12,500 lives and a cost of $4 billion. Some are due to the perhaps unconscious cupidity of a minority of greedy operators, fostered by the built-in incentives of our fee-for-service system in which most payments are made without question by third party (insurance) systems. A surgeon earns meaningful money only when he operates. His fee increases with the size of the operation. He enjoys operating just as a ballerina enjoys dancing. Other unnecessary operations are due to honest but mistaken diagnoses. There is great difference in the quality of hospitals and their staffs; this results in a greater chance of iatrogenic death or dangerous and expensive complication in those of inferior quality. We should remember that death rates in communities decrease when there is a moratorium on elective surgical interventions, as in the recent L.A. doctors' strike.

Only 23% of operations are necessary procedures without which the patient would die or suffer disability. However, 77% are *elective*, which means that although they have proper medical indications and the patient *may* benefit from them, they are not necessary for survival. The dilemma is whether the risks of elective surgery, which result in 70,000 annual postoperative deaths, are worth the wager that they will improve the quality of life. Some of the 2.4 million unnecessary operations may be ethically justified on the basis of a difficult (or impossible)—but mistaken—diagnosis.

> A 19-year-old college student suddenly developed severe and increasing pain and tenderness in her right lower abdomen, accompanied by nausea, slight fever and elevated white blood count. She was in the middle of her menstrual cycle. Although pain is common at this time in young women, her surgeon, after finding the right-sided tenderness on rectal examination, concluded that Suzy had a "textbook" case of acute appendicitis and that the risk of operating was less than that of observing. Accordingly, he opened her abdomen through the smallest possible incision, but found the appendix to be perfectly normal. Her right ovary, however, displayed a minute bleeding spot, the site of a ruptured cyst (follicle) containing an egg (ovum). If he had not operated, nothing would have happened and the pain would have disappeared spontaneously in a few days. This is an example of an operation which was unnecessary but justified, as classified by the reviewing tissue committee. There was no onus attached to this respected, conservative surgeon and no implication that he was "knife happy" or financially motivated. The committee agreed that Suzy had clinical signs and symptoms indistinguishable from acute appendicitis, which, although one of the commonest conditions requiring surgery, may be impossible to confirm prior to operation.

Estimates from varying sources indicate that of the 725,000 tonsillectomies performed annually, over 70% are unnecessary, as are 22% of both the 790,000 hysterectomies and the 225,000 prostatectomies, 17% of the 200,000 hemorrhoidectomies and 15% of the 475,000 gallbladder removals. My experience in serving on the tissue committees of several hospitals indicates that from 5 to 30% of the over 200,000 appendectomies a year are unjustified. Despite progress, 20,000 Americans still die each year from this common abdominal inflammation.

In 1981, the annual Convocation of the Fellows of the American College of Surgeons was addressed by its new president, Dr. G. Tom Shires, Chief of Surgery at Cornell Medical College as follows: "An estimated 20,000 of the 70,000 U.S. physicians who perform surgery are either inadequately trained or unqualified. . . . Many state officials believe that the unrestricted license should be abolished and that doctors should be limited to their specialties." Despite this complaint, which has been reiterated for many years, there has never been a determined, organized campaign to revamp state licensing laws. There is no way of looking into the future to predict how regulation of surgical competence will lessen the iatrogenesis engendered by surgery—requisite or elective, necessary or unnecessary, justified or unjustified. But it would be a fair assumption that the reduction of elective, unnecessary and unjustified procedures would reduce undesirable complications. In Great Britain, where surgeons are salaried, the population receives half as much surgery per capita as in the U.S., but there is no evidence that the British death rate is increased by this "neglect."

An Air Force hospital was the scene of questionable surgery, in 1978, when 25-year-old Pamela White, an Air Force sergeant, underwent operation for an anal fistula. The tract from the anus to the left leg was excised, but healing was delayed and Ms. White had difficulty in walking and having sexual intercourse. Only later did she learn that the operation had been done not by a rectal, but by an oral surgeon (who, she and her attorney thought, should not have been allowed to work at the bottom end of her alimentary canal). But the Air Force defended the practice on the dubious grounds that, in combat, oral surgeons would be required to participate in any emergency surgical procedure. Do oral surgeons serve in emergency rooms? Do anal fistulas fall into the combat category? This experience is not thought necessary in civilian training programs.

What follows is a discussion of iatrogenesis due to surgery or related procedures, without any mention of the natural complications of individual diseases requiring surgery.

Anesthesia

Melvin Smith, a 6-year-old boy, was given anesthesia in an Ohio hospital by a nurse preparatory to tonsillectomy while the surgeon was performing a similar operation in an adjoining room. The supervising anesthesiologist was called to a different room because of a patient problem after the boy was ready for his minor operation. The nurse continued to administer the anesthetic agent but did not follow the heartbeat with her stethoscope. The surgeon entered and was about to begin the operation when he noticed that the child's skin had become blue and that his heart had stopped beating. Cardiopulmonary resuscitation was begun immediately with restoration of the heartbeat to normal. The child, however, had suffered irreversible brain damage due to lack of oxygen and after seven weeks in a coma, died.

Although four out of five malpractice suits involve surgery, anesthetic accidents are the actual causes in many of these misadventures. In the case cited, the anesthesiologist would never have left the room if the operation was to be a major one such as heart or brain surgery. Anesthesia accidents in minor surgery occur in numbers out of proportion to their frequency, probably because the attending staff, not expecting difficulties, become careless, bored or fatigued.

The development of surgery paralleled advances in anesthesia. Complex, prolonged operations on seriously debilitated patients, which would have been contraindicated only a few years ago, are now possible. Anesthesia was often administered by a family doctor, intern, resident, or non-specialized assistant who gave chloroform or ether through a crude gauze face mask by open drop while observing the patient's skin color, pulse rate and blood pressure. Now, the sleep-inducing equipment and the electronic monitoring devices would crowd the surgeons out of the operating room if it were not specially designed or modified to accommodate them. Oxygen and other gases can be piped in from a central source, eliminating space-consuming tanks near the operating table but sometimes increasing the chance of mishap. Concurrently, anesthesiologists' prestige, responsibilities and income have increased. Formerly faceless, they now personally visit each patient the evening before operation. They are responsible for insuring relaxation and freedom from pain and also for pre-operative risk assessment, preparation for operation, and post-operative recovery. They have been given many duties outside the operating room; they must relieve pain, control convulsions and resuscitate patients whose heart or lung function has stopped in any area of the hospital.

The horrors of pre-anesthetic (and pre-aseptic) surgery in relatively recent history have been vividly illustrated. Surgeons in the early 19th century were shown amputating limbs, their patients liberally dosed with rum and laudanum, tied to primitive tables and "biting the bullet" while long knives and saws quickly removed arms or legs which accumulated in gory heaps. Chest, abdominal or head surgery was seldom attempted. Supportive measures such as blood transfusions or injectable medication had not yet made their appearance.

Opium, derived from poppies, was known to ancient doctors. In 1680, Dr. Thomas Sydenham, the founder of modern medicine, wrote, "Among the remedies which it has pleased almighty God to give to man to relieve his sufferings, none is so useful and so efficacious as opium." His use of its solution in alcohol (laudanum) eased many agonies, but its more potent derivative, morphine, did not appear until 1803. In 1853, the hypodermic needle and syringe were invented, increasing morphine's speed and efficacy of action. "Laughing gas" (nitrous oxide or N_2O) was the marijuana of early America and was popular at frolics and parties among the swingers of that time.

U.S. doctors were the pioneers of total general anesthesia. In 1842, a Georgia physician administered ether to remove a neck tumor. N_2O was used on a dentist in Hartford, Connecticut, who had one of his own teeth removed in 1844. The dentist then persuaded Dr. John Warren, Professor of Surgery at Harvard Medical School, to remove a tumor of the jaw with ether anesthesia in 1847. That year Dr. James Simpson of Edinburgh used chloroform in obstetrics, despite opposition from church circles. He refuted clerical critics by stating that God had put Adam to sleep while he removed a rib from which Eve was created. Dr. Simpson was later knighted because he administered chloroform to the grateful Queen Victoria during labor. All of these early agents were dangerous and caused fatalities in inexperienced hands, but the "death of pain" encouraged their use and the discovery of new drugs.

Pentothal (once used as "truth serum") appeared as an intravenous anesthetic in the 1930s. Until physicians gained experience in using it, pentothal was responsible for dangerous respiratory depression. Its improper use on patients in shock after the Pearl Harbor attack may have caused more deaths than did Japanese bombs.

Sigmund Freud, before introducing psychoanalysis, experimented with cocaine for local anesthesia and used it to wean a young physician from morphine addiction. He produced the first known modern cocaine addict. In 1884, cocaine was used for eye surgery and dentistry. Its later synthetic derivatives have become indispensable for local and spinal anesthesia.

In the U.S. during the 19th century, anyone could give anesthesia, since there were no license requirements. Operations were shorter than at present but since the toxicity was not always understood there were many sudden deaths. In the U.S. now, registered nurses may take 18 to 24 months of special training to become nurse-anesthetists. Nurse-anesthetists administer 65% of the general anesthesia in hospitals having less than 250 beds, but only 40% in larger institutions. Occupational exposure to toxic fumes causes iatrogenic disease, especially in women. Physicians may become anesthesiologists after four years of resident training. A majority of the over 11,000 certified anesthesiologists in the U.S. are graduates of foreign medical schools, which may cause difficulties in communication.

It is extremely difficult to separate post-surgical deaths due to patient disease from those due to anesthesia, but it is estimated that it causes one death in 815 major surgical cases. There are many variables: patient condition, skill of personnel and duration of operation. Although deaths are definite, complications, major and minor, are less so. For this reason, statistics are extremely inaccurate. All decisions to operate or anesthetize must take into consideration the risk-benefit ratio. Reaching this verdict is an art, acquired through experience, rather than a science founded on hard data.

Anticipating Anesthesia—Patients are given sedation before being taken to the OR. Many different drugs or combinations are used, all having undesirable effects, and must be selected to suit each patient. Although the aim is to produce relaxation, nausea, vomiting, dry mouth, low blood pressure or paradoxical agitation may result. Some may cause rapid pulse, which may be harmful in cardiac patients.

Anesthesia Choices—The first step is the application of devices to monitor the pulse, blood pressure and EKG. Current leakage or improper grounding may create a risk of burns or shock at the site of the EKG electrodes if electrical cautery is used. When the patient is in poor condition and requires arterial, venous or cardiac catheterization to obtain blood samples for analysis, complications of invasive surgery must be anticipated.

General Anesthesia

In most major operations, the patient or surgeon wishes complete oblivion. Pentothal, narcotics, tranquilizers, or other depressants are injected intravenously, singly or in combination, to get a head start by rapidly inducing sleep. Difficult respiration may be combatted with stimulants. Later, the veins used for injection may show signs of inflammation and if the drug leaks into the surrounding tissues, severe pain and swelling will result. Cases have been reported of inadvertent arterial injection which may cause gangrene of the lower arm or hand.

When the patient becomes unconscious, his muscles relax, including those supporting the respiratory channels and tongue. A tube (airway) must then be inserted through the nose or mouth into the trachea, with possible complications as described in Chapter 10. If a deformity or tumor prevents this insertion, it may have to be performed while the patient is awake or with the aid of a fiberoptic endoscope.

In extreme cases an opening must be made in the trachea (tracheostomy) for administering the anesthetic. Bleeding may result unless the tracheostomy tube fits tightly into the opening. The esophagus may be damaged, air may leak under the skin or into the chest and most dangerously, blood may be inhaled into the lungs, which can result in asphyxia (death from lack of oxygen). The most common complication of tracheostomy, however, is infection, which may be local or may extend into the lungs causing bronchitis or pneumonia. Other disasters may be obstruction of respiration by a plug of mucus or blood, or erosion into an artery with fatal hemorrhage into the esophagus or into the pleural cavity.

A week or as long as a year after the procedure, the trachea may become narrowed due to scarring from the healing process, which will cause difficult breathing and require surgical correction.

The skill of the anesthesiologist in maintaining a proper air flow to prevent brain damage and cardiac arrest by using appropriate tubes and positioning the patient is critical when problems arise. When the patient's position is changed from lying on the back to another position like the side or abdomen to suit the site of the incision, there will be major changes in the airway pattern which the anesthesiologist must control.

Nerve injuries can occur from compression or stretching of arms or legs. The most common is partial paralysis of an arm from its extension on a board while receiving intravenous medication. This is frequent after open heart surgery, but many occur with any operation. Foot drop (dropping the foot in paralysis) occurs from the pressure of stirrups under the knee in genitourinary procedures.

Circulation of the blood and blood pressure must be continually monitored and various pillow-like supports placed in proper position. When the patient is in a sitting position, which is frequent in brain surgery or whenever the incision is elevated above the heart, air may be sucked into the veins and form massive bubbles, fatally impeding blood flow through the heart.

Other vulnerable external organs are the ears, which may be crushed and folded by the pressure of the head, the male genitalia in the face-down position and the eyes, which need protection from irritation and infection.

Ether and chloroform have long been obsolete because of inflammability and toxicity, but newer agents like halothane depress the heart to varying degrees depending on dosage. Nitrous oxide, which is mainly used for minor surgery and dentistry, is also a cardiac depressant and may be dangerous in patients who have coronary heart disease.

Respiratory depression must also be carefully monitored, especially when muscle relaxing drugs are used. Mechanical breathing assistance is given by hand pressure on the breathing bag or positive pressure valve devices that may over-expand the lungs with resultant oxygen toxicity or over-accumulation of air.

> Thomas Kastle, 60, underwent surgery in 1977 for relief of a bowel obstruction due to old adhesions from previous surgery. During the operation, the surgeon noticed that Mr. Kastle's breathing was very irregular. The equipment was checked and it was found that a defective valve on the air pressure device was locked in a closed position, allowing the patient to inhale but not to exhale, thus causing over-distention of his lungs. Mr. Kastle could not be revived despite CPR, and died shortly after the operation.

The complicated equipment used for inhalation anesthesia is subject to mechanical failure, which can result in asphyxia. There may be an insufficient admixture of oxygen due to malfunction or improper setting of flowmeters. Leaks may interfere with maintenance of pressure, and Murphy's Law also applies to valves, tubing and carbon dioxide absorbers. Kidney failure, with decreased urination, can occur because of the stress of surgery.

If there is excessive oxygen ventilation, convulsions may occur, and sometimes the overstimulation of surgery after upper spinal cord injuries may cause severe hypertension. Children especially may develop hypothermia due to depression of the heat-regulating center in the brain.

Because New Zealand's medical standards are among the world's highest, the following statistics, drawn from a report of patients admitted to the ICU during the five years from 1974 to 1979, can be considered reliable: 110 or 5.7% of a total of 1,900 had post-anesthetic, life-threatening complications. Cardiovascular iatrogenesis, including irregular beating and cessation (arrest) of heart and/or lung action led the list, with 43 incidents and 10 deaths; 41 drug reactions and 22 lung infections or obstructions after airway manipulations followed. There were two strokes, one fatal, and a small miscellaneous group.

Many commonly used drugs such as sedatives and tranquilizers, alcohol, anti-hypertensives, digitalis and antibiotics will react unfavorably with anesthetic agents, which requires the anesthesiologist to have a thorough knowledge of pharmacology as well as the patient's history.

Conduction Anesthesia (local, regional, spinal)

Methods which permit consciousness and cooperation from the patient are increasing in popularity. But they have disadvantages: patient anxiety, excitation, followed by depression, of the nervous system, and an extension of the time required for the drug to take effect.

Local anesthetics, all ending in "caine" (xylocaine, for example), are administered by hypodermic injection or direct application (topical) to inflamed surfaces. They rarely produce allergic reactions, which generally begin with hives (urticaria). But if they are absorbed rapidly or inadvertently enter a blood vessel, they may cause convulsions, and rarely, death from asphyxia or brain damage. It may be difficult to distinguish reactions to adrenalin (epinephrine), which is often given simultaneously to enhance and prolong the anesthetic effect, from reactions to the anesthetic itself. Restlessness, pallor and collapse may be similar, but the initial alertness, anxiety, palpitations, fast pulse, increased blood pressure, severe headache and nausea differ.

Regional (nerve block) anesthesia requires great skill because it entails deep injection of the agent close to a nerve supplying the area to be rendered insensitive. The risks are greater because larger volumes are used and thus nerves, organs or blood vessels can be damaged. If the solution is actually injected into the nerve tissue there will be numbness and tingling and unless the needle is immediately withdrawn, paralysis may occur. For example, if a nerve in the lower neck is blocked, the pleural cavity may be penetrated, with partial lung collapse (pneumothorax). The needle and the agent may enter the spinal (subarachnoid) space, which will cause respiratory depression. Or the agent may enter a spinal blood vessel, causing convulsions. Hoarseness and difficulty in swallowing are more frequent, as in partial paralysis of the lower arm (brachial palsy).

Any nerve accessible to a needle may be blocked, and iatrogenesis will depend on the anatomic location. If a limb is shut off from general circulation by a tourniquet, the intravenous injection of a large amount of diluted anesthetic agent will produce loss of sensation. But when the solution leaks into the general circulation through a faulty tourniquet, or when the tourniquet is released, there may be ringing in the ears, dizziness or incoordination, and rarely, unconsciousness or convulsions.

Spinal and epidural (extradural) anesthesia has experienced a recent resurgence in popularity and is preferred by most anesthesiologists for themselves when they require surgery. Spinal block is performed by injecting an agent into the fluid space in the lower back just below the end of the spinal cord. The needle is inserted between two vertebrae. The local anesthetic may occasionally cause ringing in the ears (tinnitus), a bitter taste in the mouth and, in overdoses, convulsions and cardiac arrest. Low blood pressure due to blocking of nerves controlling the diameter of blood vessels with consequent dilatation may cause loss of circulation to the brain with unconsciousness and death unless it is promptly corrected. This is especially liable to occur in late pregnancy. Difficult breathing may make it impossible for the patients to cough and clear secretions from the lung.

After the operation, only a few patients complain of pain at the needle site and infection is rare unless the patient already has bacteremia (blood infection). Headache, worse and more common in young females and relieved by lying down, may persist for five days or longer and may be severe enough to be incapacitating. Older men may have painful inability to urinate for 24 hours or more, requiring catheterization.

Epidural anesthesia is performed by inserting a needle several inches below the end of the spinal cord, where only nerves and blood vessels, but no spinal fluid, are present. The needle is inserted through an opening in the back of the sacrum below the lowest vertebrae. Bleeding, especially in users of aspirin or other drugs which delay clotting, may occur, causing pressure on the lower spinal nerves with pain or weakness in the legs or inability to empty the bladder or rectum.

Problem Patients

Emergency surgery frequently must be performed with incomplete knowledge of the patient's history, often with a patient's stomach full or insufficient preparation. Preventing inhalation of stomach contents with resultant lung inflammation requires careful attention to the airway. The use of the pressure apparatus may increase the danger of vomiting because gas is being blown into the stomach. Food particles must be removed from the lungs by bronchoscopy, with its attendant complications. In cases of severe trauma, regional block is preferred.

Sickle cell anemia occurs in one black patient in 400. Blood clots can form during inhalation anesthesia in any organ or part of the body, causing pain and interference with the organ's function. The disease predisposes to gallstones, blood destruction, bone inflammation and prolonged penile erection (priapism).

Hip or shoulder replacements require the use of a toxic cement (methylmethacrylate), which causes a drop in blood pressure and decrease of oxygen in the blood in half of the patients. This effect is dangerous in elderly or cardiac patients.

After Surgery—Asleep or Awake

As pain returns, the blood pressure rises, which can cause heart irregularities and failure in patients with a history of coronary disease. The wound may bleed, encouraging later infection. Agitation and the shift from the operating table to a cart for transfer to the recovery room may dislodge still-needed monitoring lines, catheters and tubes in the trachea. Once in the recovery room, the patient may experience the after-effects of the various agents used in anesthesia and suffer respiratory depression with possible brain damage if the staff is distracted by more patients arriving. Some complications related to anesthesia may not be apparent for several days.

Lung complications occur in 5%–10% of patients, especially in smokers, the obese, the elderly and after prolonged procedures involving the abdomen and chest. A segment of lung may collapse and become airless, which can encourage the development of pneumonia.

Liver damage with jaundice, sometimes progressing to severe hepatitis and death, has been controversial since an otherwise safe, non-toxic, non-explosive agent, halothane, became widely used in the 1960s. Anesthesiologists who use halothane for long periods have seven times more risk of acquiring biopsy-confirmed hepatitis than the general population does.

A 45-year old woman was admitted to a hospital for foot surgery (bunionectomy). Following the operation she developed jaundice determined to be liver damage (hepatitis) due to halothane. However, there was no note in her medical record documenting this iatrogenic event. A month later, she reentered the same hospital for a bunionectomy on the other foot. A different anesthesiologist had no knowledge of her previous liver injury, so halothane was again administered. She again suffered liver damage, superimposed on the old hepatitis, which became more severe (fulminating) and caused massive destruction. She died approximately one month after the second surgery.

In a suit against the hospital, anesthesiologist, internist and two surgeons, it was alleged that absence of documentation in the medical record prevented the health professionals from ruling out the use of halothane in the second operation. An award of $1.4 million was granted.

This tragic case is an example of the omission of iatrogenic events from records either accidentally or deliberately. I have seen deliberate omission occur on numerous occasions to forestall possible litigation. Information essential to the continuity of her care was not available when this patient was readmitted. This placed her at great risk (10 times higher in obese middle-aged women having recent previous halothane anesthesia) and hindered the defense of all those involved in her surgery.

Six hundred and two serious anesthetic accidents (60% of all cases) with 348 deaths or incidents of damage to the brain were reported by 2,000 British anesthetists during the period 1970 to 1977: 35% were due to unpreventable accidents but 65% were due to human error. Faulty techniques, mainly involving improper insertion of tubes into the trachea, predominated. Improper postoperative care and drug overdoses were other conspicuous preventable causes of iatrogenic disasters.

Abdominal or chest operations on the stomach, bowel, gallbladder, prostate, kidneys, lungs or esophagus may all be followed by hemorrhage into the wound, forming a tender lump which may need needle drainage or, less commonly, into the peritoneal or chest cavity due to injury to a blood vessel or loosening of a ligature closing. The leakage of blood may be severe enough to cause anemia, low blood pressure, swelling or shock, and will require re-operation. Abdominal operations may infrequently injure a ureter, which is important because about half of these mishaps are overlooked at the time of surgery. Wounds may be disrupted, causing bulging of viscera out of the incision. Iatrogenic urinary infection, bacteremia, pneumonia, myocardial infarction, stomach ulcers, stroke or clotting of blood in large leg veins with fragments floating to the lungs (emboli) are often inevitable.

Sutures are commonly replaced by small metallic clips for closing blood vessels, fallopian tubes, ducts and small bronchi and for holding knots and marking tumor edges. Although these ingenious gadgets save time, they malfunction in an estimated 5% of cases. They may not completely close the duct or vessel to which they are applied and they may slip off the tissues or cut through them with resultant bleeding, erosion or damage to the tissue.

FREQUENT MAJOR OPERATIONS

The Alimentary Canal

Appendectomy. About 200,000 cases of appendicitis occur annually in the U.S. leading to 2,200 deaths. Despite its common occurrence (in one person in three living to age 70), it may be confused, especially in children, pregnant women and the aged, with many other abdominal conditions, such as "mittelschmerz." Peritonitis results when the appendix ruptures, usually two to three days after the onset of the attack.

If the stump of the appendix is not properly tied (ligated) and inverted into its site in the bulbous sac of the large intestine (cecum) with a "purse string" suture, or if the cecum is injured, a juncture (fistula) may form between the cecum and wound, resulting in drainage of feces to the exterior. Small collections of pus may form about the sites of the sutures. The trauma of operation added to infection may cause adhesions to form, which later contract, resulting in mechanical obstruction of the part of the intestinal tract affected. This may occur from several weeks to several years after the incision. The scar-like strands must be surgically severed.

Gallbladder surgery. Approximately 450,000 cholecystectomies, the most often performed and most abused non-gynecological abdominal operation, cost this nation over $1 billion last year. As the population ages, the occurrence of gallstones increases. They are found in up to 30% of autopsies, mostly in patients who never had symptoms of gallbladder disease.

When bile leaks from one of the many channels injured during cholecystectomy, it may be diluted by fluid oozing through the irritated peritoneum, accumulating as much as two gallons. Some patients suffer only distention, relieved by tapping, but others suffer peritonitis and fatal shock. If the main channel from the liver to the intestine (common bile duct) is obstructed by a small retained stone or cancer or operative injury, jaundice occurs which hampers blood clotting and increases hemorrhaging. This yellow discoloration is difficult to distinguish from that produced by the anesthetic agent halothane. Leaking bile can also find its way through the wound and drain to the exterior (biliary fistula).

Sometimes a tube is temporarily placed in the common bile duct to promote bile drainage. This can become dislocated, displaced or blocked by blood clot or minute stones. It may also become brittle and break. Such mishaps will enhance the risk of these complications, raising the mortality rate from less than 1% to over 10%. Although the principal producer of digestive juice, the pancreas, may become inflamed after any abdominal operation, pancreatitis is most frequent after surgery upon the gallbladder or its ducts.

The Esophagus

Cancer of the esophagus may occur at any point but is most common in the lower end, near or at its entrance into the stomach. A large portion of the esophagus, sometimes with the upper part of the stomach, must be removed with the tumor, and the open ends rejoined (esophagogastrectomy). During the first 10 days, leakage through the suture line is rare but has a high mortality rate. Stomach emptying must be delayed and must be promoted by making the patient sleep with the head elevated. The "dumping syndrome"—nausea, vomiting, diarrhea, abdominal pain, fast pulse, belching, sweating and generalized warmth in varying combinations—may occur in other patients. Nutritional disturbances will result. Sometimes it is necessary to suture a segment of small bowel between the stomach and shortened esophagus. This may become obstructed from narrowing caused by scar tissue, or ulcerated from the stomach acid. Lung collapse (pneumothorax) may follow.

If the diaphragm is weakened at the point where the esophagus penetrates it, the upper stomach may enter the chest cavity (hiatus hernia). This causes severe "heartburn." In its repair, perforation of the stomach or narrowing of the esophagus causing difficulty in swallowing may occur.

The Stomach

Most stomach operations produce iatrogenic effects similar to esophagogastrectomy. Partial or complete gastrectomies for ulcers or cancer produce complications following surgery in half of the cases which are fatal in 10%. Pancreatitis accounts for 1% to 2% of these deaths. Jaundice, because of injury to the bile drainage system, occurs in a varying number of cases. The suture line may leak, causing peritonitis. If a large nerve (vagus) supplying the stomach is deliberately cut to reduce acidity, intractable diarrhea may follow.

In 1982, an innovative operation was developed to reduce morbid obesity (100 pounds or more overweight): "gastric wrapping," with teflon mesh to prevent the stomach's expansion has the effect of promoting rapid satiety by early filling of the stomach. In 65 patients there was only one death reported from the procedure, due to a blood clot in the lungs. All of the other patients were successful in shedding excess weight of up to 123 pounds. Insufficient time has elapsed for the complications of this procedure to become known.

Gastroplasty, in which the stomach is partitioned or stapled to make it smaller, has been less successful. Around 50% of six thousand operations since 1977 have either failed or had serious complications. The staples may become disrupted or the remaining stomach cavity distended. It has, however, enabled patients to achieve rapid weight loss: 350-pounders can lose 30 to 40 pounds in a month and up to 150 pounds in six months! But in the series of 114 patients, nine spleens were lacerated, four requiring removal, the suture and/or staple lines leaked in 10 cases causing pain and fever, and there were three deaths, from perforation, embolism and abscess under the diaphragm.

The Small Intestine

Cancer is less common in the 20 to 24 feet of small intestine than in the stomach or colon. Most operations are done to relieve obstruction, which often occurs when scars and adhesions form after the healing of previous operations. An uncommon cause is a large gallstone, which, having eroded through the gallbladder into the intestine, blocks the intestine at a point of narrowing. If a segment of intestine is removed or its wall opened, leakage of liquid content or re-obstruction may recur. Inadvertent tampering with the blood supply may cause fatal intestinal damage. These disasters require reoperation and may all be lethal.

Small-intestinal bypass for morbid obesity has been practiced for over 20 years but is falling into disfavor because its complications include liver and kidney failure, inflammatory bowel disease, generalized arthritis, diarrhea with excessive fluid loss, skin inflammation and blood chemical abnormalities.

The Large Intestine (Colon)

This wider tube, only about four feet long including its terminal rectum, is the major location for cancer in both men and women in the U.S. Over 112,000 cases are estimated to have occurred in 1981 with 52,000 deaths. It is, however, curable in more cases than the leading cause of cancer death, lung cancer, which causes almost 100,000 fatalities annually. Like coronary artery disease, cancer of the colon is a disease of affluent Western civilization in which similar dietary factors contribute to its origin.

Multiple small outpouchings (diverticula) of the colon, which can become inflamed, certain types of colitis, and benign tumors (mostly polyps) add to the indications for surgery. Part or all of the colon can be removed with the disease. If the rectum is lost, an artificial anus must be constructed on the lower abdomen. After total colectomy, the terminal portion of the small intestine is opened to the exterior (ileostomy). If enough colon remains, a colostomy is performed. Both of these openings must be managed with care; an organization called the Ileoptimists has developed to help maintain psychological and physical support and rehabilitation for these patients. The most important adverse occurrences (in addition to bleeding and infection) are diarrhea, irritation of the surrounding skin, obstruction by scarring, or contracture or protrusion of the bowel through the opening (hernia).

BREAST OPERATIONS

Mastectomy has been called the operation women fear most. Cancer alone is frightening, but having a breast removed destroys what many women consider an important symbol of feminine identity. The psychological consequences of loss of a breast are as important as the less than 1% mortality rate of the operation.

In 1981, an estimated 110,000 American women and 900 men had newly diagnosed breast cancer. Although breast cancer increased over 60% between 1935 and 1981, its death rate of 27 per 100,000 has remained virtually unchanged. It is the greatest cancer killer of women: 7 out of 100 are expected to develop it in their lifetimes, and 23,000 of these will die. Although there has been great improvement in the early detection of breast cancer, this has not yet been reflected in an improved survival rate, which depends more on the characteristic of the cancer than on the type of intervention. If the disease is confined to the breast, 62% will survive free of cancer, for 10 years, but if the armpit (axillary) lymph nodes are involved, only 22% will be alive after 10 years. Reducing risk by early pregnancy, although contrary to modern trends in lifestyle, is, in the absence of a dramatic breakthrough, more important than illusory advances in diagnosis and therapy.

Although the radical mastectomy is obsolete, a few hard-core relics still favor this extensive, mutilating operation. If the skin incision extends into the axilla, a taut scar will form, hampering arm motion. There are many nerves and blood vessels in the axilla which may be injured, causing hemorrhage, painful partial paralysis of the arm (brachial palsy), or a protruding shoulder blade ("wing scapula"). Extensive postoperative oozing of blood may cause anemia. Blood clots may form in the arm veins and portions break off, floating to the lungs, with shock and frequent fatality. Swelling of the arm (lymphedema) due to obstruction of veins or lymph channels occurs to varying degrees in half or more of obese women, beginning several months and lasting for years after the operation. The loss of circulation will promote infection in the arm or hand, especially after burns or minor cuts.

Most experienced pathologists believe that an error rate of about 1%, depending on the nature of the tissue removed, is to be expected. A false-positive result for cancer, which can cause an unnecessary operation, is more disastrous to the patient and surgeon than a false-negative, which means only a delay until the report of the permanent section (which should be available within 24 hours) is received. Certain benign breast conditions, brain lesions and lymph node enlargements are particularly difficult to distinguish from malignancy. They constitute most of the 10% of diagnoses that the Mayo Clinic defers until the next day. Most of many reports from high-volume surgical centers, such as the hospitals of the Universities of Ohio and Texas, Columbia University and Washington University, show 98–99% accuracy. But the 1% to 2% of mistaken diagnoses can be tragic if rashly acted upon. Newer tools, such as electron microscopy and special stains require more time, but are often essential for precise classification of tumors. No harm results from such a delay.

CARDIOVASCULAR SURGERY

Surgery of the heart started with a few closed, external procedures for the correction of congenital defects, removal of a pericardium which is adherent because of inflammatory disease or radiation injury and most recently, bypassing coronary arteries closed by arteriosclerosis (atherosclerosis). Open heart surgery for the repair of congenital and acquired internal defects requires the substitution of mechanical pumping and oxygenating mechanisms for the heart and lungs, which are temporarily bypassed (extracorporeal circulation). Tubes from, and returning to, the pump-oxygenator may be inserted into a large leg artery and vein (femoral) or, now generally preferred, directly into the aorta and vena cava.

Extracorporeal circulation requires practiced teamwork among surgeons, anesthesiologists, cardiologists and nurses. Its intricate network of tubing, pumps, blood reservoirs, defoaming chambers and oxygenators creates conditions for the operation of Murphy's Law. The connections to the arteries and veins may tear or become dislodged, causing fatal hemorrhage. Before the heart can be opened, its beat must be halted, generally by passing cold solutions through its chambers by flexible pointed tubes. The blood that circulates from the artificial pump-oxygenator through the body is diluted, decreasing clotting ability. This may cause biochemical complications with kidney and lung damage. It is not unusual for the return (venous) flow of blood to be cut off by kinking or when someone steps on the pump-oxygenator tube. The pressure in the apparatus can cause injury to, or destruction of, red blood cells (hemolysis) which can result in damage to the kidneys as in a transfusion reaction.

Hemorrhage, sometimes fatal, is always a risk in preparing for open, or during closed, operations. Blood vessels may be torn or the heart itself perforated, especially if previous surgery has been performed, leaving adhesions which must be removed. Sutures may not cause perfect closure of atherosclerotic arteries. Sutures may also cut through heart muscle. If blood enters the pericardial sac it will compress the heart and restrict bleeding (tamponade), requiring immediate reoperation to drain the blood and remove clots. Fragments of fatty material, blood clot or air bubbles may enter the general circulation and permanently injure the brain.

Heart block with irregular and slow beating reduces pumping capacity and is especially likely to happen in open operations for replacing or repairing heart valves. When this happens, wires are sometimes inserted in the heart muscle and left in place to be connected to a battery-powered pacemaker. If the heart block persists, a pacemaker is implanted under the skin before the patient leaves the hospital.

Coronary Artery Bypass Surgery (CABS)

CABS is mostly a fashionable and costly surrogate for lifelong neglect of one's cardiovascular system, just as abortion is primarily an expensive substitute for contraception. In 1981, Dr. Christiaan Barnard, who performed the first heart transplant, asserted that "Without a doubt, it is the most overused operation in the world. . . . There is a public demand. It is a status symbol to have a bypass today." He added that most heart surgeons are looking for bypasses to perform and that 80% of them would be out of work without this overused operation.

The first CABS was performed in 1965 at the Cleveland Clinic, where 15 are now done daily. The Clinic claims a less than 1.0% mortality rate for selected patients. CABS was performed over 130,000 times in the U.S. in 1980 at a cost of $2 billion which continues to increase. About 80% of patients who have had CABS are still alive, but many more of these procedures are done than is necessary. In the 14 years since it has been available, CABS has been done 500,000 times in the U.S. and is now offered at 600 hospitals. The expensive and dangerous invasive procedures requiring many technical assistants which are needed for the diagnosis and surgical treatment of CAD, produces a national bill of over $4 billion for .04% of the population, exceeding that for any other operation. The cost to the individual patient varies from $11,000 to $25,000, and the surgeon's fee averages $3,000. When one considers that most cases of CAD could have been prevented by early attention to the elimination of the well-known risk factors, these expenditures are understandable but inexcusable! It is not possible to predict how new forms of medical treatment will affect the present trends in heart disease treatment. Dr. Thomas Grayboys of Peter Bent Brigham Hospital believes that most CAD patients will do very well with improved medical management, the results comparing favorably with expensive and risky surgery.

In 1981, the National Center for Health Care Technology (NCHCT) convened a Technology Assessment Forum to examine the many ethical, legal, social and economic questions which this overused operation raises. Information regarding 25,000 patients who had CABS at one of 15 centers during 1974 through 1979 showed that half of the women who had coronary arteriography showed no significant CAD; the percentage of patients with symptoms and signs of coronary artery disease who had coronary artery bypass surgery varied greatly in different hospitals and the operative mortality, which averaged almost 3%, ranged from 0.3% to 6.4%. Despite the low mortality, only 15% of patients who survive a heart attack are likely to have their lives prolonged by bypass surgery. Differences in degree of patient illness and variation of population were not sufficient to account for the above discrepancies. In general, a low volume of CABS is associated with a higher mortality rate. But better quality surgery is not guaranteed by larger institutions. By most standards, the quality of life is often enhanced by CABS, but return to work is no more frequent than with medical treatment. Strict rehabilitation programs with change in lifestyle seem sensible. However, there is still considerable controversy about whether medication, a low-fat, low-calorie diet and cautiously graduated exercise will prevent or delay progress of CAD in still open arteries or prevent clogging of the bypass graft.

A large vein in the upper leg (saphenous vein) is generally used for bypassing the clogged coronary artery. In removing a segment of this vein, nerves or lymph channels may be damaged, causing numbness and swelling which may be permanent or may gradually disappear in several months. The greatest disaster can occur when the aorta is injured as the veins are sewn into it, because atherosclerotic plaques may become dislodged, enter the blood stream and be carried to the brain. The aortic wall may be disrupted by clamps, with fatal bleeding between its layers. Suturing of the segment of vein to the aorta and to the coronary artery below the block can run into technical complications requiring great skill and experience. When the aorta is severely atherosclerotic, some surgeons prefer using the internal mammary artery instead of a vein segment. A heart attack occurs rarely in the course of this operation due to reduced oxygen supply to the heart. Irregular heart beat may occur later in up to 40% of patients.

The success rate is a compound of surgical skill and judgment, the quality of anesthesia and extracorporeal support, and postoperative management. Although 90% of patients will be temporarily—and 70–75% will be totally—relieved of pain and have their exercise capacity improved, there is no way of determining how long the relief will last. CAD is only one manifestation of atherosclerosis, which may be generalized and progressive. Around 1% of patients have had previous strokes, from closure of the large (carotid) artery in the neck or smaller brain arteries. This reduces the 5-year survival rate to 31%. With the passage of time, atherosclerosis will develop in the vein graft despite belated attempts to control risk factors. Control of these factors must be started early in life to avoid, delay or reduce the risk of the developing coronary artery disease, still our greatest killer, with a toll of 600,000 deaths annually.

In 1981, a report from John Hopkins Hospital described autopsies on 109 patients who had 236 individual CABPs. Of the 30 patients who died at operation, 99% had open grafts. Of those who died within a month 92% had open grafts, but after five years or more only 61% were open. Studies from other centers confirm this gradual closure. Angina reappears an average of six or seven years after CABP; 4% of patients having single vessel disease die in the first year unless the left main artery is closed, which increases the fatality rate from 30% to 40%. If two arteries need bypassing, 7% to 10% of patients die and if three or more require bypassing, 50% will not survive five years.

More encouraging results were reported from St. Lukes' Hospital in Milwaukee in an analysis of almost 300 patients who received chest (internal mammary) artery instead of leg-vein grafts. Seven to nine years after surgery 91% were still alive. Thirty percent had coronary angiograms showing that 94% of these were open up to nine years postoperatively. There was much less atherosclerosis than in a comparable number of venous grafts. The cardiologists there believe that motivated patients who are able to improve their life-style will have better prognoses.

Replacement of Heart Valves has been performed since 1960 and requires open surgery. The mitral valve between the left atrium and left ventricle and the aortic valve between the left ventricle and the aorta may be widened, causing regurgitation, because of old rheumatic or other inflammatory damage, or narrowed because of atherosclerosis. This causes the heart to overwork, causing enlargement (hypertrophy) and eventual failure. In the 1940s, the mitral valve was widened by a simple insertion of a finger or a knife, but this simpler process is seldom used in the 1980s. The new (prosthetic) valves are bioengineering marvels of metal and plastic. Some are obtained from pigs and specially treated, but are of doubtful durability. Yet their implantation does not assure cure, since nearly half who have survived the operation are dead or have serious complications within 10 years. During the operation, sutures may tear through the heart muscle, causing hemorrhage, or may encircle and occlude a branch of a coronary artery. The mortality rate from the operation varies from 3% to 10%.

A 64-year-old welder, complained of mild chest pain and shortness of breath when he ascended the single flight of steps leading to his shop. His doctor found that his heart was enlarged and that he had a loud murmur in his upper chest. After x-ray, EKG, and other studies it was determined that his aortic valve was narrowed by localized atherosclerosis. Replacement of his stenotic valve with a ball valve prosthesis was successful, but a month later, he developed paralysis of his right side and was unable to speak. His doctors believed that a clot had broken off from the artificial valve and lodged in his brain. After several months he gradually recovered the use of his arms, legs and facial muscles but, although mentally sound, he is still not able to speak coherently because of damage to his speech center.

Thus, having survived the operation, pitfalls persist. Some 2% of prosthetic valves develop inflammation from staphylococci, streptococci or less common organisms acquired during surgery or already circulating in the blood. The sutures may be disrupted or the opening narrowed. Clusters of bacteria may break off and particles may be carried to the spleen, kidneys or skin with minute hemorrhages in the area where they lodge. The patient will have chills and fever and the blood culture will be positive in 90% of all cases. Antibiotics are effective in less than half of the patients and progressive heart failure will ensue. In 1981, 3 out of 5 patients who had aortic valve replacement at a Boston hospital developed bacteremia, while 230 patients with infected artificial valves at the Mayo Clinic had a mortality rate of 55%.

Blood clots form on the prosthetic valves in 2% to 5% of patients each year, resulting in closure of the valve opening or small to massive strokes if they break off and reach the brain. Treatment or attempted prevention by drugs given to prevent clotting may result in generalized hemorrhages, fatal in up to 1%. A quarter of the late deaths and complications are caused when the prosthesis fails to operate because of clots or a mechanical breakdown of the ball-valve mechanism. Heart failure will result and immediate reoperation may not save the patient.

Blood turbulence about the prosthesis may cause the red blood cells to break down (hemolysis), resulting in anemia with mild jaundice and occasional kidney damage, in 5% to 15% of the cases.

Pacemakers are worn by, or inserted in, 200,000 Americans. It has been estimated that in 1980, 80,000 new pacemakers were installed. Their use is increasing by 9,000 each year. They are indicated in severe, irregular heartbeat or complete block, especially when there is fainting because of insufficient blood supply to the brain. When properly used they can increase the quality and duration of life. The power device, with a mercury, zinc or lithium battery or a nuclear unit, if the patient has a longer than 10-year life expectancy, is scarcely larger than a pack of cigarettes. It is usually inplanted under the left rib cage in a closed pouch. Following heart surgery, wires are inserted into the heart muscle. If the chest has not been opened for previous heart surgery, the wires, controlled by a fluoroscope, can be wormed through an arm or shoulder vein to be set in the heart.

A 59-year-old construction worker in apparent good health except for infrequent dizzy spells, suddenly collapsed on a hot summer day while smoking during his lunch period. He was rushed to a nearby hospital emergency room, where his pulse was found to be 34 per minute. He was admitted to the hospital and after testing, his doctors decided that he had complete heart block because of an injury sustained at work. The natural pacemaker in the nerves of the heart had failed. When his pulse fell below 40, he fainted from lack of circulation to the brain. A plutonium powered pacemaker firing at 70 beats per minute was inserted. Unfortunately, he developed painful hemorrhages under the skin of the pacemaker pocket. These healed and were absorbed in three weeks. Mike returned to work but has had to avoid strenuous labor. His power source will outlast his life expectancy.

In older patients with coronary disease whose life expectancy is less than that of Mike's, battery powered-pacemakers may run down prematurely and need recharging or replacement. If the patient is involved in an accident, the power source or electrode may be dislodged and must be reinserted before brain damage or heart arrest occurs. Wires may fracture at any point along their length. The unsightly midriff bulge may concern cosmetic-conscious patients and cause psychological problems. The plutonium-powered pack must be bullet and heat-proof to avoid possible environmental contamination.

A 1981 study of patients in coronary care units by a committee at the Brooklyn Hospital found that pacemakers were used far too often. After the report was submitted, the number of insertions of pacemakers fell by 50%. Peer reviews at other hospitals have resulted in less dramatic but still significant decreases. A study at Harvard Medical School determined that eight of 20 cardiac patients with pacemakers did not need them and the devices were removed. Many of these patients had terminal cancer or other incurable and painful illnesses, which of course presents ethical and moral problems. At an average cost of $15,000 per pacemaker, millions of dollars are thus wasted each year, including up to $1 billion in Medicare cost.

Blood Vessel Surgery

An aneurysm is a localized ballooning of the wall of an artery forming a pulsating sac or symmetrical swelling. It is usually due to atherosclerosis, although a minority are still rooted in syphilis, once the greatest cause. Less common are dissecting aneurysms caused by blood separating the layers of an artery wall, and traumatic aneurysms.

Excision of aneurysms located in the chest (thoracic aorta) requires a temporary bypass to prevent brain or spinal cord damage due to loss of circulation. The artery wall may be repaired or a dacron prosthetic graft inserted. A congenital narrowing of the artery, causing deficient circulation to the lower part of the body, may also be excised and its ends rejoined, or it may be replaced by a graft depending on its size.

Brain or spinal cord injury can cause confusion, paralysis or coma. Death may result from shock caused by low blood pressure. If debris from atherosclerotic plaques enters the blood stream, or blood clots become dislodged, the particles may enter any branch, causing loss of circulation with probable gangrene anywhere from the intestine to the extremities. The lungs may be encroached upon by the aneurysm or compressed during the operation, resulting in collapse, or air or blood entering the pleural cavities. This may require additional operative intervention, as will postoperative hemorrhage. The sutures may fail to seal the ends of the graft to the arterial wall, which is already weakened or frayed because of the destructive process causing the aneurysm.

Massive hemorrhage is a common complication of operations on aneurysms of the abdominal aorta which may be the cause of unnecessary premature death. Since the small intestine must be manipulated to expose the aorta, it may be injured by pressure or by sutures inserted to hold it in place. The large veins of the abdomen or the ureters, which are close to the aorta, must be dissected away and may be injured or perforated. The lining of the aorta above the excised aneurysm may be covered with soft, shaggy material or a clot. These may be disloged and block the leg arteries unless removed by suction through a catheter.

It has been estimated that from 5% to 15% of hypertension in many millions of people in the U.S. is caused by narrowing of a branch of the abdominal aorta which supplies the kidneys. This can be proven by arteriography, which itself has complications in almost 1% of cases. A bypass graft can correct the deficient circulation in the affected kidney, but clots, which occur in 5% of all cases, or contraction due to scarring at the suture lines, may restore the narrowing and require reoperation.

Carotid Endarterectomy in people who have had small strokes (transient ischemic attacks—TIAs) is one of the most utilized operations for restoring blood flow in a blocked artery or vein. (Almost any blood vessel can be widened or bypassed.) The artery is opened through a longitudinal incision and clamped off, and all atheromatous material is peeled off and flushed out. Small fragments may enter the circulatory system of the brain when the clamp is removed, or blood clot may re-occlude the artery. Blood leakage may occur after the artery is sutured.

Shiela Jones, 59, an apparently healthy housewife, developed multiple TIAs in 1979 manifested by temporary weakness of her left arm, forgetfulness and occasional fainting. Angiography revealed that her right carotid artery was over 90% narrowed. Endarterectomy caused relief of her weakness, but during the next year she had severe headaches and frequent fainting with bleary eyesight and a "pins and needles" sensation in her right arm. A left carotid endarterectomy gave relief for three months, but TIAs recurred in her left arm, thought to be caused by reclosure of her right carotid and possibly accompanied by fragments of atheromatous plaques or small clots carried to her brain. Exploration of the right carotid revealed injury to its lining. The surgeons believed that this was caused by the clamps applied during the original operation. Such damage had been observed previously in other endarterectomy sites. The injury was repaired by a delicate operation and Mrs. Jones has had no further TIAs.

In almost 1,200 carotid endarterectomies, the Mayo Clinic had a surgical death rate of 1.5%, principally from heart attacks, in patients with known coronary disease. Iatrogenic complications occurred in 2% of these cases. Strokes, convulsions and headaches predominated. In 1982, the Clinic reported a six-year follow-up of 109 selected patients, all operated on by the same surgeon. Reduction in the number of strokes was "better than the natural history and better than alternative treatments." However, their neurologists were "not sure that we've improved the overall mortality, although the presumption is that we've decreased deaths from stroke." All experts do not agree that the procedure's value has been proven in the long term. In the first postoperative month, 3% of these patients had strokes, one-third fatal. During the next six years, strokes occurred in 2% of the survivors each year, a better outcome than the expected 6% in patients with TIAs not endarterectomized. However, 30 of the 109 patients died, 70% because of heart disease and only 2% from strokes. Since atherosclerosis affects all arteries, "If a patient has carotid disease, the probability of having coronary disease is about 100%, even if the patient has no cardiac symptoms."

Pericardiectomy

The post-pericardiectomy syndrome may occur during the first few weeks or months after the pericardium, or sac surrounding the heart, is removed. One in five patients will experience severe chest discomfort, fever, EKG disturbances and pain in the pharynx and ears, more likely if the heart muscle has been cut into.

Heart Transplants

Donald Bird, a fortyish citizen of Princeton, Illinois, had a heart attack (MI) in 1980. Angiograms showed that several branches of his coronary arteries were narrowed. A bypass relieved his severe disabling angina for only one month, when Mr. Bird suffered another MI. This time he had a quintuple bypass, again with only one month of relief. The angina became more intense and he developed heart failure with extreme shortness of breath. He was considered to have terminal, "end-stage" heart disease. As a last resort, he was sent to Dr. Norman Shumway at Stanford University Hospital in February of 1981 and had a heart transplant in March. He was also given a new drug, cyclosporin A, to prevent rejection. During a TV interview on November 29, 1981, Mr. Bird enthusiastically stated that he plays golf and runs and that his initial impotence had disappeared.

In February of 1980, the trustees of the Massachusetts General Hospital (MGH) decided that heart transplants would not be done at their institution. In February of 1981, the Mayo Clinic inaugurated its program with its first cardiac transplantation, 14 years after Dr. Christiaan Barnard's initial attempt. In the interim, over 200 replacements had been performed and 100 recipients are still alive. Mr. Bird is one of these survivors and his operation was the 206th. Why did two renowned institutions arrive at opposite decisions?

The MGH estimated that of the 4 million Americans with symptomatic heart disease, up to 40,000 each year would be candidates for transplantation. But since we are not blessed with two hearts, donors would fall short of the demand. And the problem of rejection remains unsolved. As in Mr. Bird's case, patients must be carefully monitored and receive cyclosporin, which might cause cancer, tremors, increased hair growth and kidney damage. A transplantation program would benefit only a few patients, and the resources expended would curtail care for many others. The Intensive Care Unit would be overloaded with apprehensive potential recipients, many of whom would die while waiting for a suitable donor heart.

The Mayo Clinic on the other hand, believes that retention of transplanted hearts has improved with advances in immunosuppression and by 1979, 48% of transplant patients had survived five years. At the clinic, the operation is offered to selected, motivated patients from 15 to 50 years old. Two-thirds are expected to be living after a year and 90% of these can return to work. The cost, including rehabilitation is less than $60,000 per patient. Bypass patients are generally older and it has been estimated that it costs $150,000 to return the average patient to work. Therefore, in terms of "competing for 'effective' national health dollars, cardiac transplantation becomes a bargain," according to the clinic's reasoning.

Heart-Lung Transplants

Four of these massive operations were performed in 1981 by Dr. Norman Shumway at Stanford University Hospital. All of these patients were terminally ill with combined heart and lung disease. Three are alive and active and one is dead from kidney and liver failure. During the late 1960s and early 1970s three of these operations were attempted, but all of the patients died within 23 days. The recent success is believed due to cyclosporin A. Signs of rejection must be sought by invasive biopsy of heart muscle via a wire, terminating in a small clipper wormed through the jugular vein. Lung infection must be combatted by large doses of antibiotics.

PLASTIC (AESTHETIC-COSMETIC) AND RECONSTRUCTIVE SURGERY

Plastic surgeons, whose field is one of the fastest growing specialties, are consulted by "people from every social and economic background—more than half earn less than $25,000 per year," according to a recent report by the American Society of Plastic and Reconstructive Surgeons (ASPRS). Most of these operations were hand surgery (150,000), tumor removals

(106,000), and breast augmentation or reduction (104,000). Only 40% were aesthetic—breast surgery, face lifts and "nose jobs." Sixty percent were reconstructive, 25% were for congenital abnormalities such as cleft palate and hair lip; 20% for trauma rehabilitation, including burns and dog bites; and 15% for tumor-related surgery.

30-year-old Sophie Saunders of North Carolina was afflicted with neurofibromatosis ("Elephant-man" disease). Disabling, painful and deforming tumors grew on the nerves of her neck, over her eyes, arms, spinal cord and brain. In 1976, a plastic surgeon removed a wrinkled, orange-sized mass from her right lower neck. The next day, Sophie was distressed to discover that she could not move her right arm or shoulder. A neurologist showed that a nerve bundle had been injured (brachial palsy) during surgery, requiring further costly treatment but with only partial recovery, which led to liability litigation.

Hand Surgery

The human hand cannot be duplicated by a robot. Because it is crucial for skilled craftsmanship and creative art, the hand is responsible for the evolution of our brain. The hand is vulnerable to injury in industry and recreation and its function may be lost because of naturally occurring strokes, polio, or local muscle, nerve, bone or supporting tissue disease.

Some orthopedic surgeons restrict their practice to lucrative hand surgery, competing with plastic surgeons. To correct deformities, contractures and loss of strength, a variety of operations have been devised. Tendon transfers to bones for which they were not originally intended or the grafting of a portion of a less used tendon may fail because of scarring which restricts movement of muscles or joints. After improper treatment of injuries, poor alignment may result, with deformity and loss of function. Sometimes dislocations of finger joints are mistaken for sprains, which results in swelling, pain and limitation of motion.

Partially or completely lost or useless thumbs can be replaced by other fingers, generally the fifth, which permits the important pinching and grasping maneuvers. Problems relating to inadequate blood supply, deformity, excessive length or insufficient or excessive mobility of the substituted finger may require additional, delicate and costly tinkering.

When nerves are severed, their repair requires intricate, sometimes microscopic, surgery for best results. Bleeding between the rejoined ends, loss of moisture from overly long application of a tourniquet, or premature movement may destroy the juncture. Because some nerves control movement and others, sensation, mixing up their ends may result in oversensitivity to cold. In hasty repairs after accidents when anatomical landmarks are hard to locate, a nerve may accidentally be joined to a tendon.

Tumor Removal

Tumors may be located anywhere. Therefore, benign or malignant tumor surgery may be performed by a general surgeon or one specializing in the regions involved, such as the ear, nose and throat, the orthopedic or the gynecologic area, etc., unless the lesion is in an exposed area.

"Black cancers" (malignant melanomas) and other skin tumors are predisposed to occur in areas exposed to sunlight. Because of the wide excision deemed necessary and the desire to have as inconspicuous a scar as possible, they are frequently removed by plastic surgeons. Complications are much like those of any surgical incision.

Breast Augmentation, Reduction and Reconstruction

Bad results might be expected in up to 25% of all augmentation mammoplasties.

> A 26-year-old woman had silicone implants at an ambulatory surgical facility under local anesthesia. The next day she noticed pain, swelling and increased firmness. It was obvious to her cosmetic surgeon that bleeding had occurred around the implant, which called for reoperation, removal, curbing of bleeding and reinsertion with a slightly pressurized dressing. Antibiotics had to be given to prevent the infection which sometimes occurs after such manipulation.

If the gel implant should leak, a dense fibrous scar will form around the irritating substance, causing undesirable lumpiness and woody firmness. Rarely, the implant will become visible through a gap caused by skin erosion from pressure.

Some women whose breasts are excessively large may suffer from chronic backache as well as psychologic problems. Removal of pounds of breast tissue and overlying skin is performed through an incision under the breast. After suturing the incision, redundant skin may protrude leaving "dog ears" which require further treatment. Swelling caused by fluid accumulation may cause the breast to become excessively taut, posing the danger of the sutures tearing out and a delay in healing, possibly requiring a skin graft. An unexpected cancer could complicate the operation but because it will be detected early the patient may be considered lucky. If major portions of tissue are removed there will be a loss of nerve fibers, which will cause loss of sensation. Unless great care is exercised the nipple may be too high or too low or may point sideways. Reoperation will be required, with additional unsightly scarring.

Pendulous breasts, which tend to become exaggerated from frequent nursing and age, may also be enlarged. The pull of gravity will stretch the skin, and when combined with skin tension, will make the scar of the repair (mastopexy) wider and weaker, with wound edge separation possible.

Although radical mastectomy is now obsolete, reconstruction may be desired years later, or soon after simple breast removal. Prostheses are available in many shapes and sizes for placement under the skin grafts which are initially required. The pigmented areola may be replaced by dark skin from the vulva, which is aesthetically objectional to some women, who prefer tatooing. The possibility that reconstruction will make a recurrence of cancer difficult to detect is under debate.

Face Lifts

The cult of youth has led men, as well as women, to desire unlined faces. This parallels the rise in expensive hairstyling salons, hair transplants and health clubs. Vanity may not be the only reason. To rekindle marriage, promote job security, start a new career or to delay retirement while facing younger competition, may require enhanced self-confidence.

> Although still pretty and possessing a trim figure, 59-year-old Mrs. Baxter's face and neck showed deep wrinkles and "wattles." As the principal of a junior high school, surrounded by young people, she thought she looked older than any of her colleagues. During the Easter vacation she had a face lift under local anesthesia. "The next day," she said, "I had pain under my chin and a fever of 103°. I really felt rotten. I went back to my surgeon. He was very upset. He opened the incision and fluid came out. He put a rubber drain in and gave me some antibiotic. The next day he put in two more drains. Pus continued to seep out for two weeks but I felt better. I had to go back to school with a scarf to hide the bandages, but now I'm satisfied with my appearance."

Mrs. Baxter's infection is a rare occurrence because of the excellent blood supply to the face. Too much tension will cause a mask-like, "china-doll" look, especially after repeated face lifts, because the limits of elasticity are reached. Gravity will win in the end. Each smile will stretch the skin. Lying recumbent on the face and on the ears will hasten the return of wrinkles, first on the lower cheeks and neck, after ten years or more, depending on the genetic endowment, while the forehead remains smooth. Areas of loss of sensation may occur because of nerve involvement.

Nose Jobs (Rhinoplasties)

Not all rhinoplasties are performed for reasons of vanity. After trauma to the face from falls, blows or accidents, gross deformity with breathing difficulty may result, as with deviated septums. Still, many patients bring pictures of people they would like to resemble. Older patients have difficulty in adjusting to their new appearance and the relative inelasticity of their skin may make reconstruction difficult, as it is in younger patients with thickened skin due to acne. Infections are more common than with face lifts. After surgery, the nose is packed with gauze and toxic shock syndrome has been reported. The patient is often not satisfied with the results because of the many subtle variations possible. Repair of a hump may leave a depression, a saddle-nose or ski jump profile. Others may have residual "parrot's beaks," or "polly tip" deformities. All of these will require secondary correction. Much depends on the patient's psychological status and the doctor-patient relationship.

Baggy eyelids are repaired by blepharoplasty. They may be due to thyroid disease or allergy and require more than cosmetic surgery. After the operation, bleeding may cause swelling and discoloration. The eyes may appear sunken or asymmetric or the upper lid may droop due to excessive removal of fat.

Dog Bites. Over 700,000 Americans are bitten each year, but only one in 10 on the face. Many of these wounds require multiple cosmetic operations, causing permanent disfigurement. About 80% of the bites are inflicted on people familiar to the dog. Since the iatrogenic complications are those of wound repair in general, I will not discuss canine carnage further.

Dermabrasion and Chemical Peeling. The removal of deep, pitted scars from acne, smallpox, injuries, tatoos and multiple small tumors can be accomplished by a rotating steel wire brush, resembling dental apparatus. There is considerable bloody spray and the operator's face must be protected by a plastic shield. Permanent redness of the face, minute cysts called milia, infection, or deeper local scarring, especially in skin already damaged by x-rays or exposure to the sun, may result.

The same lesions may be treated by chemical peeling, usually with a solution containing carbolic acid (phenol). Complications are similar to dermabrasion but there may also be blotchy loss of color, increased sensitivity to sunlight and contracted scars. A recent tragedy occurred in Chicago when a patient died of phenol poisoning because of excessive absorption through the skin.

Cleft Lip and Palate. These congenital defects come in many combinations. There may be two clefts, one on each side of the lip, and one or both nostrils may be included. Almost everyone has seen poor results of such operations: depressed scars, "whistle defects" and exaggerated cupid's bows. After repair of the defect in the palate, some patients will still have speech, hearing and dental defects.

Abdominoplasty. Distorted abdomens may not be due solely to obesity. They can occur after multiple pregnancies or in cases of poorly positioned umbilicus. Many pounds of fat and tissue may be removed. Besides the usual risks of hemorrhage and infection, there may be giant scars, deformed and displaced navels, and blood clots (emboli) entering the lungs which are sometimes fatal.

Hair Transplantation

During the past 20 years approximately one million people have had plugs of their own hair transplanted from the sides and back of their heads to bald areas. Complications such as infection and bleeding are rare, but itching and intermittent twinges of pain may occur. Numbness in the donor and recipient areas may persist for several months. A few predisposed people, particularly blacks, may develop unsightly scars. When the graft heals it may be slightly elevated, creating a "cobblestone" appearance. Small dilatations of arteries due to trauma to their walls (false aneurysms) or abnormal communications between arteries and veins forming minute, blood-filled sacs are rare occurrences. Unsightly results may be caused by poor technique or improper spacing or by trying to transplant too many plugs in too short a time.

Less commonly synthetic acrylic fibers are used, but the insertion is not as safe as its proponents claim. Deterioration and loss of color will occur in a few years. The procedure is generally performed by a technician using a slotted implantation needle. All of the above complications may occur here, as well as tumor-like swellings due to a foreign body reaction. Disastrous, permanent loss of the remaining natural hair may be an aftermath.

The complications of thigh, arm and buttock lifts, repair of protruding ears, forehead and eyebrow lifts and correction of receding chins differ insignificantly from the more common cosmetic operations described in this section.

GYNECOLOGIC SURGERY—THE RAPE OF THE PELVIS

Hysterectomy

Hysterectomies win first place among major operations. Around 800,000 are performed annually in the U.S., with 1,000 deaths, at a cost of $1/2 billion. The delicate manipulations of the urologist have been contrasted to the less subtle surgery of the gynecologist, whose mishaps are less likely. Unnecessary hysterectomies, estimated at 25%, are a greater concern. One-third are removed for dropping of the uterus (prolapse) or bulging of the bladder or rectum (generally via the vagina), the rest for fibroids, sterilization, cancer and intractable bleeding.

In 1980, a survey of 5,500 major gynecologic operations revealed that injuries to the bladder and ureter were the most common iatrogenic misadventures after hemorrhage and infection. Bladder and ureter injuries occur in four out of every 1,000 cases. Ureteral injury was much less frequent, but more serious and difficult to repair. Other studies revealed complications in up to 2% of all such cases.

Thirty-two-year-old Marcia Sorenson had lower back pain for many years. Her family doctor sent her to a hospital, where an orthopedist could find no evidence of organic disease after a series of tests, including x-ray. A gynecologist found an irregularly enlarged uterus and a hysterectomy disclosed a benign tumor (fibroid), three inches in diameter, within the uterine wall. Her hospitalization was prolonged by wound infection and incomplete recovery of vigor. Her back pains continued and later, foul-odored urine leaked from her vagina. She also had difficulty controlling the urine flow through its natural opening and was continually wet. Another gynecologist was consulted, who confirmed that her bladder had been perforated during the operation, resulting in an abnormal juncture (vesicovaginal fistula) with the vagina. A complicated and costly second operation was required to repair this damage.

Inflamed leg veins, birth control pills and cancer increase the danger of blood clots breaking off and traveling to the lungs with fatal outcome. Injuries to the intestine and abscess formation following infection are rare. There may be a decrease or loss of sexual drive (libido) or painful intercourse, which may require prolonged therapy.

Radical hysterectomy for cervical cancer involves removal of the pelvic lymph nodes and the upper third of the vagina. Depending on the stage of the disease, it may be extended to resection of the tubes, ovaries, bladder, lower colon and rectum. An artificial anus (colostomy) and bladder must be constructed. The mortality rate is from 10% to 15%.

Myomectomy. Young women with fibroids who desire children may have the benign tumor removed from its uterine bed. Strangely, this conservative operation may be more dangerous than hysterectomy because of the greater likelihood of postoperative hemorrhage.

Mini-Laparotomy for Sterilization. This procedure, which entails a small incision one-half to one inch long above the pubis done under local anesthesia, does not require the expensive and complex equipment needed for laparoscopic sterilization. Since the early 1970s, the Agency for International Development (AID) has distributed over 30,000 kits to 36 countries, where 10 million sterilizations are done annually.

While complications occur in over 2% of laparoscopies (see Chapter 9) and are more serious, in mini-laparotomy or closure of the fallopian tubes by synthetic rings or clips, iatrogenesis is half as common. Most important, although unusual, are perforation of the uterus and tearing of the tubes. The procedure may be technically impossible in extremely obese women or those who have adhesions from previous operations.

Mini-laparotomy involves less equipment and training than laparoscopy. It is more appropriate for non-specialists working with ambulatory patients away from large, well-equipped hospitals.

Oophorectomy and Salpingectomy (Ovaries and Tubes)

The only significant complication of removal of the ovaries is premature menopause. The tubes may not only be removed but also repaired (tuboplasty) if their blockage causes sterility. Although inflammation due to gonorrhea is the principal cause, viral infections or adhesions due to a previous case of appendicitis or pelvic surgery may also result in closure. Tuboplasty will fail to achieve fertility in 2/3 of its attempts and increase the likelihood of a tubal pregnancy, which may rupture with dangerous hemorrhage.

Dilatation and Curettage

D & Cs are performed for diagnosis or for abortion. In a study of almost 3,000 diagnostic procedures, the uterus was perforated in over six cases per thousand. This is especially likely to occur in cases involving cancer, pregnancy and old age. Injury to the bladder or intestine by the sharp instrument will require immediate operative repair. The cervical opening may be permanently widened, predisposing the patient to spontaneous abortion in later pregnancies, or it may be narrowed or closed, causing missed menstrual bleeding and sterility.

An alternative or addition to D & C for the diagnosis of uterine cancer is the Gravlee jet-wash, introduced in 1964. There are conflicting reports of its diagnostic accuracy. A Finnish hospital found two cases of widespread cancer of the peritoneum following this procedure in 80 cases, with the malignant cells flowing through the fallopian tubes.

Cervical Biopsy and Conization. When the cervix appears abnormal or the "Pap" smear is positive or suspicious, a small fragment from, or circular excision of its opening is obtained for microscopic confirmation or removal of a small superficial cancer. After healing, scarring may shorten the cervix, promoting later miscarriage, or narrow its opening to a pinpoint. Cancer, invasive or non-invasive, may recur and become manifest months or years after this conical excision.

GENITOURINARY SURGERY

The relief of obstruction to the free flow of urine and/or semen by overgrowths, tumors, stones, inflammation or injury is the principal function of this specialty. Approximately 300,000 prostates are removed and 250,000 urethras dilated in the U.S. annually. Surgery of the male sexual system is more delicate but less frequent.

Prostatectomy

Although the usual removal through a cystoscope of an enlarged prostate blocking the flow of urine (transurethral resection) is a major operation, it was discussed in Chapter 10 as an invasive procedure because a skin incision is not needed unless the urethral opening needs widening to admit the cystoscope. Healing may result in a deformed opening causing a dispersed "watering can" urinary stream. Cure of dribbling may be disappointingly incomplete.

A few prostatectomies are performed via the skin between the scrotum and the rectum (perineum) or through the lower abdomen, especially if they are unusually large or cancerous. The operations may be simple or radical. The muscle and nerves which control the bladder neck may be injured, resulting in loss of control and dripping of urine. Conversely, narrowing of the urethra may partially close the flow. The ureters may be inadvertently blocked, causing pain and failure to urinate. The testicles and the attached small epididymis through which spermatozoa glide will be inflamed in one in 24 cases. Impotence is almost universal when cancer is present, but although delayed, erections and orgasms persist in most men when benign prostates are removed.

Kidney Surgery

A kidney may be removed (nephrectomy) if it has lost its function because of inflammation, multiple cysts or blockage of a ureter, or if it contains a tumor. If cancer is present in the urinary collecting system, the ureter is also removed. Rarely, urine may leak through the wound, particularly if only a segment of a kidney is excised for a benign cyst or a stone in one end.

Kidney stones, which hospitalize 200,000 Americans each year, may become stuck in a ureter if they are small enough, causing agonizing pain (renal colic). Most can be removed by a long catheter with a grasping device. Larger stones may need surgery and recur in one case in seven. Lung collapse (pneumothorax) is more common in this procedure than in most other operations, since the pleural cavity may be inadvertently entered. Kidneys that have been damaged because of the obstructing stone may require removal. The mortality rate is less than 1%.

When both kidneys have ceased to function because of progressive, irreversible inflammatory or immunological disease, uremia results. Waste products accumulate in the body and will inevitably cause death. Dialysis can rid the system of these toxins but requires perpetual enslavement to a costly and dangerous chemical mechanism. When a kidney from a suitable matched donor, preferably a close relative, can be transplanted, the patient is freed from bondage. But perils persist. During the operation, the recipient, usually anemic and hypertensive, must be carefully monitored to anticipate cardiac or respiratory failure or muscle paralysis from relaxant medication. The junction with the ureter may heal poorly, with leakage of urine due to the drugs given to prevent rejection, the central problem in these cases.

Rejection may be immediate (hyperacute), with loss of blood supply. This disaster requires prompt removal of the disintegrated kidney and a return of the patient to dialysis. Transplantation may be tried again but the risk of rejection recurring is increased.

A 1981 report by the American Society of Transplant Surgeons, reviewed the results in 881 transplants in 879 recipients: 95% of those under 50 who received kidneys from relatives were alive and functioning after a year, but survival was reduced to 90% if the kidney was obtained from a cadaver. In patients over 50, the survival rates were 77% and 82% respectively. This is a great improvement over that of the previous decade and it is certain that the benefits, despite iatrogenesis, exceed the risks.

Bladder Surgery

Most benign tumors and chronic inflammatory conditions of the bladder can be removed or treated through a cystoscope. But cancer requires partial or complete removal of the bladder, depending on the extent and depth of invasion. An artificial bladder can be constructed of a detached segment of small intestine into which the ureters are inserted (ileal conduit). It is attached to the abdominal wall, through which an opening is made for the urine to drain into a sealed plastic bag. But this is such a complex operation that complications are common occurring in up to 80% of all cases. Urinary or fecal leakage through any of the half-dozen junctures of bowel, ureters, abdominal wall and skin, will lead to an almost 50% fatality rate. Intestinal obstruction, degeneration of the intestine substituting for a bladder and closure of any opening due to contraction by scarring have significant mortality rates and require additional treatment. Kidney infection and/or stones occur in approximately 5% of all cases. The likelihood of inflammation and encrustation of the skin around the external opening (stoma) requires meticulous preventive care.

Mrs. Janet Scalzi was referred by her gynecologist to a urologist for removal of a small out-pouching (diverticulum) of her urethra. After the operation, a perforation (fistula) into her vagina developed, causing uncontrolled leakage of urine and making sexual relations disagreeable. Two additional operations failed to completely close the fistula. This unpleasant complication is more common in males, draining to the outside or into the rectum.

Sexual Organ Surgery

A multitude of operations for congenital deformities, from plastic reconstruction to amputation for cancer or sex change, may result in narrowing or closure of the remaining urinary opening (meatus).

Impotence, a metaphor for any deprivation of power, is not loss of desire but failure to initiate or sustain an erection.

Inflatable cylinders or solid plastic splints can be inserted into the penis to correct non-psychogenic impotence, mostly following spinal cord injury with or without paraplegia. A bulb-like pump sewn into the scrotum squeezes fluid into the prosthesis, producing a reasonable facsimile of a natural erection in over 80% of all cases. Leakage, erosion into the urethra, premature decompression, fracture, and penile scarring due to rejection of the foreign material have been reported, requiring additional treatment. Concealing erections simulated by solid splints when not in use is not completely achieved by taping or athletic supporters. Partners have complained of excessive size and hardness, requiring excess lubrication and buckling and bending.

A testicle may not have descended into the scrotum by age five. This requires surgical correction (orchiopexy) because the risk of traumatic damage, malignancy, or twisting, with consequent gangrene or loss of production of male hormone and sperm, is increased. The testicle may lose its vitality from accidental disruption of its blood supply. If already shrunken, as often occurs if orchiopexy is delayed until puberty, it may be removed and replaced by a plastic implant, which in rare cases can ulcerate through the scrotal skin.

Tumors of the testicle run the range from the benign to the virulently malignant. The latter may require not merely removal, but also radical operation with dissection of the lymph nodes in the groin and lower back. One or both kidneys may be lost because of injury to their blood supply or ureters. Many of these patients are given chemotherapy before operation, which greatly retards their recovery from the operative trauma.

Circumcision

The ritual of circumcision, a minor operation, is an unnecessary expense usually added to the bill for delivery of a male child. Unless performed as a religious ceremony, how can one justify the strange but accepted practice of looping off the protective foreskin of an organ so vital to future social approval and ego gratification? This $75–100 operation is performed about 1.5 million times annually in the United States, or on 80% of newborn sons.

The usual medical advice is that circumcision can prevent phimosis, a condition in which the foreskin cannot retract from the penile head, causing infection. However, most circumcisions are performed before the infant's foreskin can be completely retracted, which generally cannot be accomplished until the age of three. Why not wait to see if this problem develops?

Another widely accepted belief is that the presence of the foreskin increases the risk of cervical cancer in spouses of the uncircumcized, as well as the relatively rare penile cancer in these men. Statistical analysis in the 1960s revealed cervical cancer in 2.2 per 100,000 Jewish married women with circumcized husbands, and in 4.4 per 100,000 of non-Jewish married women with uncircumcized mates. This seemed to indicate that the mere fact of circumcision halved the likelihood of cervical cancer. But this evidence was clouded by the discovery that 5.5 per 100,000 of women whose husbands were circumcised but did not practice genital hygiene contracted cervical cancer.

Ceremonial circumcision is widespread in undeveloped countries. Studies of Hindus, Fijiians, Parsees and Moslems indicate that the degree of sexual hygiene, promiscuity and general cleanliness are more important than circumcision in the risk of cervical and penile cancer. Statistical evidence in both developed and undeveloped countries supports the claim that circumcision is not necessary for good health when modern sanitation is employed.

The complications of circumcision, although rare, invalidate any real or imagined benefit. Occasionally, partial closure of the urinary opening follows, with later ulceration requiring prolonged medical care. It has been estimated that in the U.S. one newborn male in 500,000 dies from complications of circumcision, a risk comparable to infant appendectomy.

The American Academy of Pediatrics concluded in 1971 and again in 1975 that there is "no valid reason for routine circumcision of the newborn." If every newborn male in America were circumcised, the national bill would reach $200 million a year. My research of the world literature concurs; the operation's counterproductivity outweighs its minimal advantages and the phallus should remain intact in the absence of specific disease. The operation should be replaced by education in personal hygiene. To remove the foreskin for the possible prevention of cancer is as logical as removal of the infantile appendix to prevent future appendicitis.

Hernias

Over 750,000 annual hernia repairs (herniorrhaphies) put this operation in second place among major operations in the U.S. Although we commonly think of hernias as protrusions of the peritoneum, sometimes including a loop of intestine, through an opening or rupture in the groin or umbilicus, they may occur anywhere a part of the body or an organ bulges from its normal position—for instance, hiatus hernia, the entrance of part of the stomach into the chest cavity through a widening of the esophageal slit in the diaphragm.

Groin herniorrhaphies, the most frequent variety, total about 550,000. They can cause an unsightly bulging and, if complete, may extend into and swell the scrotum. Intestinal obstruction may occur due to compression, followed by strangulation with gangrene of the intestine if the blood supply is compressed.

At operation, the seminal canal (vas deferens), the nerves serving the abdominal wall, or rarely, the root of the penis may be severed. Sutures may transfix the intestine with subsequent obstruction or abscess. An opening into the bladder may cause leakage of urine and, like the other mishaps, must be repaired immediately. If the herniorrhaphy is uneventful, it is sometimes advisable to remove the appendix simultaneously because the benefit exceeds the risk of additional complications.

HEAD AND NECK (ENT) SURGERY

The Thyroid

Unsightly, smooth or lumpy thyroid enlargement may be accompanied by overactivity with protruding eyeballs (exophthalmos), mental impairment (cretinism) or local pressure on the trachea. It may originate in inflammation, cancer of varying virulence, or benign tumor. Sometimes only a solitary nodule is observed or felt.

If the thyroid is totally or partially removed, there is a slight but serious risk of nerve injury which may result in hoarseness or in paralysis of the vocal cords requiring emergency airway opening (tracheostomy). Decreased thyroid function (myxedema) may produce mental sluggishness, overweight and quick fatigue upon exertion. Taking frozen sections to determine the presence of cancer may be misleading because the malignancy may be missed in the sections selected or be misinterpreted as benign. The parathyroid glands, small button-like nodules on the thyroid capsule, may be inadvertently removed, lowering the level of calcium in the blood and causing spasms or convulsions, cataracts, or psychological disturbances. If the vocal cords become spastic, suffocation may occur.

Insufficient removal of thyroid tissue may result in recurrent overactivity or malignancy. Air may enter the large veins in the neck and be carried to the heart fatally cutting off the circulation. The trachea may be compressed by hemorrhage or swelling, with resultant respiratory obstruction.

Tonsillectomy and Adenoidectomy (T&A)

This "bread and butter" ritual has fallen from 1.2 million in 1965 to 500 thousand in 1979, thanks to alternative treatment with penicillin and the realization that over 70% of T&As are unnecessary. This procedure is second to circumcision as the most abused operation in the U.S. Unscrupulous operators in small private hospitals have been "ripping off" Medicaid: At a hospital in south Chicago, two sets of five children from low income families had T&As within two weeks, a sordid scheme to increase income by wholesale volume. None of the children had abscesses, breathing or hearing loss, or ear drainage which might have necessitated this procedure.

During my internship, I had a belated tonsillectomy followed by a streptococcus infection that put me out of action for three weeks. My chief resident, after similar surgery, bled profusely at home and required readmission and transfusion. Sometimes this surgery has its chief iatrogenic effect on the pocketbook of the patient or the family.

Deviated Septum (Submucous Resection)

A 43-year-old businessman had had difficulty in breathing through the right side of his nose for many years. He was told by an ENT specialist that the partition between his two nasal cavities was deviated to the right and that a simple operation, in which a portion of the out-of-line bone cartilage is removed under the nasal lining, could correct it. Joe consented, and the minor operation was performed without difficulty under local anesthesia. As in a cosmetic nose job, the nasal cavities were packed with gauze strips to hold the bone in place. The next morning, a nurse was horrified to find Joe dead in bed. Somehow, the pin below the nostrils which held the packing in place had become loose, and he had inhaled (aspirated) the gauze packing into his larynx above the vocal cords and had been asphyxiated. I had been told that similar unpublished tragedies due to careless postoperative observation have occurred.

A less deadly cosmetic complication is "saddle-back" deformity (sunken nose) due to excess removal of supporting cartilage. Since toxic shock syndrome has been reported after rhinoplasty (nose job), there is no reason why this risk should not occur with submucous resection, from infection of the nasal packing with the same newly evolved toxin-producing staphylococcus.

Tracheostomy is cutting an opening (stoma) into the trachea into which a tube is inserted. It can be life-saving when breathing is obstructed.

"Proud flesh" (granulation tissue) may grow in the wall of the trachea above the stoma up to a year later, causing the coughing up of blood and re-obstruction. The stoma may become blocked by later scarring. With this condition, inhaling blood into the lungs may result in bronchitis and pneumonia. The esophagus or the pleura may be perforated or air may be sucked under the skin or into the chest. Employment problems and marital disharmony are frequent because the unsightly opening in the neck is difficult for some to accept.

Radical Neck Dissections. Cancers of the mouth, breathing passages, the parotid and other salivary glands and the overlying tissues, if extensive, are often massively removed with surrounding soft tissue, cartilage and bone. The lymph nodes of the neck, which perhaps are invisibly involved, are dissected away down to the collar bone (clavicle). The lower jaw may be wholly or partially removed in a mutilating operation with nearly 3% mortality and doubtful survival value.

Tubes carrying air and anesthetic agents are inserted into the trachea and may become kinked or blocked by mucus. Brain damage may occur within several minutes if this is not corrected immediately. There may be grotesque swelling of the tongue and face due to lymph channel compression, occasionally permanent, which bestows a "chipmunk-like" distortion. Narrowing of the airway after operation by blood, mucus, displacement of the tongue or compression by a bandage over swollen tissues may be slow and imperceptible and require tracheostomy. Low blood pressure may result from stimulation of regulating neck nerves, causing a shock-like state.

Parotid and mastoid surgery have the common risk of severence of the facial nerve or one of its branches.

After many ear infections, a 6-year-old girl developed swelling and pain behind her right ear with high fever. Her pus-containing mastoid bone was chiseled away, but she was left with permanent right facial palsy causing distortion of her mouth and inability to close her right eyelid. She must wear a patch to protect her eye and has of course developed personality problems.

ORTHOPEDIC SURGERY (Bones and Joints)

Arthritis

Arthritis strikes in many guises. Its varieties affect more people in the U.S. than does any other disease, causing universal misery. Fortunately, it is seldom fatal. The national bill for lost work and medical care as a result of arthritis is almost $3 billion annually. Most forms of arthritis, such as the several forms of rheumatoid arthritis (not to be confused with the acute transient inflammation of joints accompanying rheumatic fever) and gout, are generally not surgical problems. Degenerative joint disease (osteoarthritis), a slowly progressing disorder of later life occurs primarily in the weight-bearing joints, causing pain, deformity and limitation of motion. This dividend of the "golden years," although incurable, can be aided by surgical replacement of useless joints. Many patients, including some children with hips disabled by rheumatoid arthritis, have been able to discard their walkers and wheelchairs. Good results in the short term can be expected in all but 5% of patients; and their generally advanced age makes the inevitable mechanical and biologic deterioration of little consequence. Insufficient time has elapsed for late adverse effects to become manifest. Results in over 60% are now considered satisfactory.

Many patients undergoing total hip-replacement surgery experience sudden collapse. The cement used in bonding the synthetic plastic joint to bone is highly toxic and causes depression of blood pressure. During surgery, the cement is forced into the marrow cavity and the prosthesis hammered in. Small particles of fat from the marrow (emboli) are carried to the brain and lungs. More recently, there has been experimental and clinical proof that air emboli to the heart (sometimes fatal) occurs in 30% of all hip-replacement cases. Urinary infections occur in 15-30%.

The Lower Back

If arthritis is the most common incapacitating disease in the U.S., its offshoot, chronic lower back pain, is the single most prevalent, non-lethal, incapacitating ailment. There are dozens of derangements among the complicated bones, muscles, tendons and nerves of the spine. The patient's attitude toward his or her symptoms adds to them.

A prominent surgeon was unhappy about his chronic lower back pain and waddling gait, which were aggravated by long hours of standing at the operating table. His orthopedic colleagues decided after x-ray studies that he had forward displacement of his spine upon his sacrum (spondylolisthesis). A fusion was recommended and the lumbar spine was solidly attached to the sacrum by bone grafts. But six weeks of postoperative immobilization in bed encouraged the development of bilateral pneumonia, consequently ending the doctor's life.

Spinal Disc Surgery

The disc, a rubbery cartilaginous structure, lies between the bodies of all vertebrae to absorb the shock of movement and jarring that walking, running and jumping cause. The disc's outer layer is dense and fibrous, holding the spongy center in place. If the fibrous capsule ruptures, the softer core will herniate, generally sideways, and press upon the sciatic nerve, causing severe pain radiating down the leg aggravated by coughing and sneezing. The diagnosis is confirmed by x-ray examinations of the spine using contrast media to outline the surrounding subarachnoid space. The adverse effects of this chemical have been described in Chapter 3 (Radiation).

Although the operation for the removal of a herniated disc (laminectomy) is generally successful, it is very bloody. In order to save time, some orthopedic surgeons have allowed free bleeding, replacing the loss with transfusions. This pernicious practice is not only costly but dangerous and has occasioned rebuke by hospital surgical review committees. Operative trauma is severe, requiring several days of private nursing.

After a day in which she played five sets of tennis, 19-year-old Susan Petersen awoke the next morning unable to get out of bed because of an excrutiating pain radiating down her left leg. A myelogram confirmed a herniated disc and laminectomy was performed. Several days later Susan became nauseous, vomited several times and was dismayed to discover blood in her urine. Intravenous contrast media showed leakage from a perforated ureter at the level of the laminectomy. The perforation was drained by a catheter and healed in less than two weeks. Other cases have been reported of more serious, complete severance of a ureter with difficult and sometimes unsuccessful surgical repair.

It has been estimated that 200,000 laminectomies are performed each year in the U.S. The average cost including time lost from work is $20,000 (the surgeon's fee is $2,500 or more), with an annual total of $4 billion. Insurers believe that nationally this is the most expensive of all operations. A new drug, chymopapain, derived from papaya juice is utilized by injection in Canada and is on clinical trial by the FDA in the U.S.; it can halve the cost and reduce hospitalization from eight to four days. It is expected to be available during 1982 (meanwhile, many Americans have gone to Toronto, Vancouver or Montreal). Adverse effects other than those expected from any large needle puncture occur in 1% of patients who suffer hypersensitivity shock. The patient can safely return to work 50% sooner, and can perform light work in two to three weeks and heavy work in six weeks.

Chiropractic or Osteopathic Manipulation

A 25-year-old office worker complained of a "catch in the neck" one morning and went to see a chiropractor who performed a series of maneuvers including head rotation and tilting. He felt dizzy during the treatment and an hour later had severe headache and nausea. The manipulation was continued until he suddenly lost consciousness and stopped breathing. A physician was called, who administered CPR and had him admitted to an ICU where he was placed on a respirator. Six hours later, John was in deep coma and unresponsive. His EEG was repeatedly devoid of brain electrical activity and after two days he died. Autopsy revealed clotting in the large arteries at the base of the brain and parallel to the spinal column. The brain was soft and swollen and portions appeared to be degenerating.

Manipulation of the neck is performed so commonly that there is no information regarding the risk of complications from injury to the vertebrae or spinal cord or blood clotting in the large blood vessels of the neck and skull. Stroke, sometimes fatal, paralysis of all four extremities (quadriplegia), and brain hemorrhage or disintegration, over one-third fatal, have been reported 27 times in the English medical literature. It is certain that other unrecorded injuries have occurred.

The Treatment of Common Fractures and Dislocations

It is difficult, in many cases, to distinguish complications due to the trauma itself from those caused by treatment. For our purposes, damage that could have been prevented but was not prevented will be considered iatrogenic.

Fat embolism traveling from the bone marrow to the brain, kidneys and lungs occurs in most major fractures. Its severity and mortality rate depends on its magnitude. It can be minimized by gentle handling, prompt at-the-scene splinting and by applying tourniquets during operative fixations. Pulmonary embolism by blood clot is more likely in the elderly, diabetics, users of oral contraceptives, paraplegics, cancer patients and the obese. Although there is no guarantee, the odds can be shifted in the patient's favor by early stabilization of the fracture and by getting the injured person out of bed for exercise as soon as possible. The same measures plus avoidance of edema by elevation, and careful smooth casting and padding to prevent constriction will reduce the risk of pain and withering (atrophy) of the limb, local death (necrosis) of bone, delayed nerve paralysis, loss of joint motion, pressure, bed sores (decubitus ulcers), non-union of the fractured ends, or deformity.

Compound (open) fractures may become infected by pus-forming or tetanus or gas-gangrene-producing, bacteria. Cleaning and cutting away of devitalized tissue (débridement), and administering penicillin or newer antibiotics (cephalosporin) and tetanus antitoxin will prevent most of these dreaded sequelae. The same precautions are needed when fractures must be joined by operation (open reduction), especially when nails, pins, screws or plates are required.

LUNG SURGERY

Because most operations for removing a lobe or entire lung are performed on heavy smokers, the patient may be endangered by tobacco-induced pre-existing emphysema, fibrosis (chronic obstructive pulmonary disease) or coronary artery disease. Despite the danger which should be evident when smoking-caused cancer or emphysema kills family members, friends or well-known personalities, the public remains apathetic. Smoking, in absolute terms, has increased, although it has diminished slightly relative to population growth. Unfortunately, the media seldom mention lung cancer when deaths are reported, and instead use such euphemisms as protracted illness or unspecified cancer.

Cancer of the lung killed 90,000 Americans in 1977 and is expected to top 120,000 when 1982 figures are compiled. Deaths from all smoking-related causes approach 400,000 annually, making the tobacco industry which promotes this noxious addiction the single greatest mass murderer in history. At the present rate of increase, there will be 300,000 new cases in the U.S. annually by the year 2,000. Despite the cost of tobacco products, nationally estimated at $28 billion, there is more smoking and more lung cancer and emphysema in lower income groups and blacks.

Iatrogenic effects of preliminary bronchoscopy have been discussed in Chapter 10 (Invasive Procedures). Sometimes, if only a single lobe is removed, hardened mucus, a misplaced airway tube, or a fragment of tumor may obstruct the main bronchus, preventing lung reinflation and requiring bronchoscopic or surgical removal. The opposite lung may fail to re-expand for similar reasons. Several hours to three days after surgery, the heart may twist on its supports and herniate into the empty pleural cavity. This may obstruct the main blood vessels and cause death. A remaining lobe may rotate on its root with strangulation and gangrene.

Leakage of inhaled air from the end of the severed and sutured or clipped bronchus (bronchopleural fistula) occurs in almost 3% of these cases. An extraordinary case was reported in which a metallic clip slipped off and was coughed up by the patient. Air under pressure will cause tension against the opposite side and fluid, often infected, may accumulate. There is danger of drowning if the remaining lung is submerged. Further surgical repair is necessary and convalescence in survivors will be prolonged for years.

When the empty pleural space fills with purulent fluid, drainage by wide tubes or by creating an opening which can be closed months later after healing, is indicated. This is a lengthy, expensive and not always successful process. Less than 5% of victims are cured despite advances in surgery, radiotherapy and chemotherapy. It is a dreadful prospect for a disease which is—with associated emphysema—*at least 90% preventable.*

12.

IATROGENESIS IN OBSTETRICS

The most accurate indicators of a highly civilized standard of living are the infant and maternal mortality rates. Although our maternal mortality rate is only one death per 8,000 deliveries nationwide (14.1 newborn deaths per 1,000 maternal deliveries), the U.S. is 16th among all nations despite great improvement during the past 15 years. The lowest national infant mortality is in Sweden, with 7.8 per 1,000 despite its high percentage of unwed mothers! Norway is 5th with 9.2 and both are lower than any of our states. New Hampshire, Idaho and Wyoming have the best records, all just under 10 per 1,000. But even our Caucasian population averages a high 12.3 per 1,000 and non-whites, 21.7 per 1,000. These figures point to cultural and socioeconomic factors in our high infant mortality, principally the unthinking neglect of many young parents and their unwillingness to use available facilities for prenatal care.

A whopping 99% of pregnant Swedes obtain excellent prenatal care which *they learn in school*. Many use well trained midwives who generally devote more time to their charges than do physicians. The quality of obstetrical care is excellent, even at smaller hospitals. The few immigrants to Sweden from countries with high infant mortality rates share the native Swede's advantages.

Paradoxically, the chances of a mother and her newborn child not surviving are greater in large teaching hospitals than at small community hospitals. Although this may be because low income and unmarried women who have had inadequate prenatal care and a poor lifestyle are more likely to enter them, it is also true that these large hospitals are perhaps more apt to interfere with the normal process of maternal delivery in the course of training students and residents.

The complications attending amniocentesis, anesthesia, planned parenthood, hormonal prevention of miscarriage, infection, childbirth in older women and prenatal x-rays have been discussed in earlier chapters.

Misdiagnosis: Although pregnancy is an almost universal female experience, its diagnosis may be missed or delayed by the presence of large uterine fibroids or ovarian cysts which may be confusing by their size. Premature menopause, skipped periods because of endocrine abnormalities, and extreme obesity may also retard recognition. During my embryonic years of family practice, an obese teenager was brought to the emergency room because of nausea and severe abdominal pain. The initial impression of appendicitis was rectified when she gave birth to a 6-pound boy.

An obstetrician was sued for pain and suffering resulting from the mistaken diagnosis of spontaneous abortion which was actually a ruptured pregnancy in the right fallopian tube. Expert testimony showed that he was negligent in not having a pathological examination of the bloody tissue his patient had passed and in not examining her birth canal or doing a physical examination after she had called him in extreme pain.

Iatrogenesis in Obstetric Operations

Infections and excess hemorrhage resembling those occurring in gynecologic procedures are more likely to occur in women in poor health but may follow operations to facilitate delivery.

Incision of the Perineum (Episiotomy) is the most common obstetric operation and is done to prevent a ragged tear when the fetal head stretches the birth canal. After the mother gives birth the incision is sutured, but pain and hemorrhage into the tissues may follow. Sensitive scars may form long after delivery causing painful intercourse. Plastic reconstruction may bring relief.

Operative Vaginal Delivery may be necessary in difficult cases, such as those with poor uterine contractions, narrow pelvis or wrong position of the fetus, for instance, hip or shoulder presentation. It includes the use of forceps or a vacuum extractor, manual manipulation, rotation of the head (or rarely, destruction of the fetus). Eye injury, fractures, damage to the spine or brain causing permanent spastic palsy (in around one of 200 children), or death may result.

Complications in the mother comprise tearing of the cervix and lacerations of the vagina which are readily repaired by sutures. The vagina can be tightened by "husband stitches."

Cesarean Delivery. Unfortunately, this major operation is increasing 10% each year in the U.S. In 1972, it was not among the ten most frequently performed operations, but in 1979, it was third, with 600,000 performed (1 of 6 deliveries). Although older women are now giving birth, often with complications leading to cesareans, more teenagers are also undergoing this abdominal surgery. The conventional assumption of cesareans having to be repeated is being challenged by the American College of Obstetricians and Gynecologists in order to reverse this trend, and new guidelines have been suggested for physicians and hospitals. The complications are those of hysterectomy, but there is greater danger of perforating the bladder or causing permanent loss of muscle tone in the uterus. In later pregnancies, vaginal delivery, if attempted, may fail or cause rupture of the uterus through the old scar. This results in an infant mortality rate of 15% to 29%, although the maternal mortality is low. Rupture is less likely with a low horizontal incision than with the "classic" long vertical scar. Delayed cesarean may have a tragic aftermath.

Estelle Wolf noted labor pains in the early morning and was admitted to a maternity service where her "bag of water" ruptured spontaneously. At 8 a.m. a nurse noticed that the amniotic fluid had an abnormal brown color from staining with fetal intestinal content (meconium). Labor did not progress all that day and she begged her physician to perform a cesarean delivery but he refused. The next day after 24 hours of continuous, unproductive labor, she felt feeble fetal movement and her contractions ceased. A nurse could not hear a fetal heartbeat. The doctor arrived at 6 p.m., confirmed that the fetus had died and tried to induce labor through medication but was unsuccessful. A cesarean was eventually performed; autopsy revealed that the fetus had died of inhaling amniotic fluid and meconium. This might have been prevented by heeding the warning discoloration *two days previously.*

Tubal (Ectopic) Pregnancy: When the tube is removed, the blood supply of the ovary may be restricted and it too may have to be excised. Later pregnancies may also be ectopic, occurring in the opposite tube or on the same side if repair has been attempted. In rare cases, an abdominal pregnancy may occur if a tubal pregnancy ruptures and the placenta attaches itself to the surface of another organ.

Other Operations During Pregnancy: Any surgical procedure may enhance the risk of miscarriage, especially those involving the lower abdomen or genital tract, and should be performed only in emergencies.

Plastic Surgery After Pregnancy: Stretch marks (striae) on the breast and abdomen cannot be eradicated but can be made less visible. After many pregnancies the breasts and abdomen will be enlarged and the skin distended, but the sagging may not be visible until the age of 60. The abdominal muscles will be torn and cannot be restored by exercise. They can, however, be repaired, with the possible complications described in the previous chapter.

Miscellaneous Mishaps. pHisoHex (hexachlorophene), a powder or liquid detergent used in the 1960s as an antiseptic on newborns, was discontinued for this purpose by the FDA in 1972 because it was found to be absorbed through the skin, causing occasionally fatal brain damage with convulsions. But it is still used for hand-washing by nurses and in general care areas. A Stockholm study showed that many nurses washed their hands as often as 10 to 60 times daily with pHisoHex or used it in a hand cream; 66 of 460 offspring of these nurses had malformations, 25 were severe involving the esophagus, heart, central nervous system, cleft lip and palate. There were 41 "minor" defects, such as extra fingers or congenital hip dislocations. Experiments on rats with hexachlorophene, which should have preceded its use by humans confirmed this iatrogenesis.

The reputedly purest food in the world, breast milk, whose use is advised by pediatricians and obstetricians as best for mother and baby, is losing its pristine image. Not only have toxic DDT and PCBs been found in it in polluted areas, but cytomegalovirus (CMV), formerly thought to be transmitted to the fetus via the placenta or vaginal secretions, has been isolated. CMV can cause hepatitis and brain damage. Thirty-eight of 278 (13%), low-income Alabama mothers were found to have CMV in cultures of their milk; 11 of 19 of their breast-fed infants (58%) acquired CMV infections, while none of 9 bottle-fed offspring became infected. Nevertheless, the investigators concluded that the "small risk is outweighed by the well established values of breast feeding." A note of caution was raised regarding wet nurses and the use of unmonitored milk banks for premature babies who have little immunity against CMV. If the milk is stored in the frozen state for a week or more, the danger of infection will be eliminated.

If an expectant mother takes large doses of aspirin or a labor-delaying, anti-arthritic drug called Indocin®, the life of the child can be endangered, according to researchers at the University of California Medical Center. These drugs interfere with the baby's ability to switch from maternal blood and oxygen circulation to its own, resulting in "blue babies"—oxygen-starved infants who die if their circulation cannot adjust. Although the manufacturer warns against this use of Indocin®, obstetricians have prescribed up to 10 aspirin tablets daily with "alarming" increased frequency in the final weeks of pregnancy for women prone to premature labor.

Are Deliveries Safer if Performed by Nurse-Midwives?

Twenty years ago there were less than 300 nurse-midwives in the U.S. Today, almost that many are graduated each year from 25 training programs and 2,500 have been certified. Most doctors support this concept but believe that nurse-midwives should be part of physician-directed teams. Nurse-midwives emphasize prenatal counseling, family-centered childbirth, and limited intervention in the natural process. They have persuaded hospitals to allow family members to attend labor and delivery, to allow mothers to hold their infants immediately after birth, to eliminate fetal monitoring and confinement to bed in uncomplicated births. Costs are one-third to one-half of physician deliveries. With proper selection and back-up utilizing anesthesia and blood transfusions when needed, results are at least as good despite continuing controversy.

Avoiding Iatrogenesis by Natural Birth—Fact or Fiction?

The attempt to avoid the suffering of labor by medical intervention in hospitals with drugs and other medication, anesthesia, x-ray examination, sophisticated monitoring equipment and instrumentation has hazards. To find a middle-road, women and their husbands have turned to natural childbirth.

Dr. Fernand Lamaze, a follower of Pavlovian conditioning techniques which he observed in the USSR in the early 1950s, postulated that women could be programmed to dispense with drugs which have harmful effects upon the fetus. By the early 1970s, hospitals across the nation had been persuaded to inaugurate Lamaze training as part of their prenatal preparation.

About 700,000 expectant couples are now trained in Lamaze methods each year. Advocates assert that the nearly 17% of cesarean births can be reduced to 5% by the Lamaze technique. But it is no panacea, as those beleaguered mothers who have required epidural anesthesia or narcotics or cesarean deliveries can attest!

Hazards of Home Delivery

Until 1920, most births in the U.S. occurred at home. Maternal mortality was forty times and infant mortality three times the present rate. Half of all gynecologic surgery was caused by maternal injury at delivery. Today the rate is less than one in 10. In the 1940s, hospital deliveries had increased to over 50%. Now, only slightly over 1% of all births in the U.S. take place at home, but the growing movement for natural childbirth and humanization of medical care has led to a revival of the desire for home delivery.

Births outside of the hospital may be accidental due to delay, or a result of religious taboos, or poverty, especially among rural migratory workers. Or they may be deliberately chosen as the ultimate extension of natural childbirth. The outcome of only the last category can be logically compared with that of hospital delivery. If the family has a clean, comfortable home, if high standards of prenatal care are maintained, if there have been one or more previous normal deliveries, if no complications are expected, if birth is attended by a trained nurse-midwife or physician, and if obstetric and pediatric back-up support is quickly available in the event of unexpected problems, studies of large numbers of cases can produce data justifying a verdict. During the past four years, records from Denmark, Holland, England and 47 U.S. states, have shown that infant mortality at home is *two to five times that in hospitals* despite iatrogenesis. Even in some advanced European countries where home delivery has been more common than hospital delivery, the trend is shifting in the opposite direction toward the hospital.

The English experience is instructive. With selected mothers and support by obstetricians transported in elaborately outfitted ambulances bringing intravenous fluids, incubators, oxygen, blood and plasma, and equipment for forceps and cesarean deliveries, the costs were found to exceed that of hospitals. Many of these "flying squads" are being discontinued because of decreased demand. There is no way that mobile facilities can match those available in well-run hospitals. Canada, which has no such program, has a lower infant mortality rate than England.

Even a few minutes' delay may mean the death of the infant or mother. Those who advocate home births in the U.S., which does not generally provide such facilities, must be made aware of its risks when unanticipated complications occur. A recent statement of policy by the American College of Obstetricians and Gynecologists aptly summarizes the present position:

> Labor and delivery, while a physiologic process, clearly presents potential hazards to both mother and fetus . . . These hazards require standards of safety which are provided in the hospital setting and cannot be matched in the home situation. We recognize, however, the legitimacy of concern of many that the events surrounding birth be an emotionally satisfying experience for the family. The College supports those actions that improve the experience of the family while continuing to provide the mother and her infant with accepted standards of safety available only in the hospital.

13.

VACCINES—IATROGENESIS OF IMMUNIZATION

Vaccinations have saved millions of lives. Those of us who remember the 1920s recall the frightened but fruitless exodus of families from cities before the annual summer polio season, the iron lungs, the friends and relatives with withered, paralyzed limbs and the dramatic struggle of FDR, stricken with polio at his secluded Campobello retreat. Until the 1920s, infectious diseases were the greatest killers of Americans, although their victims had decreased from 785 per 100,000 in 1900 to 489 per 100,000. Armies suffered greater losses from bacteria than from bullets.

The toll of infectious disease fell to 285 per 100,000 in 1930 when it was overtaken by heart disease and stroke, with 436. Except for pneumonia and influenza, which have retained fifth place, the contagious scourges yellow fever, smallpox, scarlet fever, cholera, diphtheria, typhus, typhoid, tetanus, tuberculosis, plague, poliomyelitis, whooping cough, measles, and meningitis can all be designated disappearing diseases. Although years of painstaking research are required to develop new vaccines, once marketed their use is simple and inexpensive. In terms of years of life saved, they outweigh all of our sophisticated technology by an overwhelming margin.

We cannot give antibiotics and immunization *all* the credit for this human salvage. Infections originating in the hospital (Chapter 6) still take their toll of research and hospital technicians. But typhoid and tuberculosis started their declines before specific vaccines and "miracle drugs" were developed. Poliomyelitis decreased before the introduction of the Salk and Sabin vaccines as did cervical cancer before the application of "Pap" smears. Natural increase in human resistance or decrease in aggressiveness of the bacteria or viruses, as well as sanitary disposal of wastes, may be of equal importance.

There are seven diseases for which vaccines are routinely administered in childhood in this country: diphtheria, measles, mumps, whooping cough, poliomyelitis, rubella and tetanus. In 1977, however, 20 million of the 50 million children under 15 lacked at least one dose of the recommended vaccine. That year, a $128 million nationwide Childhood Immunization Initiative was launched by HEW. The results are impressive. By 1980, 96% of children entering school were immunized against diphtheria, tetanus and whooping cough, measles, and rubella; 95% were vaccinated for poliomyelitis and 92% for mumps. These diseases were at or near record low levels in 1981. All 50 states require documented immunity as a condition of first entry into school. Only four cases of diphtheria and six of paralytic polio were identified in 1981, and all others showed substantial decreases from the previous year.

As always in medical intervention, we must consider the harm-benefit ratio in the application of prophylactic immunization to populations. There will always be unanticipated consequences and unfortunate accidents due to lapse in quality control. These lead to lurid anecdotes, exploited by self-promoting publicity seekers, which frighten the gullible public. Despite their evident benefit, which far exceeds their harm, adverse effects of vaccines, either dangerous or merely uncomfortable, will always furnish fuel to those who make a career of attacking advances in disease prevention for financial or ego-gratifying gain. All vaccines have some degree of risk attached, and most produce sore, swollen injection sites and mild transient fever. The ominous global population explosion is an iatrogenic consequence of mass immunization without countervailing contraception.

DPT (Diphtheria, Pertussis and Tetanus-Triple Shot Vaccine)

In April of 1982 there was a flurry of alarming telecasts that must have made millions of parents tremble with fear. Children were shown who had suffered brain damage resulting in convulsions and permanent retardation following DPT injection. But many children died of strangulation or heart failure caused by diphtheria, or pneumonia after having had pertussis (whooping cough). During the 1920s, hundreds of thousands of children in this country suffered from these diseases which caused thousands of deaths. Contagious disease hospitals were full and the population of schools was decimated during epidemics. During my overseas army service I observed several cases of diphtheria of the skin contracted by unimmunized young soldiers in North Africa, which resulted in fatal heart inflammation.

The main concern at present is with the pertussis portion of the triple vaccine. Because it is made up of the entire bacteria, no one yet knows which component causes immunity. Almost all American schoolchildren are vaccinated with this substance, which is 80% effective. In 1979, four Tennessee infants died within 24 hours and four others within a week of inoculation from the same lot of vaccine, prompting the state to halt its distribution. Cause and effect was not accurately established, because the age at which DPT is administered, between two and six months, is precisely the age at which the risk of sudden infant death syndrome is greatest. But, *the risk of disease is far greater than the risk of immunization*. This recurring theme must be emphasized lest children be left in limbo between injection and aggressive bacteria.

Hepatitis B (HB) Vaccine (Licensed by the FDA in 1982)

The CDC reports that 200,000 cases of HB occur in the U.S. each year, 50,000 with jaundice and 10,000 requiring hospitalization, at a cost of over $4.3 million weekly. Of these, 12,000 to 20,000 (6–10%) become carriers. There are 4,000 deaths from cirrhosis and 800 from liver cancer secondary to HB annually. There are 750,000 carriers in this country (.3%) and an estimated 200 million globally, especially in Africa and Asia. There the carrier rate is 10%–20% (30–60 times higher than that in the U.S.); and the most common cancer is that of the liver, 10 to 20 times greater per capita than in the U.S. Approval of the Hepatitis B Vaccine by the FDA thus marks an important milestone.

HB infections can cause more than hepatitis: serum sickness syndrome with rash, and arthritis, kidney, blood vessel and skin disease. These can be detected by tests for the Australia antigen (first found in the blood of an Australian aborigine), which is part of the HB vaccine. The vaccine is prepared from the blood of asymptomatic carriers whose blood contains the Australia antigen.

Safety tests were performed on chimpanzees and on over 4,000 human subjects. Among them were over 1,000 homosexual men, who are at high risk for HB infection. Ninety-six percent became immune after three doses in a 6-month period and not a single case of HB developed among them. Thus far only local tenderness and slight temperature elevations have been found in a minor percentage of those vaccinated. The test for susceptibility costs $10, 3 doses of vaccine $100. Booster shots may be required after five years.

HB vaccine is indicated for HB-susceptible persons. Dentists, oral surgeons and hygienists are at greatest risk. Others include patients on kidney dialysis, inmates of institutions for the mentally retarded, recipients of multiple transfusions, medical staff exposed to blood or its products, male homosexuals, sexual partners and children of carriers, and travellers, including military personnel, in areas where HB is highly prevalent.

A modified HB vaccine will be released in 1982. Used in combination with other drugs, it is now under study to determine its ability to eliminate the carrier state. This has great beneficial implications to the 800,000 carriers in the U.S. alone, especially for those medical and dental professionals whose careers are clouded by the threat of infecting patients.

Influenza Immunization—Preventing Pneumonia

Influenza in the U.S. has been relatively infrequent in 1981–82. Nevertheless, there have been several outbreaks in schools and nursing homes, totalling 200 cases. During the past December and January, 30 persons, or 25% of the aged residents of an Atlanta nursing home developed Asian influenza, with nine deaths among the unimmunized. No immunized residents died, and only 16% became ill. There were 12 cases of pneumonia, some of the influenzal (viral) type and others bacterial. Similar relative protection was demonstrated in later outbreaks. Authorities advise that all persons over 65, as well as those under 65 with chronic underlying illnesses, should have annual influenza vaccinations. But influenza may also occur in the young, demonstrated by an outbreak in an elementary school in Michigan in February of 1981, affecting 38 of 161 students and several siblings.

During the ill-fated immunization campaign by the government against swine flu in 1976, 10 of every million adults developed a 5% fatal paralytic skeletal disease, Guillain-Barré syndrome (GBS). A receptionist in a pediatric clinic had a sudden onset of disabling arthritis 10 days after her flu shot and has been bedridden 90% of the time. She has had both hips replaced by artificial joints and will require additional surgery on her knees, hands and ankles. The U.S. government was ordered by the court to award her $1.5 million.

GBS, which occurred 5–6 times more frequently in those vaccinated for influenza in 1976 than it did in the unvaccinated, has decreased in the recipients of the newer lots of influenza vaccine. Their risk was increased by only 4% in 1978–79 and is even lower now. The Congressional Office of Technology Assessment (OTA) reported in February of 1982 that the flu vaccine is inexpensive and effective and that during 1972–78, 150 million vaccinations were responsible for 13 million more years of life at a cost of $63 for each year. During this period, influenza caused 127,000 deaths and cost $2 billion for treatment. Only 22 million (20%) of U.S. adults now receive influenza vaccine each year. But the vaccine can cause temporary, dangerous overreactions to common medicines, such as those given for blood clots or asthma, by causing them to remain in the body longer. Several of those vaccinated suffered stomach hemorrhages, one after 12 stable years following aortic valve replacement and anti-clotting medication.

Pneumonia Vaccine for Everyone?

Pneumonia from all causes is the fifth largest killer in the U.S. With 3.2 million cases—50,000 of them fatal—accounting for 7 million hospital days and 24 million days of disability annually, a workable vaccine would be desirable. But we must distinguish viral and other pneumonias, which often follow influenza, from the less common pneumococcal pneumonia which can be primary or secondary to pneumococcal bacteremia. The incidence of pneumococcal pneumonia is probably in the range of one to two cases per 1,000 each year, or 200,000 to 400,000 in total. Despite antibiotics, it can be fatal in those weakened by chronic illness or old age. A vaccine was licensed by the FDA in 1977 after it was found effective in trials with South African gold miners, who are particularly susceptible. However, controversy exists regarding the benefit of the vaccine to those at highest risk in this country. The OTA does not believe there is enough evidence of general benefit, and it will be several years before enough data are amassed for a verdict to be reached. Except for children with sickle-cell anemia, diabetics, those with kidney or lung disease or cirrhosis of the liver, "There is no convincing evidence to support widespread immunization" even for chronically ill persons or those in nursing homes. Adverse reactions including weakness, muscle pains, headache, chills and fever, light sensitivity or nausea are rare and occur in one of 100,000 vaccinations.

Measles Vaccine (Attenuvax)

Measles, one of the most contagious of all infectious diseases, was expected to occur in all families in the past generation. Its serious complications, such as middle ear infection, pneumonia or encephalitis, are fatal in one of 3,000 cases. Along with smallpox, it was one of the destroyers of the susceptible American Indian and Polynesian populations. Before vaccine was available in 1963 over 400,000 cases were reported annually in the U.S. causing 364 deaths. Now its incidence has been reduced 99%, with only 3,000 cases recorded in 1981. Nevertheless, 423 school children who had been vaccinated contracted the disease, since there is a 5% failure rate. The live-but-weakened, egg-grown virus vaccine, administered at the age of 15 months, may cause flare-ups in children with tuberculosis. It should not be given to those who are known to be allergic or hypersensitive to chicken products or to the antibiotic, neomycin; pregnant women; and patients receiving steroids, irradiation or chemotherapy.

In approximately 130 million doses, encephalitis with mental retardation and/or impaired hearing has occurred 130 times. However, this reaction has not definitely been proven to be due to the vaccine. Encephalitis complicates natural measles 5 to 10 times more often.

Measles, Mumps and Rubella (German Measles) Virus Vaccine

This combined vaccine has the same complications as that for measles. There may also be transient sore throat, headache, fever, rash, swelling of the lymph nodes, parotid, and testicles, hemorrhagic spots over the skin, arthritis, and neuritis.

The importance of vaccinating children against rubella was demonstrated by the epidemic of 1964–65 which resulted in 20,000 infants with heart ailments, deafness, cataracts, and/or mental retardation (chronic rubella syndrome-CRS), and 30,000 stillbirths in the U.S. The cost of care has been estimated at $1.5 billion. Priority is given to preschool and school children to decrease the risk of exposure to the vaccine of a pregnant, non-immune female. By 1981 a record low of 2,000 cases of rubella was reported, mostly in young adults, down from 3,900 in 1980. But only a small minority of susceptible women have been vaccinated and an average of 39 CRS cases occurred each year between 1975–79. In Chicago alone, there were 31 cases of CRS in 1978 and 1979. None of these children's mothers had been vaccinated against the disease or had had prenatal screening, although a simple test is available to determine their immunity.

Poliomyelitis—The Dreaded Disabler

Poliovirus vaccines have been used since 1955. Although their benefit has been denied by some religious cults and dissenting doctors, they have dramatically decreased paralytic disease from 18,000 in 1954 to an annual average of less than 13 in 1973–1980. Most unvaccinated adults in the U.S. are immune, but some are not and have the slight risk of acquiring vaccine-associated poliomyelitis.

Oral Polio Vaccine (OPV), the product of years of research by Dr. Albert Sabin, was licensed in 1963 and rapidly supplanted the previous vaccine, which required injection. Over 95% of its recipients become immune. But OPV is a live virus and there is a remote risk that it will cause the disease it is intended to prevent. In the 12 years between 1969–1980, 290 million doses were given, resulting in 92 cases of paralysis (one in 3.2 million doses). Of these cases, 25 occurred in healthy recipients, 55 in healthy close contacts, and 12 in persons who had immune-deficient conditions. There is no way to predict which individuals will suffer this remote risk.

Inactivated Polio Vaccine (IPV), the fruit of Dr. Jonas Salk's investigations, was licensed in 1955. Four injections produce immunity in 95% of all recipients; 428 million doses were given in the U.S., mostly before 1962, when the Sabin OPV proved more convenient. When first used in 1955, before purification was perfected, a few polio cases (one in 37,000) resulted, but this has not recurred. An improved IPV, developed in Europe, has produced virtually 100% immunity after two doses. Serious complications have not occurred in the short period of its use. However, IPV contains traces of neomycin and streptomycin, and there is a remote possibility of hypersensitivity reactions to these antibiotics.

Smallpox Vaccination

In May of 1980, the World Health Organization declared that smallpox had been globally eradicated. The last case appeared in 1977. Smallpox vaccination of civilians is now indicated only for laboratory workers directly in contact with smallpox or related viruses. Military personnel are still being immunized because of the possibility of biological warfare.

Although routine pre-school smallpox vaccination in the U.S. ceased in 1971, 500,000 doses were distributed in 1980. Without evidence substantiating its benefit, it has been inappropriately used for treating shingles, and herpes of the lip and genitalia. In 1981, a California physician's license was revoked because he administered smallpox vaccine to a leukemia victim who also had herpes. The patient's vaccination site became swollen, his illness worsened and blisters appeared over many other areas. This complication (generalized vaccinia necrosum) occurs only in persons with underlying immunologic defects; it has a 20% fatality rate.

Brain damage due to post-vaccinial encephalitis occurs in two to six unlucky cases in each million vaccinations. Other rare iatrogenic events following smallpox vaccination are: inflammation of the spinal cord, generalized vaccinial blisters and rashes, infection of the vaccination sites, and accidental contraction of the disease, which has caused several cases of blindness when the eyes were involved. These mishaps may cause permanent disability or even death. The risk-benefit ratio has now shifted to favor elimination of vaccination except in special cases. What will occur in the future when the global population loses its immunity is a matter of speculation. Laboratory-maintained viruses must be held in maximum security to prevent accidental infection of a susceptible population.

The New Rabies Vaccine

Despite its infrequency, with only a few cases recorded in humans in the U.S. each year, rabies is one of the most feared of diseases. It is considered to be uniformly fatal, but a few cases have recovered after heroic anticonvulsive treatment. Most human and animal cases die after agonizing convulsions. Bats, however, may be healthy carriers. The biting animal may be observed for 10 days and, if not ill or dead by that time, the danger is believed to be over, but it is best to administer a single dose of human rabies immune globulin and daily doses of vaccine, before the results of animal confinement or new laboratory tests are known. If the animal shows no signs of illness or if tests are negative, the vaccine should be discontinued. The incubation period in humans is from 10 days to a year, averaging 30–50 days. Therefore, there will be time to build immunity, except in bites on the head.

Two types of vaccine have been available. One is made from ultraviolet-killed nerve tissue, the other is grown in duck embryos (DEV). The advantage of the latter is that it does not contain the factor which has caused occasionally fatal paralysis in recipients of the nerve vaccine. But it will often produce severe hives, breathing difficulty, cramps, nausea, vomiting, diarrhea, and rarely, shock, paralysis or brain damage (encephalitis). Although these vaccines are dangerous and uncomfortable, the decision to use them is based on the risk-benefit ratio. Up to 40% of persons bitten by a rabid animal will develop the disease, and serious iatrogenesis with the vaccine is less frequent or deadly than the infection in the unimmunized. Unfortunately, the vaccine must be given in 21 doses at different sites on the abdomen, lower back and thighs.

Persons at high risk include veterinarians, delivery people, spelunkers, and laboratory personnel working with rabies vaccine. These groups should receive preventive immunization before being bitten despite the slight risk of iatrogenic complications. A new intradermal vaccine has been developed and used on 1,500 people. Redness and swelling have been the only aftereffects. Because of the hazards and inconveniences associated with the use of the older vaccines, new agents have been developed from human cells—human diploid rabies vaccine (HDRV)—and rhesus monkey lung cells—rhesus diploid rabies vaccine (RDRV). RDRV is much less expensive and requires only two injections for immunization superior to that produced by DEV. Reactions are similar but less intense than those with DEV. Further tests using smaller doses with air-injection guns are now underway on members of the U.S. Army's Green Berets.

Tetanus

A dreaded complication of deep wounds, especially those received in manured battlefields, in burns, and in addicts, tetanus is easily prevented by DPT or toxoid vaccine. The World Health Organization estimates 500,000 annual deaths globally, overwhelmingly in undeveloped countries. The U.S. toll is now only about 60 cases per year, but the mortality rate approaches 50%. Clinical tetanus does not confer future immunity, therefore active immunization with toxoid is indicated for those who recover.

In January of 1982, a report from the U.S. Air Force showed that in over 700 recipients of tetanus toxoid, no serious complications occurred. Hypersensitivity responses, such as transient hives and wheezing, were mild. Even though it is probable that no person who ever received four doses of toxoid or DPT with boosters every ten years ever developed tetanus, additional toxoid and hyperimmune tetanus human globulin should be given immediately following any deep puncture wound. The instructions given with the preparation must be followed, since there are frequent changes with new advances.

14.

TRANSFUSIONS

Blood carries oxygen but does not (as was once thought) transmit personality, those physical or mental qualities which make us individuals. In the 17th century for example, it was speculated that blood from a mastiff, transfused into a bloodhound, would dilute the bloodhound's keen scent.

The classification of blood seemed simple, when, at the turn of the century it was discovered by a German-born American, Karl Landsteiner, that it could be divided into four groups: A, B, AB and O. But the Rh system, found in the early 1940s, and numerous other subgroups restored its complexity. Except for the Rh factor, most of these do not affect transfusion because their ability to cause reactions is very weak. The survival time of the transfused red cells in the recipient is all-important and depends on precise techniques of typing, matching and storage.

The prime indication for the transfusion of blood is anemia, which can be acute or chronic or secondary to accident or injury, with oxygen-deprivation in body tissues and a loss of blood volume producing shock. Whole (homologous) blood collected from donors in plastic bags and prevented from clotting by a small amount of anticoagulant is generally utilized. If large quantities are needed, packed red cells are preferred because twice as many can be given in an equal volume. In the process of concentrating the red cells, platelets, white cells, antihemorrhagic factors, albumin and plasma protein fractions can be obtained as by-products for special purposes. New developments include the freezing of blood, a difficult, expensive process which permits storage and shipment, and autologous blood, obtained from the recipient for later use and blood substitutes.

Since over 5 million transfusions, mostly of two or more units of blood, are administered annually from over 11 million donations of approximately a pint (500 ml), the iatrogenic effects amount to a substantial total. The use of blood is increasing because of the ease with which it is obtained.

IATROGENIC EFFECTS OF HOMOLOGOUS TRANSFUSIONS (From Donors)

Hemolytic Reactions

The dangers of infection with bacteria, HBV and NA/NBV have been discussed in Chapter 4 (Nosocomial Infections) and administrative, human and clerical errors were included in Chapter 7 (Hospitalitis). Mistakes in typing and cross-matching, can result in destruction of the donor's cells by antibodies present in the patient's plasma, and can cause serious or fatal (hemolytic) reactions. These reactions occur when the broken down cells and their released hemoglobin damage the kidneys and other organs. However, mishaps due to identification errors are far more common.

Although the American Association of Blood Banks, the FDA and the College of American Pathologists all require strict adherence to safety regulations for accreditation, mishaps due to mechanical and electrical breakdown and human error are inevitable. Failure of fail-safe procedures can involve the patient, the specimen drawn for typing and cross-matching with the donor blood, and the record of the transactions. The patient may not be correctly matched up with the blood sample, the report of its compatibility with the donors blood, the issuance of the blood from the refrigerator or finally, the administration of the transfusion.

> Wilbert Bronson, a 30-year-old barber, was given type B blood instead of A while under anesthesia for a back operation. Ten days later he died of a hemolytic reaction which caused deep jaundice and kidney failure.

The chain of events which may lead to mistaken identification begins with the admitting and floor clerks, and involves nurses, residents, attending physicians, operating room personnel and laboratory clerks and technicians. The wristband may have an incorrect or misspelled name. The age and sex listed may be erroneous. Patients with similar names may occupy the same or adjoining rooms. Problems may be compounded by language and hearing difficulties. A semiconscious patient mutters the name Joseph Smith and this is transcribed on his record and identification. Later it is discovered that Joseph Smith is a friend he had wanted to notify, but that his own name is Max Brown.

Despite mandatory disaster drills, when numerous casualties are received from a train, bus or aircraft accident, the emotional strain may cause personnel to mislabel specimens and patients' tags. The laboratory ceases all activity except that related to blood-banking, and some technicians engage in testing and recording processes with slackened skills from lack of practice. When a physician gives an oral order to a nurse because he cannot leave a patient, the nurse may in turn transmit a garbled requisition to the blood bank.

In extreme emergencies it may be necessary to give blood to patients in shock before completion of typing and crossmatching, which requires at least 15 minutes. Packed group O, Rh negative blood is used for this purpose. After the crossmatching is completed, group-specific cells may be used. But errors have occurred. Two of 44 fatal reactions reported between 1976 and 1978 resulted from blood being mistyped as O. If a person requires massive transfusion, i.e., 10 units of blood, he will have only about 28% of his original blood remaining. Therefore, the pretransfusion sample is no longer valid for additional crossmatching and new samples must be drawn for this purpose. Sensitization of a woman of childbearing age will cause new antibodies to develop in her blood, which may result in destruction of fetal blood during pregnancy.

Because patients with the same or similar names may be in the hospital at one time, wristband number identification may avoid tragedy. In 1968, two patients were admitted to a hospital at the same time with hip fractures on the same side, attended by the same physician, and born in the same month. Both required transfusions. But Ruth *Harris* Rogers was Rh positive and Ruth *Smith* Rogers was Rh negative.

The notoriously illegible handwriting of most doctors may be misinterpreted, but even the stamped addressograph print may be partially obliterated. The blood sample tubes may be wrongly labeled and interchanged. When serum is transferred to a second tube, another mix-up is risked. Multicopy forms and labels will not help if the original is incorrect.

The best patient identification is the wristband. But sometimes surgeons and anesthesiologists cut the band if it interferes with venipuncture and attach it to the bed or chart.

> An experienced blood-banker found that her hospital number was not on her wristband when a blood sample was being withdrawn for testing. She related that "the omission was corrected, but when she returned from surgery she found that her wristband had been cut and attached to the bed." Her surgeon was upset when she refused transfusion.
>
> Two men of the same age and ethnic origin with identical first, middle and last names were admitted to the same service of a Veterans hospital. Blood was ordered for both. Their hospital numbers were 429756 and 429956. Cursory examination of their wristbands failed to note the different 4th digit and a fatal reaction resulted.

The first report of a hemolytic (red cell destruction) reaction dates back to 1667. Because of many fatalities, it was not until blood groups were discovered that the use of blood in significant quantities became common. When typing and compatibility testing (cross-matching) made transfusion reasonably safe, its adverse effects were often overlooked.

The Mayo Clinic studied 47 hemolytic reactions in the transfusion of 268,000 units of blood during the 10 years between 1964 and 1973 (1 per

5,700). This was a 10-fold improvement over the collected experience of the previous 24 years, with 80 in 43,000, or 1 per 541. In all studies, females were at almost triple the risk of males because of obstetrical complications requiring more emergency transfusions with hasty, incomplete or absent crossmatches. The risk of sensitization by the fetus' blood adds to the odds of hemolysis. Older persons have more reactions because they are more likely to have been sensitized by previous transfusions. Surgical patients who need additional blood exceed those with medical conditions in exhibiting the early signs and symptoms of hemolysis; fever, chills, chest pain, nausea and low blood pressure may be masked by anesthesia.

Later untoward reactions were: diminution of urinary output with pink or brown discoloration, jaundice, anemia and failure of blood clotting. Eight, or 17% of the 47 patients with hemolytic reactions died, at a rate of one death in 33,500 units transfused. The improvement is spectacular considering that older studies showed a mortality rate from hemolytic reactions of 35% to 40%. Transfusion deaths reported in 1942 were one in 1,300; in 1953 they were one in 13,000. Twenty-four of the 47 reactions (51%) at the Mayo Clinic could be traced to one or more of the human errors previously described in the tortuous trial of transfering the blood from donor to patient.

An even more comprehensive 1981 British report of 44 deaths in 422,000 units showed that 72% were due to hemolytic reactions. The source of error was found in 38 cases: blood was given to the wrong patient in 17 cases, an administrative error occurred in nine, the wrong patient sample was tested in seven and a technical error occurred in four. In one case incompatible blood was given without testing. Recapitulating previous studies, over half the deaths (24) were due to failure to identify the patient or the blood sample, errors which are not correctible by computers.

In Vietnam it was found that one unit in 1,000 was mismatched by military blood banks, but the errors were rectified by retyping with automatic blood grouping apparatus before administration. These errors were not due to overworked technicians, since each performed only 40 blood grouping and matching tests daily.

The best prevention is reducing the use of blood transfusions without proper indications. Because of the ease with which blood is obtained, it is greatly overused, sometimes for cosmetic reasons. Medication containing iron would often serve as well.

Hospitals have organized committees to monitor transfusions, especially those in which only a single unit is used which the patient could dispense with in at least 70% of the cases. If blood is really needed, larger quantities are generally required.

Pseudo-Hemolytic Reactions: Many transfusion reactions caused by blood destruction are not due to incompatibility. The recipient cells can be disrupted by drugs, congenital cell fragility, infections, irrigation of the bladder by water, collections of blood in cavities or tissues (hematomas) or mechanical trauma from artificial heart valves or blood vessels. The donor cells will be weakened by freezing or overheating, mechanical trauma from heart-lung machines used in open heart surgery or bypass, infection, mixing with drugs, or aging.

Immunologic Reactions. Although reactions due to hemolysis are the most dangerous, other iatrogenesis may be caused by a newly discovered white cell clot-promoting particle or fluid-component protein imcompatibility. A survey of 70,000 transfusions in 13,000 recipients found adverse responses in 6.6% including fever, chills, allergy with hives, or other, more rare reactions. When an infant develops a febrile reaction it does not shiver, but may have diarrhea and refuse feedings. Herpes of the lips occurs infrequently.

Other Reactions. If large amounts of cold blood straight from the refrigerator are administered, the recipient's temperature may fall, causing cardiac arrest in debilitated patients. The blood is usually kept from clotting by the addition of a small amount of citrate solution. In massive transfusions the citrate will inactivate the blood calcium and increase the chances of cardiac arrest, especially in patients with liver disease.

Particulate and Foreign Material. Despite filtration, small clumps of white cells and platelets may enter the recipient's blood and, if in large quantities, may damage the lungs. Small amounts of air from the plastic tubing are harmless, but larger amounts from glass bottles (no longer used) were once a hazard.

Damage to Veins. If the needle or catheter remains in place over 12 hours, inflammation and clotting will occur which not only destroy the usefulness of the vein for further blood or fluids but may also cause a dangerous infection (septic thrombophlebitis) with bacteremia.

Pyrogens. Even if bacteria are destroyed by sterilization, the dead organisms or their chemical products remaining in tubing or its connections may cause mild fever, which lasts a few hours and has no permanent adverse effects. Disposable plastic equipment has greatly reduced this problem.

Transmission of Disease

Malaria: Bertha Dodds, a 65-year-old sufferer from cardiac valve disease, had never left the U.S. In 1978, she had open heart surgery during which eight units of blood were utilized. Recovery was uneventful and she was discharged in two weeks. At home, she became mentally confused, lost her appetite and vomited several times. She returned to the hospital three days after discharge. Malarial parasites were unexpectedly found in her blood smear. She did not respond to standard antimalarial drugs, but recovered after exchange transfusion with over five quarts of blood plus additional antimalarial agents. The records of the blood bank revealed that one of the donors of the blood administered during surgery had come from Ghana six years previously. Although he gave no history of malaria at the time of donation, further questioning elicited a history of possible malaria during his childhood and a flu-like illness after a trip to Ghana in 1977. His blood was positive for malarial antibodies.

Up to 1975, less than one case of malaria in each million transfusions was diagnosed in the U.S., discounting the Vietnam war years (1967 to 1972). The donor in Mrs. Dodds case was eligible according to the standards of the AABB and the Red Cross, which require a waiting period of six months after a visit to a malarial area. But 3-month-old, prematurely born, Stephen McDonald, who received several transfusions after his birth in Boston, developed anemia in 1982 and also had malarial parasites in his blood. None of his donors had malaria and none had been in a malaria-infested country recently. However, malaria may remain dormant in the human body for many years.

A review of 2,000 cases of transfusion-acquired malaria, predominantly in tropical countries, revealed that the great majority of cases had been contracted from blood stored less than five days, but in rare instances, blood stored over two weeks. Because there has been a recent resurgence of malaria in parts of the world where it had been controlled, there is need for a reevaluation of standards for donors.

Syphilis: Forty years ago, transfusion-acquired syphilis was a serious problem because blood was transferred directly to the patient. Now all donors are tested and spirochetes carrying syphilis do not survive storage temperatures 4–6°C. However, the reactive factor (reagin) is transferred and in the unlikely event that it is present in the donor's plasma, the recipient may have a positive test for as long as 20 days.

Cytomegalovirus (CMV): This virus causes serious varieties of pneumonia, hepatitis and infectious mononucleosis, especially after multiple transfusions; these occur most often in heart but occasionally in other surgery, in infants, in organ transplants or in patients undergoing chemotherapy for cancer. A San Francisco hospital had five cases in nine months in non-cardiac surgery. Nine other cases were found in the literature. The risk of CMV infection, which is usually manifested first by fever three or more weeks after any surgery, increases proportionately with the number of transfusions given.

Iron Overload: When hundreds of transfusions are given over a period of years, as in the chronic anemias which occur in Mediterranean people, iron will be deposited in most parts of the body and can result in liver and heart failure, which may be fatal.

Wastage of Blood: Once blood is crossmatched for a specific recipient it is reserved for that person and cannot be used for other patients. The reserved period varies from 24 to 48 hours. If not used it may become outdated and must be discarded at considerable loss of time and money. Many elective operations, such as plastic and orthopedic procedures, which seldom require transfusion, could dispense with crossmatching, which sometimes requires four or more times the number of units actually used. The crossmatching could be delayed until it is actually needed. It is generally considered that an acceptable ratio of crossmatching to actual use should be no more than 2.5/1. This would reduce inventory problems, the risk of misidentification, loss of technicians' time and overall costs.

AUTOLOGOUS TRANSFUSION—Resurrecting an Old Art
(This literally means transfusing oneself; homologous transfusion is from other persons)

Autologous Transfusion During Operations

The first effective transfusion ever recorded was performed in 1818 in England. The crude technique of returning blood to a patient was sometimes performed during massive operative bleeding into the abdominal cavity or during amputations. The blood was merely sponged, ladled or caught into a container, filtered, and reinfused into a vein. Although it was successful and lifesaving in several circumstances, it was not used in the U.S. until 1917. Because of the primitive apparatus, complications and hazards included breakdown of blood, generalizing blood clotting and fat and air bubbles in small vessels. As blood became more easily available and safer with wartime organization in the early 1940s, the art disappeared. However, in the 1960s, because of expense and renewed awareness of complications, it seemed reasonable to recycle blood shed in surgery or trauma back into the patient without risking incompatibility or hepatitis or requiring expensive storage with the chance of misidentification. This technique is acceptable to groups like Jehovah's Witnesses who do not permit the use of homologous blood (from others). Several commercially marketed devices are available. The state of the art is not yet perfect—trauma to the cells induces blood breakdown, loss of platelets and blood clotting components, and the risk of fatal air bubbles when the blood is reintroduced under pressure—but improvements may be expected as demand increases.

The reinfusion of shed blood is unwise when the wound is contaminated, since bacteremia may occur. Malignant cells may also be disseminated. It is also undesirable in severe brain or multiple traumatic injuries where the anticoagulant may promote further bleeding. Well-trained technicians are required and for economic feasibility, at least two units of blood must be recoverable.

Preoperative donation and storage: A practical method of avoiding many complications is the donation of one's own blood for future use. The blood is processed in the usual manner although the patient need not meet all the standards of the AABB unless the surgery is cancelled and the blood is to be used for another recipient. Most healthy people will replenish a unit of blood in 72 hours to a week as the bone marrow is stimulated into action.

Typing and crossmatching are unnecessary, although often performed to prevent misidentification. The risk of acquiring a new disease and other reactions is eliminated. It is interesting that many surgeons in my acquaintance who do not take time to explain this seemingly paradoxical procedure to patients awaiting elective surgery insist on using autologous blood for their own families. It is particularly suitable for young, healthy persons requiring orthopedic or plastic surgery, or other operations such as hysterectomies or mastectomies for benign conditions and for pregnant women or patients with CAD. Because new preservatives permit a 35-day shelf-life, patients can deposit up to five units of blood by weekly donations, the last not less than three days before surgery. Many hundreds of autologous transfusions amounting to almost 85% of the requirements for plastic and orthopedic procedures, 50% of heart and blood vessel operations and a third of patients undergoing bypass, have been successfully administered in various centers, with reduced complications.

If the surgery can be delayed, the blood can be stored in a frozen state for up to three years. Anyone can in theory keep a six-pack or more of blood for oneself to be used if needed later, but the expense is great and organized facilities for this purpose are not generally available. Other shortcomings are: the usual delays in acceptance of unaccustomed procedures; the unwillingness of physicians to spend extra professional time in explanations and in getting informed consent; the additional paperwork, the labeling of blood FOR AUTOLOGOUS USE ONLY; and the anxiety of patients.

Sometimes, in spite of all precautions, patients who have predeposited their own blood are still given blood from other donors because of communication failures. Laboratory or clerical errors can occur just as with homologous blood. Another difficulty arises when there is last-minute cancellation of surgery when the blood is nearing its expiration date. Unless suitable for another patient, it must be discarded, adding to expense. These difficulties should be overcome as its advantages, which far outweigh its disadvantages, become manifest and as technology improves.

Danger to Donors

Although the public is urged to contribute blood and receive satisfaction from helping others as well as the self-benefit of receiving a return if needed, donations are not entirely without risk. Most common is a transitory fainting reaction, probably psychogenic and occurring predominantly in first-time donors. If frequent contributions are made, iron stores will be depleted before the simple hemoglobin test shows a fall, mostly in women, with secondary anemia resulting. Air embolism, for which there was a real risk when blood was collected in glass bottles, is no longer a danger with the use of plastic bags. Accidental puncture of an artery will cause leakage of blood into the surrounding tissues and the possibility of damage to the arterial wall.

A procedure called leukapheresis is used 50,000 times annually in the U.S. to obtain white blood cells (leucocytes). These are separated from the red cells and given to patients whose leucocytes have been depleted in certain leukemias receiving chemotherapy and marrow deficiencies, risking serious infection and bacteremia. The leucocytes are also used in the manufacture of interferon.

After the white cells are separated, the red cells and plasma are returned to the donors, who may undergo the procedure frequently because they are paid or are helping to prolong the life of a family member. The FDA found that 5.5% of donors suffered adverse reactions, many of which are not associated with other blood donations. The blood is spun in a centrifuge to separate the leucocytes; it can result in blood cell breakdown or air bubbles. A citrate solution may be added to the blood to prevent clotting before it is returned and can cause fever, chills, strange sensations (paresthesias) about the mouth and a feeling of tension. Other facilities use heparin to prevent clotting which may cause more serious symptoms. One donor in four experiences fatigue for several days following the procedure. Chills, nausea and vomiting, and lower abdominal pain have been reported in varying percentages.

Leucocyte Transfusions

If a patient is expected to recover from depletion of leucocytes with bacteremia because of restoration of bone marrow function, leucocyte transfusions may improve the chances of survival. But if the marrow is permanently destroyed, the procedure is useless. Increased temperature will result in 5% to 40% of these procedures. Pulmonary distress is more serious but less common, manifested by wheezing, cough, fluid in the lungs and areas of x-ray density. When this complication occurs, the transfusion must be discontinued. Another indication is anemia due to bone marrow failure or cancer chemotherapy. Leukocyte transfusion would add 11% to the hospital bill of the average leukemia patient and cost $18 million nationally.

Platelet Transfusions

These clot-promoting particles are concentrated by an intricate process and are indicated whenever a patient has an extremely low platelet count and is actively bleeding. The defect of continued transfusions of platelet concentrates is that the patient will eventually fail to respond. Severe headache and low white cell count may occur with the usual risks of viral infections.

Bone Marrow Transplantation

Since marrow is removed by needle and syringe suction from various spaces in the pelvic bones, passed through screens and after mixing with an anticoagulant, given to the patient intravenously, it is really a transfusion. The cells pass through the lungs and enter the marrow cavities via the blood stream. It has been used in over a thousand patients who have leukemia or aplastic anemia. Immunosuppressants must be given, as with all transplants, and chemotherapy and total body radiation added. Rejection occurs less often than with solid organ transplants.

At the University of Washington Medical School in Seattle, out of 26 patients with acute leukemia who obtained marrow from identical twins, six (24%) are alive and free of the disease after 5 years; 110 patients received marrow from non-twins with 14 survivors (13%). A major cause of complications was a syndrome called graft-versus-host disease (GVHD) with skin, liver and intestinal involvement. Recurrence of leukemia occurred in most cases but there was significant improvement in duration of survival. The use of cyclosporin A has reduced rejection.

A 1981 report of 24 children with acute leukemia showed encouraging progress. Five years after marrow transplantation, 11 were alive and apparently free of the disease, compared with two out of 21 utilizing chemotherapy alone. In their struggle, 20% developed life threatening GVHD with skin rashes and liver involvement. Others had brain damage and/or cataracts. But apparent cure in a previously incurable disease is a good portent for future progress.

Substitutes for Blood

The many hazards and the time consumed in obtaining, typing, matching, storing and administration of blood and the tragic results of inevitable misidentification have cried out for an oxygen-carrying stable substitute applicable to all recipients.

Fluosol: Several years ago the Green Cross Company of Japan developed this teflon-like substance which has the property of transporting and releasing oxygen. Unattractively resembling skim milk, it is an emulsion of minute particles of varying size in a liquid medium. In 1978, one of its originators, Dr. Ryoichi Naito, received a small injection with no adverse effects. Later, a man having severe bleeding after prostate surgery was given Fluosol and since then over 500 Japanese patients have received the substance.

The disadvantages of Fluosol are that its effects last only 72 hours and it lacks the clot-promoting, infection-fighting and immunologic qualities of natural blood. It is stored in the frozen state and its shelf-life is not known. The inevitable iatrogenic effects have not yet made their appearance, but will eventually after use on thousands of recipients. Biopsies have shown that it creates a foreign body reaction causing large, fat-laden cells to form in the liver tissue.

The FDA permits only eight pints for a single recipient. In 1982, a Jehovah's Witness was badly injured in an auto accident from which his wife died after refusing a blood transfusion. He received eight pints of Fluosol but needed more circulatory support and the court approved the request of his doctors to give him additional whole blood since he had five children depending on him for support.

Hemoglobin: This compound is the actual oxygen carrier of blood. It is produced from stale red cells, carries oxygen and is now under experimental animal investigation in cases of shock due to hemorrhage. In crystalline form it can be stored for years and in liquid solution, cold or frozen, for 18 to 24 months. Its chief advantages are that it can be produced from outdated blood which would otherwise be discarded at great economic loss and needs no typing or crossmatching, thus avoiding reactions due to misidentification. However, it can carry Hepatitis B virus and its other possibly iatrogenic effects await its release by the FDA for human use.

15.

DIALYSIS

In the early 1960s, when dialysis began to be applied to patients whose kidneys had failed, it was hailed as a humane, heroic and dramatic life-saving procedure. Dialysis was preferable to the then-often unsuccessful kidney transplants which were followed by the death of 40% of patients within a year. Blood from the patient's arm vein was circulated through an artificial kidney apparatus that removed accumulated toxic substances. The blood was then returned to another vein to recirculate through the body. At that time the cost was $40,000 per year for each patient. Facilities were insufficient to match the demand and anonymous committees were formed to decide who would live and who would die.

When the Senate passed an amendment to the Social Security bill in 1972 extending Medicare coverage to patients with kidney failure, a new era began. The End Stage Renal Disease program (ESRD) has changed the character of the dialysis population. In 1972, the average age of the people under treatment was between 37 and 43, with less than 20% over 50. Most had little wrong with them apart from their kidney failure and could be rehabilitated to lead productive lives at a total cost of $250 million. It seemed futile for the elderly and very sick to undergo dialysis. The program now reaches over 50,000 people and costs the nation over $1.2 billion dollars. The annual increase since 1972 has been 5,000 to 6,000 each year with no sign of a leveling-off at a stable number. Although many patients are alive who would have died of kidney disease, they are often far from well.

There are great differences among western European countries and the U.S. in the number of patients per capita who are on dialysis programs, varying from six to 144 per million population in Europe, compared to over 205 per million in the U.S. Socioeconomic factors are more important than medical considerations, since the most affluent countries (and states in the U.S.) have the largest numbers of patients under treatment.

Rehabilitation efforts vary according to the policy of the dialysis center. In an Ohio facility, only one of 40 patients was working. Dr. Richard Rettig, Senior Social Scientist of the Rand Corporation, who has been investigating dialysis centers, recalls, "This patient said that the other patients found it amazing to think that it was possible to return to work." Another center, in Washington, D.C. discouraged rehabilitation when they moved the starting time from 7:00 to 5:30 P.M., not allowing many patients time to get there from work. It had originally been envisaged during the senatorial debate in 1972, that most ESRD patients would be productive if they received dialysis.

Physicians and psychologists who have observed patients find that many are hypochondriacal and depressed. They feel that they are prisoners of the medical profession and linked to a robot by an umbilical cord. Their suicide rate is seven times the national average. Some deliberately miss appointments and fail to follow the strict low sodium, low potassium and low fluid regimen dialysis requires. Others use more direct methods. Before the ESRD program, most patients expected to die but were young and had positive attitudes toward life.

Normal lives are impossible for patients on dialysis. If they do not comply with their prescribed diet, chemical imbalances develop, with extreme weight gain, nausea, cramps, diarrhea and weakness. But even if the patients follow directions, they become anemic, develop a rise in blood pressure and fragile bones, and are often impotent. Their schedules are disrupted by the lengthy 4-hour, 3-times-weekly sessions. Although a few patients can be dialysed at home with the help of a trained aide, friend or family member, most must go to central facilities owned privately or by corporations. As it is very difficult to switch to other centers, they become dependent on the doctors and staff, whom they are afraid to offend with complaints since they feel their lives depend on the good will of those who serve them.

A recent published survey by doctors at Duke University School of Medicine found that half of the dialysis patients in the U.S. were not working and were less happy and more debilitated than expected. One in five was unable to lead an independent existence.

The government, which pays for the ESRD program, does not adequately monitor the quality of care, although its agencies maintain quantitative data on the number of transfusions, hospitalizations and complications each patient undergoes annually. The U.S. is the only country in which a system has developed for dialysing terminally ill or incompetent patients. This has disturbed many kidney specialists and aides concerned with the program. The Act of Congress authorizing ESRD has made it legally and morally difficult to reject even vegetative subjects, who are not even considered for dialysis in England and other countries.

Ethical impasses to dialysis are presented by patients who have severe, incurable, chronic diseases in addition to kidney failure. These include victims of widespread cancer, heart failure and blind, depressed diabetics. But no one wants the government to be God-like in deciding who shall live and who shall die. In my opinion, it is time for doctors and patients to act on the realization that not everything is curable or even treatable.

The ethical and moral implications concerning dialysis permit no easy answer. According to Dr. Bernard Adelman, a kidney specialist at Northwestern University Medical School, "The final decision about the care of this patient must come not from the vote of a committee . . . not from the dictates of governmental policy, board or directive, no matter how compelling the economics, but rather from the I-thou relationship of a physician with his patient."

Survival on hemodialysis meets with environmental and iatrogenic obstacles, although half of all young adults can be maintained for 10 to 20 years. Two percent will die of a human error accident every 10 years, but as technique improves, an increase in over-20-year survivals is happening. The principal causes of death are coronary artery disease and infection. With hundred of liters of water circulating through the apparatus, some may ooze into the blood stream carrying calcium, magnesium, copper, fluorine, sodium, zinc, cadmium and other elements which will be concentrated in the blood because of deficient kidney excretion. Aluminum in excess concentration has caused brain damage (encephalopathy), with speech difficulty, hallucinations and dementia. Twenty-one university-associated centers reported an average illness episode rate of 4% between 1972 and 1978, sometimes accompanied by softening of the bones with spontaneous rib and pelvic fractures. A single Chicago center suffered an outbreak affecting 20 persons. This may occur less often, since aluminum is now removed by deionization, although the effectiveness of deionization has not been proven. Organic and plastic particles from the tubing, as well as silicones, lodge in the liver and can cause cirrhosis-like scarring, many with clinical evidence of liver disease. Formaldehyde, used to sterilize component parts of the equipment, will also find its way into the blood stream and will be toxic to body cells. Numerous gastrointestinal disorders have recently been noted, particularly colitis, with occasional perforation, ulcers and diverticulitis.

The most common infection in long-term hemodialysis is hepatitis. Studies by the Center for Disease Control from 1975 through 1978 showed that 55% of patients and 34% of the staff were infected in 78% of the centers. Strict isolation procedures resulted in a decrease in incidence. Up to this writing, we have no figures on the effect of the newly approved HBV vaccine, but it will probably be a partial solution. When patients discover that they harbor HBV in addition to having renal failure, they may react more negatively to the hepatitis than to their kidney disease. Many experience leper-like alienation. Others deny the added illness and fail to take measures to protect contacts. When tested, up to 60% of family members are found to harbor HBV.

Cases of viral inflammation of the membranes surrounding the heart (pericardium) have appeared in patients undergoing hemodialysis.This may cause scarring and adhesion of the pericardial layers, impeding the heart's pumping action and requiring pericardiectomy, a dangerous operation. Five such cases occurred in several weeks at the Veterans Administration Hospital in Washington, D.C.

There is an increased tendency to bleed during dialysis because of platelet abnormalities and anticoagulants introduced through the circulating blood. Blood and clots can occur over the brain, in the stomach or intestine, the pericardial sac, the eye, the soft tissues and muscles of the back, the pleura, the liver, and the space between the lungs and heart (mediastinum), causing severe shortness of breath.

A comprehensive study of 154 children, aged one to 16, on the ESRD program showed an incidence of 1.6 per million population in this age group. Although complications similar to those described for adults occurred, they were fewer in number, and dialysis was more frequently terminated by successful renal transplantation (see Chapter 11).

Home treatment can be accomplished by continuous ambulatory peritoneal dialysis (CAPD), in which fluid is circulated into and out of the abdominal cavity through a permanently implanted catheter. The many square yards of intestinal covering serve as a membrane through which toxic wastes are removed. The process is not as efficient as machine hemodialysis and is subject to the same iatrogenic effects as abdominal taps, with peritonitis predominating (see Chapter 10). Other problems include loss of body protein and excess accumulation of sugar and fats, creating a diabetes-like condition, severe itching, anemia, bone disease and impotence. Only an unknown percentage of scrupulously careful patients can successfully accomplish CAPD. Nevertheless, its use is increasing.

Machine hemodialysis can also be done at home, but costly questions regarding the reimbursement of aides, the training of family members as assistants, and maintenance arise. There are also, as with CAPD, psychological problems with spouses and other family members.

The dilemmas of dialysis remind us that the ancient Greeks enshrined the attributes of man and nature and the human predicament in the myths of the Gods. Hubris—the arrogant defiance of fate ordained by Zeus—led to punishment by the Goddess Nemesis who exacted revenge on anyone who upset the balance; like Prometheus, who, consumed by pity for the sad lives of humans, stole fire from heaven to brighten their lot. For this defiance he was chained to a rock. During the day, his liver was eaten by an eagle and it regenerated during the night. Nemesis has demanded retribution from every nation of the ancient and modern world, when hubris exceeded humility. Iatrogenesis is our retribution.

16.

REDUCING THE RISK OF IATROGENESIS

"The only thing necessary for the triumph of evil is for good men to do nothing."

—Edmund Burke

A lessening of adverse effects has been suggested in the preceding chapters describing various medical and surgical interventions. This chapter summarizes the state of the art of protection from iatrogenesis, the epidemic of modern medicine. This is not an easy task for the consumer, who is subjected to the overpowering and too often dehumanizing routines of the medical citadel which we have permitted or even eagerly invited to dominate our lives. We have abdicated our individual responsibilities in preventing disease and learning about our most precious possession, our bodies.

An intelligent businesswoman complained to me recently about pain, weakness, numbness and tingling in both hands. Although I am not an expert in skeletal or nerve disease, it seemed very likely that Louise had "carpal tunnel syndrome," a condition in which the nerve supplying the hand is compressed by a narrowing of the bony canal through which it passes, closely crowded by tendons which flex the fingers. I recommended an orthopedic surgeon whom I thought competent. Dr. Lakey released the constricting ligament to decompress the nerve and she is now free of symptoms. But Louise hadn't the ghost of an idea of what was happening to her wrist or why the minor surgery was necessary, although the anatomical relationships are simple and easily understood by looking at a diagram. Although there were no adverse effects, I am sure she would have a better idea of what was wrong if her sailboat, car, or Mixmaster malfunctioned than she had about her own supporting structure. Despite all cautions about informed consent, she did not understand the doctor's brief, hurried explanation.

Another example of how difficult it is for most people to absorb medical information is the memory of a television program about hospital infections in April of 1982, based on the data assembled in Chapter 6.

During this telecast, I made three separate appearances, and experts from the CDC as well as surviving victims of nosocomial infections were interviewed. Only one of a number of acquaintances had any recollection of the important subject matter which seemed unable to reach to the grassroots level.

When a patient signs an informed consent form prior to operation or invasive procedure, he or she is sick, worried and anxious. It is less probable that he would understand all the hazards possible than would a person who is well and alert. The physician must take time to explain to the patient or family exactly what risks and benefits may be expected.

Most people think that surgery presents the greatest risk of iatrogenesis. But with powerful new drugs, life-support systems and invasive procedures, internal medicine in diagnosis and treatment may be more hazardous because more patients are involved. There are many risks that must be taken on the basis of *probability* of benefit—without any guarantees. No doctor can have complete knowledge or experience about all the possible results of treatment of a given disease. This was illustrated by the many case reports of new complications of illnesses that have been treated for years with approved standard methods, as in the recent discovery that the deadly Reyes syndrome may be associated with aspirin usage. It is now potentially dangerous for patient and doctor to tell a mother to give her child an aspirin and "call me tomorrow."

THE DOCTORS' DILEMMA

Although the new generation of doctors are better trained than their fathers, they have not had time nor will they ever have the opportunity to acquire experience of the natural, untreated course of many prolonged, remittent and/or self-limited diseases. Varieties of pneumonia, anemia, tuberculosis and indolent malignancies and many diseases of muscle and supporting soft tissues may *not* require drastic drug therapy with inevitable adverse effects.

The thousands of choices available in diagnosis or therapy cannot all be juggled simultaneously, since the human brain can handle only five to seven ideas at one time. Computers are being programmed to store, analyze and return to the clinician information on myriads of possibilities, forestalling the likelihood that a doctor may overlook possible complications of a disease or its treatment and thus delay correction. Short courses of a week or less are offered in many centers on utilization of a new invasive or operative procedure. After completion of such quickie training, the doctor may rashly use the new information or method on his patients, even though his theoretical knowledge exceeds his experience and deftness. Even when skill is acquired in the use of an invasive procedure such as cardiac catheterization, diagnostic and therapeutic enthusiasm may cause the doctor to overestimate its applicability and effectiveness and underestimate the risk of adverse effects.

The aging of the patient population poses new problems. Doctors are trained to find a single underlying cause for a patient's illness and to treat it vigorously. But geriatric patients often have multiple disorders and are more fragile and more likely to experience iatrogenesis when multiple and sometimes incompatible diagnostic and therapeutic agents are used. These high-cost users of medical care constitute 13% of in-patients with complex illnesses, but occupy 50% of hospital facilities and consume most of the U.S. medical services.

Geriatric medicine has been a much neglected specialty in this country and will require rejuvenation as demand increases. Most of its efforts will be expended on the management—mostly palliation—of unpreventable, incurable or untreatable disease. While the major causes of death in the middle and later years, heart disease and stroke, have been drastically reduced since the 1960s, other infirmities of the aged, especially cancer and bone and joint disease, will need care if not cure.

Most doctors are trained in crisis care of established illnesses. But to reduce iatrogenesis, major medical efforts must be diverted to prevention by reducing risk factors promoting premature development of atherosclerosis, with its major manifestations of CAD and stroke; cirrhosis of the liver; cancers of the lung, skin, liver, large bowel, breast and uterus; pneumonia; and accidents—all major and common killers. Too much time and too many funds are spent on researching the diagnosis and treatment of obscure and uncommon diseases which affect only a small percentage of the population, and in improving the care of hopeless terminal cases. The problem is that the benefits of prevention may not be manifested for 20 or 30 years, while the patient must be weaned from deeply entrenched pleasurable habits.

One of the most difficult dilemmas confronting a doctor is determining the validity of a new diagnostic, surgical or medical procedure. The new is not necessarily better than the old. The best way to find out is through a controlled clinical trial, comparing the old with the new in terms of patient benefit, after-effects, risks, and cost. This method is often lengthy and expensive as well as inconclusive. Only after a procedure or medication is used on thousands of patients for many years will all of the iatrogenic effects be exposed. When prisoners or mental defectives are used for this purpose, ethical and moral considerations also arise.

For example, the value of coronary artery bypass, 130,000 of which are done annually in the U.S. at a cost of $2 billion, is still being argued. At an NIH-sponsored conference in 1981, a panel of medical and surgical cardiologists, economists, statisticians and philosophers debated the indications, preparations, morbidity and mortality after surgery of CABP and its long-term effect on the quality of life. They concluded that CABP is a major advance in the treatment of coronary artery disease, with the caveat that it is not indicated in every case, and that there are different expectations for different degrees of arterial narrowing along with the number and positions of the arteries affected. The NIH has organized similar conferences on breast cancer screening and chemotherapy of malignant disease.

It is an apparent paradox that, on the whole, more iatrogenic events occur in the largest and most specialized centers than in the smaller but well organized community hospitals. But it is obvious that the most difficult, unusual, and hard-to-manage medical and surgical cases are referred to these institutions. Proprietary hospitals operated for profit are accused of "cream-skimming," meaning that they try to exclude very sick patients who are liable to have life-threatening and costly complications or fatal outcomes. This gives them the specious reputation of obtaining better *statistical* results.

What is the patient's good? In discussing ethical dilemmas in the care of the ill, Leon R. Kass, M.D., PhD., of the Committee on Social Thought of the University of Chicago argues that physicians should: "Keep their eye on their main business, restoring and correcting what can be corrected and restored, always acknowledging that death will and must come, that health is a mortal good, and that as embodied beings we are fragile beings that must snap sooner or later, medicine or no medicine. To keep the strings in tune, not to stretch them out of shape attempting to make them last forever, is the doctor's primary and proper goal."

In terminal cases, the first thought of the doctor should not be "will this intervention prolong life," but "will it increase or decrease the patient's pain, discomfort and suffering?" In practical terms the doctor should have the courage to withhold intravenous medication, antibiotics and artificial resuscitation while administering whatever narcotics are necessary to achieve relief even at the risk of depressing respiration. To make these judgments requires wisdom obtained only by long experience, which is not teachable in medical schools.

THE CONSUMER'S ROLE IN REDUCING IATROGENESIS

By definition, iatrogenesis is caused by doctors, medical personnel or hospitals. It logically follows that the less you have to do with them the less risk you run of adverse effects. This means that you must assume as much control of your health as possible, while avoiding the risk factors. Although some iatrogenesis is inevitable, its risks can be decreased.

But you will need a doctor and a hospital sooner or later.

How do you choose a doctor? Do you need a family physician (or "primary care specialist")? One can never be sure that the best choice has been made, but as in all medical matters, a calculated risk must be taken, considering those factors which should yield a better chance of obtaining a proficient, honest and humane doctor. He too may be a victim of our vast expanding medical-industrial establishment, for he must conform to its mores.

When ill, choose a specialty board-certified internist and for your children under 16, a certified pediatrician unless you live in a small village or rural area where a primary care (or family) physician is the only one available. If you know a doctor or registered nurse, find out from whom they or their families receive their medical care. Professionals are more likely to have reliable information regarding proficiency than are gossipy neighbors. If not, you can find your doctor's training and qualifications in the Directory of Medical Specialists or the American Medical Directory, available in public libraries.

At one time it was to be expected that a graduate of a prestigious medical school such as one of the "Ivy League" schools in the East, Johns Hopkins in the South, the University of Chicago or Washington University in St. Louis in the Midwest, or Stanford in the West would have a superior endowment of talent. This is no longer necessarily true, since curricula and qualifications are standardized. More important is the hospital in which your doctor spent his residency—where he was actually prepared for independent practice.

Again there is no certainty, but a teaching hospital affiliated with a medical school and offering approved residencies in many specialties is most likely to offer good training. The past few years have witnessed greater emphasis on the human and interpersonal aspects of the doctor-patient relationship. Directories of hospitals offering such training are also available at public libraries. Do not be influenced by scary articles or half-true books. You are looking for competence, and the selective process of the best hospitals in choosing their house staff is more likely to obtain intelligent young men who will work hard to perfect their skills.

Eighty percent or more of disorders are self-limited or not improvable by any intervention. In only 10% will the doctor's ministrations cause improvement; the final 9 or 10% will end with serious iatrogenic problems because of wrong treatment or bad luck. Therefore, the doctor's efforts are important in under 20% of his cases, but in these they may make the difference between life and death, as well as ensure good quality of life without iatrogenesis. Skill and intelligence do make a difference in many touch-and-go, life-threatening illnesses and operations. (Do not be misled by rumors from neighbors: Some physicians with the best public relations and reputations may actually be charlatans or relative incompetents.)

Your new doctor should not be too young or old. If over 60 he may retire while you still need help, but will be able to transfer you to the care of a competent younger man. Avoid pompous doctors who convey the impression of God-like certainty. You should be asked to participate in decisions about your care. If difficult choices must be made or doubt exists about the diagnosis, are you informed and is a second opinion sought by you welcomed or resented? In uncertain cases the doctor should not wait for you to ask for another consultant but should originate the request.

How do you relate as a person to your doctor? Does he treat you warmly and unhurriedly, as a human being with problems other than the ailment for which you consult him rather than as a composite of separate organs? Does he appear tired and irritable from overwork or personal problems? Too many physicians are impaired by strain and tension which they try to relieve by drugs and alcohol. Is the office suite like an assembly line in which the doctor flits from patient to patient in numerous examining rooms, often interrupted and distracted by phone calls while you wait in exasperation? This annoyance is generally due to poor scheduling by the office staff or by taking on more patients than can be handled. Good medical care takes time, concentration and close attention to details. Are you left bored and shivering, on a cold examination table, covered only by a thin sheet instead of a blanket while your examination is delayed? This could raise your blood pressure. The doctor should explain what is found on examination. If he does not, ask. If you don't understand why surgery is proposed or what it is expected to correct, a diagram of the anatomy should be drawn or shown from a textbook. The doctor sets the tone for his office staff. You should be greeted courteously and feel that they care about you. The staff should also answer your questions fully.

Practical matters like accessibility, parking, transportation and the efficiency of the doctor's scheduling should be considered. The closest competent doctor will save you travel time and traffic annoyances and permit house calls when necessary. Does the doctor set an example by maintaining his own health and fitness? Avoid doctors who imply, "Do as I say, not as I do." Does he take time to advise you about preventing disease, inquiring about your health habits, lifestyle, diet, exercise, smoking and drinking, as well as your occupational hazards? Find out who covers him when he is on vacation or out of town and check the surrogate's credentials carefully.

If you develop a specific condition such as a urologic or orthopedic disorder, your internist will be able to refer you to a competent specialist. Do not take anything for granted. Make sure the new expert has credentials from an approved residency program and has been certified by his specialty board. DO NOT BE AFRAID TO ASK if you do not see the certificate displayed in the office. Ask your doctors about their hospital staff memberships and privileges. The kind of hospital where you would like to be treated for common procedures which cannot be done on an outpatient basis, such as appendectomies, mastectomies, cholecystectomies, some hernia repairs, are the well-run, fully accredited, smaller community hospitals, preferably close to your home. Large teaching hospitals will bring you a plague of unnecessary examinations by medical students and residents who tend to overorder expensive, fruitless and sometimes risky, diagnostic tests. That is why these larger hospitals are more expensive. You are also paying for the upkeep of the residents and for research projects which may not be covered by government grants. Of course, if you are to undergo open-heart or brain surgery, you will have to accept these annoyances, common to specialized teaching hospitals. I hope readers will not consider me chauvinistic when I advise them to go to hospitals staffed primarily by American residents. Experience has taught us that the best-trained young American doctors are admitted to hospitals of the highest caliber. Those of lesser reputation must select less desirable, foreign, possibly non-English-speaking and inferiorly trained residents. This is not prejudice but a fact of (your) life.

Unless you are unconscious because of an auto or other accident, do not let yourself be taken to a city or state institution. You should remember that these have the highest infection rates and the most incompetent paramedical personnel. If you should be so unfortunate as to be taken there by the police while helpless, insist on being transferred as soon as possible to your doctor's community-run hospital, which may not be free of all dehumanizing influences but is bound to give better personalized care. (Stab wounds of the heart are a probable exception because most inner-city hospitals have teams alerted for such violence.) Your doctor will know where you should be transferred if specialized treatment is needed for orthopedic rehabilitation, massive burns, transplants, or open-heart surgery, all of which must be concentrated in larger teaching hospitals.

An increasing number of procedures are now being done on an outpatient basis and you must insist that your surgery be "in-and-out" whenever possible. You will not only save money but also reduce your risk of infection and other iatrogenesis. If you must enter a hospital, do not be awed by its overpowering environment. Make sure that all preliminary tests are done prior to admission in line with your intention to spend as little time in the hospital as possible. When multiple tests are ordered requiring blood to be drawn from a vein, ask about their absolute necessity, and insist that samples be obtained no more than once daily unless you are being monitored for constantly changing chemistry (as in insulin-dependent diabetes).

If you are otherwise healthy, but are to have pelvic, abdominal, orthopedic or other local surgery, try to refuse multiphasic chemical screening, the routine chest x-ray exam and EKGs. You may not succeed, as these procedures may be mandated by staff bylaws, and it is not advisable to leave the hospital for this reason. But you will add your voice to those who object to useless, costly mumbo-jumbo and hasten the revocation of obsolete regulations.

Object firmly, preferably in writing, if you are awakened at 5 A.M. to be weighed, or if at any time you are awakened to be given a sleeping pill or sedative (this actually happens). Many nurses may be inexperienced trainees, unsure of themselves and capable of making mistakes in dispensing medication. *Know what you are being given and why.*

Do not permit major surgery like mastectomy to be done on the basis of a diagnosis obtained solely by frozen section while you are under anesthesia. This will prevent anguish when on awakening you find that a breast or limb has been summarily removed. Sometimes many less-than clear slides must be prepared to evaluate your problem (usually a tumor). This is one of the few instances in which I advocate spending an extra day in the hospital awaiting the more definitive diagnosis which should be available next morning from the pathologist's examination of permanent paraffin sections.

Do not allow yourself to be given single unit blood transfusions. If you really need blood, two or more units will be necessary. And know your blood type so you can check the label on the blood bag. Remember the horror stories you have read of patients being given the wrong blood type with fatal consequences!

When your surgical wound is healing and you have recovered from the initial postoperative weakness, or when maximum hospital benefit is reached in medical conditions, insist on being discharged. Your recuperation will be enhanced at home. Every extra day you remain exposes you to additional risk as well as cost. If for any reason, especially on weekends or holidays, you feel your discharge is being unnecessarily delayed while you require no further hospital treatment, use discretion in signing yourself out against medical advice.

If you feel you were not treated properly by any staff member, it is not only your right but your duty to send a letter of complaint to the administrator or executive vice-president of the facility. This will stimulate better quality control and improve training in personal relations. Conversely, if you were given tender loving care over and above routine duty, a letter of appreciation would be most welcome.

Although I have not discussed drug reactions at length in this book because they have been published in other volumes and the information is readily available by consulting the Physicians' Desk Reference, they constitute the majority of iatrogenic events. Question your physician about dosage, timing, and interactions with other drugs, and explain any previous drug or allergic reactions you or your family members may have experienced. If you are pregnant, avoid all drugs except in life-threatening conditions.

Finally, scrutinize your bill carefully and insist on an itemized account. Because of their special understanding, most doctors find errors when they are hospitalized. Tests and medication that were never performed or administered are frequently charged for. Your insurance does not cover everything and even if it did, excess costs come out of the pockets of all of us.

You have legitimate privileges embodied in the "Patient's Bill of Rights." Although these have not been officially codified, most are recognized by law.

THE PATIENT'S BILL OF RIGHTS

You are entitled to:

1. Impartial access to needed treatment including hospitalization regardless of race, creed, national origin, age, or source of payment.

2. Not be subjected to malpractice—procedures of doubtful validity performed by a physician untrained or inept in their application or impaired by illness, alcoholism or drugs.

3. *Informed* consent—a reasonable amount of information regarding nature, purpose and risk in any procedure—even if you don't ask for it. The decision to intervene should be made by you on the basis of understanding this.

4. Knowledge of who is personally responsible for your care if it is shared by several physicians.

5. Communication with those responsible for your care.

6. Diagnosis and prognosis given with candor in understandable language.

7. Reasonable privacy while hospitalized; your consent should be obtained if you are the subject of teaching rounds.

8. Confidence in the provider of your care or be permitted to change to a different doctor.

9. Not be subjected to experimentation without consent.

10. Continuity of care by the same physician or group.

11. If of sound mind, freedom to leave the facility, even if the bill has not been paid.

12. Not be discharged except on criteria established by your doctor regarding maximum hospital benefit.

13. Access to information in your medical record. After all, you own this information.

14. A bill for services to be seen and itemized on request.

Although the principles of this Bill of Rights seem straightforward, some elements have engendered controversy. What is informed consent? Although it guards individual rights, can all patients really understand their condition? And do they all really *want* to be told? Many will inwardly deny that the risks apply to them. Patients generally read or have a document read to them, but the disclosure is couched in general terms. All the details cannot be explained.

A study recently made regarding angiography risks showed that only one-third of patients really wished to be informed. Over a quarter were made more uncomfortable by learning of the hazards, and this produced fear and anxiety which may be detrimental to success. There was also incomplete recollection of the information four to six months after surgery. Despite attempts to avoid technical wording, the specialized medical language is too complex for most people. In many cases when patients are very ill, the decision to proceed must be made by proxies—family or friends.

Diagnosis and prognosis should be given with candor and with judgment. Must this right be modified? The doctor often does not know the true diagnosis, nor can the outcome always be predicted. The most prestigious physicians, backed by the resources of renowned centers, will inevitably make mistakes. We have seen how records may even be switched and patients misidentified. But will the art of communication with candor have a harmful or beneficial effect on management of the disease? Are not some physicians so obsessed by the fear of malpractice litigation that they tell *too much*? No generally applicable rules can be made. The wise doctor should impart to each patient, as gently as possible, information which will aid cure or improve the quality of remaining life. Remissions are always possible and spontaneous cures, although rare, have been recorded.

The distinguished Norman Cousins, who survived an undiagnosed but supposedly fatal disease, said, "There are two parts to every serious illness. One is the illness itself. The other is the panic it produces. The illness and panic are in a state of ominous interaction. Panic adds acute stress to existing disease. Anything that impairs the usefulness of treatment—including truth-telling—ought to be avoided or appropriately modified."

When a doctor rashly misinforms a patient that he has cancer of the prostate, his entire family is needlessly inflicted with anguish. But even if the truth is unequivocably known, the manner in which it is presented can have important effects.

> During my residency it was the hospital's policy to have blood counts performed on all its junior medical staff. I was in the laboratory when a technician audibly gasped, "Oh my God! Dr. Darrow has leukemia!" I rushed to her microscope and confirmed the presence of the cancerous cells. The chief pathologist immediately verified my diagnosis. We were now faced with the question of what to do? Morgan Darrow was one of our most intelligent, hardworking and popular interns. Only now did we consider that he had recently appeared slightly pale and tired, which was attributed to overwork. We had a conference with the administrator and the chief of medicine and decided that under the circumstances it would be best to tell him nothing because treatment at this stage would be futile, and he was about to enjoy a month's vacation as a ship's surgeon. We thought it would be most humane to let Morgan have a period of happiness before symptoms demanded intervention. Although the hospital personnel all knew, the doctor left for his vacation and it was not until almost a year later that increasing weakness, enlargement of his spleen and lymph nodes, with joint hemorrhages required full disclosure and palliative treatment. It is unlikely that this extension of quality of life would be possible today because of the threat of a malpractice suit.

In fatal diseases the physician is obliged to treat the patient, not with intent to save life but to make the last weeks, months or years as comfortable as possible. Remembering that will to live, hope, and confidence in the doctor are important factors influencing the patient's ability to relish the life remaining, it seems reasonable to impart or omit whatever information will aid this end. It is known by anthropologists that people can die if they violate a taboo against tribal mores and that voodoo actually kills because the victim strongly believes that it will. Modern doctors can use the will to live as a tool enhancing meaningful survival. A hopeless prognosis can jeopardize this effort. It is unfortunate that information designed to thwart malpractice litigation may protect the physician but harm the patient.

Morale is most important in helping the patient cope with his final battle. The truth ought to be told at a time and in a manner that will ease the path into infinity.

The patient's Bill of Rights must be supplemented by an obligation to avoid risk factors which increase the chance of needing medical care or of being hospitalized with all the iatrogenesis-promoting hazards. Eating sensibly; avoiding tobacco; moderation in the use of alcohol; exercising regularly; sleeping seven or eight hours nightly; and keeping weight within normal limits are all part of a rational lifestyle within human control despite peer group pressures. Studies have shown that the average health of persons who observe these practices is the same at 70 as that of persons 35 to 44 who did not. Virtually universal insurance spreads the cost of voluntarily acquired illness upon the entire community. We need a new ethical code requiring that all of us assume responsibility for reducing heart disease, cancer, stroke, accidents and cirrhosis, our leading and most costly causes of diminishable disease and death.

BIBLIOGRAPHY

Chapter 1

Spain, D.M. Complications of Modern Medical Practices. New York, Grune and Stratton, 1963.

Gregg, A. Challenges to Contemporary Medicine. New York, Columbia University Press, 1956.

Illich, I. Medical Nemesis. London, Calder and Boyars, 1974.

Carlson, R. The End of Medicine. New York, John Wiley and Sons, 1975.

Mendelsohn, R. Confessions of a Medical Heretic. Chicago, Contemporary Books, 1979.

Morbidity and Mortality Weekly Report. Leading Causes of Death, September, 1981.

Chicago Sun-Times. April 27, 1982.

Chicago Tribune. October 10, 1981.

Thomas, L. *In* Dorsey, D.: Dissertation on Riding Tigers. CAP Bulletin:167, March, 1978.

Rang, M. The Ulysses Syndrome. Canadian Medical Association Journal 106:122, 1972.

Hardison, J. The Sky is Falling. American Journal of Medicine 68:163, 1980.

Curtier, T. Bibliography of Oliver W. Holmes. New York, University Press, 1853.

Thorup, O. Jefferson's Admonition. Mayo Clinic Proceedings, March, 1972.

Slaughter, F. Conquest of Childbed Fever. New York, Collier Books, 1961.

Moliere, J. Le Medicin Malgre Lui; L'Amour Medicin, 1666.

Thaddeus, V. Voltaire, Genius of Mockery, 1928.

Cluff, L. Clinical Problems with Drugs. Philadelphia, W.B. Saunders, 1975.

Crile, G. A New Look at Biopsy of the Breast. American Journal of Surgery 126:117, July, 1973.

Codman, E. The Product of a Hospital. Surgery, Gynecology and Obstetrics, 1914.

Luft. Should Operations be Regionalized? New England Journal of Medicine 302:996, 1980.

Barr, D. Hazards of Modern Diagnosis and Therapy - The Price We Pay. Journal of the American Medical Association 159:1452, December, 1955.

Schimmel, E. Hazards of Hospitalization. Archives of Internal Medicine 60:10, 1964.

Seidl, L. Adverse Drug Reactions. Bulletin of the Johns Hopkins Hospital 119:299, 1966.

Thorup, O. Mayo Clinic Proceedings, 1971.

Mulroy, R. Iatrogenic Disease in General Practise. British Medical Journal 2:407, May, 1973.

Couch, N. Cost of Mishaps in Colonic Surgery. American Journal of Surgery 135:641, 1978.

Couch, N. Surgical Mishaps. New England Journal of Medicine: 304, 1981.

Steele, K. Iatrogenic Illness in General Medical Service. *Ibid.* 304:639, 1981.

Vaisrub, S. Probing for Causes. Archives of Internal Medicine 139:397, April, 1979.

Morgan, P. The Periodic Health Examination. Canadian Med. Assn. Journal 121:1161, 1979.

American Medical News, December 4, 1981.
Romm, F. The Periodic Health Exam. Southern Medical Journal 74:265, 1981.
Roe, B. The UCR Boondoggle. New England Journal of Medicine 305:41, 1981.

Chapter 2

Grand Rounds. Northwestern University Medical School, July 16, 1978.
Charap, M. The Periodic Health Examination: Genesis of a Myth. Annals of Internal Medicine 95:933, 1981.
Fletcher, S. Canadian Task Force Approach to Periodic Health Examinations. *Ibid.* 92:253, 1980.
Schor, S. Evaluation of the Periodic Health Examination. *Ibid.* 61:999, 1964.
Spark, R. The Case Against Regular Physicals. New York Times Magazine, July 25, 1976.
Fries, J. Take Care of Yourself. Reading, Mass., Addison-Wesley, 1975.
TIME. July 26, 1976.
Morgan, K. The Annual Fiasco. Medical Journal of Australia 2:923, 1969.
III World Congress for Cervical Pathology. Obstetrics and Gynecology Survey 34:781, 1979.
Caspi, E. Malignancy in Jewish Women. Israel Journal of Medical Science 13:299, 1977.
Walton, R. Cervical Cancer Screening Programs. Canadian Medical Journal 114:1003, 1976.
Gardner, J. Preventive Medicine, December, 1977.
TIME. Flap about Pap. November 13, 1978.
American Cancer Society. Cancer Related Checkup 30:195, 1980.
Coppleson, L. Prevention of Carcinoma of the Cervix. American Journal of Obstetrics and Gynecology 125:153, 1976.
Medical World News. Volume 20, May 30, 1977.
Medical World News. Pound of Prevention—Ounce of Cure? May 15, 1978.
Wall Street Journal. February 26, 1980.
Olsen, D. Multiphasic Screening. New England Journal of Medicine 294:925, 1976.
Delbanco, T. The Periodic Health Examination. Annals of Internal Medicine 92:251, 1980.
Rubenstein, L. Baseline EKGs. Journal of the American Medical Association 246:1770, 1981.
White, P. Half a Century of Running. New England Journal of Medicine 265:988, 1961.
Alsofrom, J. Kenneth Cooper—Aerobics. American Medical News, Volume 17, Aug. 25, 1978.
Paffenbarger, R. Physical Activity. American Journal of Epidemiology 108:161, 1978.
Morris, J. Vigourous Exercise in Leisure Time. Lancet, 1207, December 1980.
Redwood, D. The ST Segment During Exercise. Circulation 54:703, 1976.
McHenry, P. Abnormal Exercise EKG-False Positives. American Journal of Cardiology 47:1152, 1981.
Bruce, R. Exercise Tolerance Test. New England Journal of Medicine 306:1112, 1982.
Harell, F. Evaluating Medical Tests. Journal of the American Medical Association 247:2543, 1982.

Noakes, T. Coronary Atherosclerosis in Marathon Runners. New England Journal of Medicine 301:86, 1979.

American Medical News. 1981.

American Medical Association Council on Scientific Affairs: Exercise Test. Journal of the American Medical Association 246:1015, 1981.

American Medical News. Volume 7, January 16, 1978.

Bruce, R. Exercise Tolerance Test. New England Journal of Medicine 306:1112, May, 1982.

American Medical News. 1981.

Brand, D. X-rays in Musculoskeletal Trauma. New England Journal of Medicine 306: 333, 1982.

Farnsworth, P. Routine Pre-op X-rays. Journal of the American Medical Association 244:582, 1980.

American Heart Association Cookbook. New York, David McKay Company, 1980.

Boucet, K. Is Curable Lung Cancer Detected by Semiannual Screening? Journal of the American Medical Association 224:1361, 1973.

Gifford, R. A Bit of Heresy. Archives of Internal Medicine 138:1207, 1978.

Bartha, G. Routine Chest X-ray and EKG. *Ibid.*:1211, 1978.

American Medical News. March 12, 1982. *In* Colloquium, March, 1982.

American Cancer Society. Breast Cancer Incidence. Cancer, Volume 32, 1982.

National Cancer Institute. Lung Cancer Mortality. Journal of the American Medical Association 241:1582, 1979.

American Cancer Society. Pregnancy and Breast Cancer. Cancer Abstracts 23:180, 1973.

American Cancer Society. Breast Cancer Detection. Cancer 28:182, 1978.

Bailar, J. Mammography. Annals of Internal Medicine 84:77, 1976.

American Cancer Society. Minimal Breast Cancer. Cancer 28:144, 1978.

Mahoney, L. Mammography. New England Journal of Medicine 302:60, 1980.

Foster, R. Self-Examination Practices. New England Journal of Medicine 299:265, 1978.

Greenwald, P. Breast Self-Examination. *Ibid.*:271, 1978.

Yonemoto, R. Breast Cancer in Japan and U.S. Archives of Surgery 115:1056, 1980.

Robbins, S. and R. Cotran. Pathologic Basis of Disease. New York, W.B. Saunders, 1979, p. 1257.

American Cancer Society. Risk Factors for Breast Cancer. Cancer 30:276, 1980.

American Cancer Society. Incidence of Colonic Cancer. Cancer, Volume 31, 1981.

Burkitt, D. Colonic Cancer Epidemiology. Journal of the American Medical Association 231:617, 1975.

Kurnick, J. Colorectal Cancer Detection. Journal of the American Medical Association 243:2056, 1980.

Greegor, D. Colorectal Cancer. *Ibid.* 245:571, 1981.

Fowler, D. *Ibid.*

Kurnick, J. Colorectal Cancer. Journal of the American Medical Association 246:1772, 1981.

American Medical News. February 16, 1979.

TIME. Volume 57, August 31, 1981.

TIME: Dying Autopsy. Volume 90, September 18, 1978.

Roberts, W. The Autopsy. New England Journal of Medicine 299:332, 1978.

Bloom, M. Second Thoughts on Continuing Medical Education. Medical World News, Volume 53, November 12, 1979.
Grubb, A. Hospital Education and Training. Hospitals 55:75, 1981.
Berg, A. Continuing Medical Education. Journal of Family Practice 816:1171, 1979.
American Medical News. Volume 17, December 18, 1981.
James, J. Impact of the Medical Malpractice Slowdown in Los Angeles. American Journal of Public Health 69:437, 1979.
Curran, W. Retaliatory Actions in Malpractice. New England Journal of Medicine 304:211, 1981.
Golin, C. Malpractice Crisis. American Medical News April 28, 1978.
Malpractice Rates Hurting Patients. Council of American Physicians Bulletin, Volume 349, June, 1977.
Hines, W. Medi-Fraud. Chicago Sun-Times, February 8, 1981.
O'Connor, P. *Ibid.* October 4, 1981.
Rowan, C. *Ibid.* April 2, 1982.
Council of American Physicians Bulletin. Volume 287, May, 1981.
Natof, H. Ambulatory Surgery. Journal of the American Medical Association 244:1116, 1980.
American Medical News. October 23, 1981.
Fraumeni, J. Cancer Among Nuns. Journal of the National Cancer Institute 42:455, March, 1968.
Chicago Tribune. January 3, 1975.
Phillips, L. Emergency Room Skull Radiography. Health, Education and Welfare Department Publication 78–806, July, 1978.
Frame, P. O.P. I.V. Antibiotic Therapy. JAMA 248:356, 1982.

Chapter 3

American Cancer Society. Radiation and Cancer. November, 1980.
College of American Pathologists. February 1980.
Warren, S. The Pathology of Ionizing Radiation. Bioastronautics Data Book (2nd Ed.) Washington, D.C., 1973.
Chicago Sun-Times. March 23, 1978. (FDA report)
Family Health, January, 1981.
Committee on Biological Effects of Radiation: Exposure to Low Levels of Radiation. Washington, D.C., National Academy Press, 1980.
Forrest, J. Radiologic Errors. Western Journal of Medicine 134:485, 1981.
Rachmaninoff, N. Tumors of the Skin Following Irradiation. American Journal of Clinical Pathology 36:427, 1961.
Bross, I. Risks from Diagnostic Radiation. American Journal of Public Health. 109:130, 1979.
Hopkins News. June, 1981.
Griffiths, J. and Ballantine, R. Silent Slaughter. Chicago, Henry Regnery, 1972.
Goffman, J. Radiation and Human Health. San Francisco, Sierra Club, 1981.
Swartz, H. Radiation Exposure for Pregnant Women. Journal of the American Medical Association 239:1907, 1978.
Duffy, B. Cancer of the Thyroid in Children. Journal of Clinical Endocrinology 10:1296, 1950.
Carroll, R. Thyroid Cancer. Journal of the National Cancer Institute 33:277, 1964.

Dunlap, C. Effects of Radiation. *In* Anderson, W.: Pathology, 5th Ed. St. Louis, C.V. Mosby, 1966.
McGregor, D. Cancer Among Atomic Bomb Survivors. Journal of the National Cancer Institute. 59:799, 1977.
Rachmaninoff, N. Sarcoma Following Irradiation. American Journal of Clinical Pathology. 36:427, 1961.
Physicians' Desk Reference for Radiology. 1979.
Weatherby, R. Postradiation Sarcoma of the Bone. American Journal of Clinical Pathology. 77:237, 1982.
Kern, W. Postirradiation Malignant Histiocytoma. *Ibid.* 76:126, 1981.
Shehata, W. *Ibid.* Illustrated Medical Journal. 159:107, 1981.
Robinowitz, M. Coronary Artery Disease in Young Women Irradiated for Breast Carcinoma. American Journal of Clinical Pathology 77:246, 1982.
Hessel, S. Complications of Angiography. Radiology. 138:273, 1981.
Eisenburg, R. Renal Failure After Angiography. American Journal of Medicine. 66:43, 1980.
Paulin, S. Coronary Arteriography. New England Journal of Medicine 305:223, 1981.
Steel, K. *Ibid.*
Meyers, M. and Ghahremani, G. Iatrogenic Gastrointestinal Complications. New York, Springer-Verlag, 1981.
Felson, B. Radiologist on the Rocks. Seminars in Roentogenology 4:361, 1973.
Mendeloff, J. Granulomatous Reaction to Barium. American Journal of Clinical Pathology. 26:155, 1956.
Stacey, J. Killed by the CAT. American Medical News 13: October 23, 1981.
American Medical News. CT Scanners Praised. November 27, 1981.
Compty, M. Acute Renal Failure with CAT Enhancement. Journal of the American Medical Association 246:1366, 1981.
Byrd, L. CT-Induced Acute Renal Failure. Archives of Internal Medicine 139:491, 1979.
Mitchell, A. Risks to Children from CT Premedication. Journal of the American Medical Association 247:2385, 1982.

Chapter 4

American Medical News. February 19, 1982, p. 14.
TIME. November 2, 1981, p. 94.
White, P. Nutrition, a Medical, Political and Public Issue. Journal of the American Medical Association 241:1407, 1979.
Fortune. December 14, 1981, p. 48.
Chicago Sun-Times (Parade). January 17, 1982, p. 32.
TIME. January 23, 1982, p. 50.
Callaway, W. Obesity, A "Culture-Bound" Syndrome. Mayo Clinic Proceedings. 57:327, 1982.
Blackburn, G. Recent Advances in Obesity Research. London, Newman Publications, 1975.
Berland, T. Consumer Guide. Diets '79, pp. 6, 27, 112.
Lantgua, R. Cardiac Arrythmias Associated with Liquid Protein Diet. New England Journal of Medicine 303:735, 1980.

Crosby, W. Improving Iron Nutrition. Western Journal of Medicine. 122:499, 1975.
Olsson, K. Preclinical Hemochromatosis in a Population on a high-Iron Fortified Diet. Journal of the American Medical Association 239:1999, 1978.
Finegold, M. Total Parenteral Alimentation. American Journal of Clinical Pathology 77:378, 1982.
DeWys, W. Enteral and Parenteral Nutrition. Journal of the American Medical Association 246:1725, 1981.
American Medical News, April 2, 1982.
Dunkerly, R. Gastrointestinal Disorders—The Role of Diet. Postgraduate Medicine 59:182, 1976.
Spellberg, M. Cancer of the Colon in Jews. International Congress of Gastroenterology. *In* Chicago Tribune, January 3, 1975.
Ballin, J. Fallacy and Hazard—Human Gonadotropic Hormone. Journal of the American Medical Association 230:693, 1974.
Rivlin, R. Therapy of Obesity with Hormones. New England Journal of Medicine 292:26, 1975.
Stare, F. The Save Your Life Diet. Chicago Tribune, July 30, 1978, p. 32 (Living).
Ibid. The Atkins Diet, p. 3.
American Medical News. October 21, 1980.
Lucas, A. "Pigging Out." Journal of the American Medical Association 247:82, 1982.
Gunby, P. Physical Changes in Runners. Journal of the American Medical Association 245:547, 1981.
American Medical News. Delayed Menarche Linked to Athletics. October 2, 1981, p. 13.
Chicago Sun-Times. Take the Stairs. January 12, 1979, p. 16.
LaPorta, M. Elevation of CPK after Exercise. Journal of the American Medical Association 239:2685, 1978.
Haycock, C. Exercise and the Cardiovascular System. Journal of the American Medical Association 247:2985, 1982.
Priest, J. Exercise-Induced Changes in Laboratory Tests. American Journal of Clinical Pathology 77:285, 1982.
Solomon, J. "Abnormal" Laboratory Results in Runners. Journal of the American Medical Association 241:2262, 1979.
Brenner, A. Portable Face Mask in Exercise-Induced Asthma. Journal of the American Medical Association 244:2106, 1980.
Gibbons, L. The Acute Cardiac Risk of Strenuous Exercise. Journal of the American Medical Association 244:1799, 1980.
Carruthers, M. Safe Sport. Lancet 1:447, 1975.
TIME. Does Running Avert Coronaries? October 6, 1981, p. 104.
American Medical News. Running Alters HDL Levels. April 2, 1982.
Jones, R. Mortality of Joggers. Journal of the American Medical Association 247:2569, 1982.

Chapter 5

Schmahl, D. Iatrogenic Carcinogenesis. New York, Springer-Verlag, 1977.
Health and Human Services. Second Annual Report on Carcinogens. April 30, 1982.
Farber, E. Chemical Carcinogenesis. New England Journal of Medicine 305:1379, 1981.

Preger, L. Induced Disease. New York, Grune and Stratton, 1980.
Noller, K. Exposure to DES. Mayo Clinic Proceedings 56:577, 1981.
American Medical News. April 11, 1979.
Yodaiken, R. Formaldehyde Toxicity. Journal of the American Medical Association 246:1677, 1981.
National Institutes of Health. Dilantin During Pregnancy—Neuroblastomas. Journal of the American Medical Association 239:1849, 1978.
Hoover, R. Saccharin—Bitter Aftertaste. New England Journal of Medicine 302:573, 1980.
Gunby, P. Cancer—Good News—Bad News. Journal of the American Medical Association, 243:1789, 1980.
National Cancer Institute. As reported in the Chicago Tribune, December 2, 1981.
Sontag, S. Illness as Metaphor. New York, Farrar, Strauss, Giroux, 1977.
Morbidity and Mortality Weekly Report. Vital Statistics, Annual Summary, 1980. September, 1981.
Thomas, L. The Big C. New York Review of Books, November 9, 1978.
Kiely, J. Antineoplastic Agents. Mayo Clinic Proceedings 56:384, 1981.
Gup, T. and Neumann, J. Cancer. Chicago Sun-Times, October 25–27, 1981.
Theiss, J. Cancer Drugs. Journal of the American Medical Association 247:11, 1982.
Hellerstein, D. Cures that Kill. Harper's, December, 1980, p. 20.
Rubins, J. Non-Hodgkin's Lymphoma Following Treatment for Hodgkin's Disease. American Journal of Clinical Pathology 74:696, 1980.
Susskind, D. Teen-Agers with Bone Cancer. Public Broadcasting System, October 13, 1981.
Henderson, C. Adriamycin and the Heart. New England Journal of Medicine 300:310, 1979.
Young, R. Antineoplastic Drugs. New England Journal of Medicine 305:139, 1981.
Epstein, S. The Politics of Cancer. San Francisco, Sierra Club Books, 1978.
National Institutes of Health. Chemotherapy's Negative Aspects. Journal of the American Medical Association 244:1084, 1980.
Goldberg, R. Depression in . . . Advanced Cancer. Journal of the American Medical Association 246:373, 1981.
Dorsey, D. Science and Technology as Ritual. Pathologist 127: March, 1982.
D'Angio, G. Costs of Cure of Children's Cancer. Hospital Practice, November, 1980.
Goldberg, I. Nervous System Effects of Cancer Therapy. Journal of the American Medical Association 47:1437, 1982.
Cohn, K. Chemotherapy from Insider's Viewpoint. Lancet 8299:1006, 1982.
Chicago Sun-Times. Interferon. November 24, 1981.
American Medical News. Interferon. April 2, 1982, p. 12.
Shottenfield, D. Cancer Risks of Medical Treatment Cancer 32:258, October, 1982.
Frei, E. The National Cancer Chemotherapy Program. Science 217:600, 1982.
Riecken, H. Informed Consent to Biomedical Research, JAMA 248:344, 1982.

Chapter 6

Chicago Sun-Times. March 3, 1982.
Feingold, D. Hospital Acquired Infections. New England Journal of Medicine 283:1384, 1970.
Rogers, D. Changing Pattern of Microbial Disease. *Ibid.* 261:677, 1959.

Thoburn, R. Infections Acquired by Hospitalized Patients. Archives of Internal Medicine 121:1, 1968.

Maranto, G. Hospital Sleuths. Johns Hopkins Magazine 35: June, 1981.

Allen, J. Trends in Nosocomial Infection. American Journal of Medicine 76:389, 1981.

Remington, J. Please Don't Eat the Salads. New England Journal of Medicine 304:433, 1981.

Albert, R. Chicago Sun-Times 23: June 11, 1981.

Givens, C. Catheter-Associated Urinary Infections. Journal of Urology 124:646, 1980.

Platt, R. Mortality Associated with Nosocomial Urinary Tract Infection. NEJM 307:637, 1982.

Hunt, T. Surgical Wound Infections. American Journal of Medicine 70:712, 1981.

Ehrenkranz, N. *Ibid.*:909.

MMWR. 31:16, 1982.

LaForce, F. Hospital Acquired Pneumonias. *Ibid.*:664.

Cross, A. Respiratory Devices in Nosocomial Pneumonia. *Ibid.*:661.

England, A. Nosocomial Legionellosis. *Ibid.*:707.

Stamm, W. and Bennett, J. Nosocomial Infections. *In* Communicable and Infectious Diseases. St. Louis, C.V. Mosby, 1981.

Maki, D. Nosocomial Bacteremia. American Journal of Medicine 70:719, 1981.

Maki, D. Nationwide Epidemic of Septicemia Caused by Contaminated IV Products. *Ibid.* 60:471, 1976.

Smith, I. Afebrile Septicemia. JAMA 248:1502, 1982.

Morbidity and Mortality Weekly Report. Nosocomial Bacteremias Associated with IV Fluid: 20, 1971.

Werner, M. Biohazards in the Laboratory. Medical Laboratory Observer: 81, July, 1981.

Klein, J. Infections in Hospital Employees. American Journal of Medicine 70:919, 1981.

Fischer, G. Pneumococcal Sepsis with False-Negative Blood Cultures. American Journal of Clinical Pathology 78:348, 1982.

Duray, P. Tuberculosis from Frozen Sections. New England Journal of Medicine 305:166, 1981.

Maynard, J. Nosocomial Viral Hepatitis. American Journal of Medicine 70:439, 1981.

Pattison, C. Hepatitis B in Hospital Personnel. American Journal of Epidemiology 101:59, 1975.

Pantelick, E. *Ibid.* American Journal of Medicine 70:924, 1981.

Krugman, S. Hepatitis B Vaccine. American Medical News, April 9, 1982.

Lamberg, L. MD Hepatitis Carriers. *Ibid.*, May 25, 1979.

Vaisrub, S. Hepatitis B—In the Doctor's Office. Journal of the American Medical Association 232:1270, 1975.

Orenstein, W. Hospital Acquired Hepatitis A. Pediatrics 67:494, 1981.

American Medical News. Queens Hospital Hit by Hepatitis. January 22, 1982.

Morbidity and Mortality Weekly Report. Viral Hepatitis in Staff of Pediatric Ward 26:77, 1977.

Yesus, J. Post-Transfusion Hepatitis. Laboratory Medicine 12:703, 1981.

Kaslow, R. Hospital Personnel. *In* Hospital Infections. Boston, Little, Brown, 1979.

Fraser, D. Systemic Mycoses. Journal of the American Medical Association 242:1631, 1979.
Sang, C. Fungal Infection Among Cancer Patients. American Journal of Clinical Pathology 72:617, 1979.
Klein, J. Hospital-Acquired Fungemia. American Journal of Medicine 67:51, 1979.
Sheldon, D. Cutaneous Mucormycosis. Journal of the American Medical Association 241:1032, 1979.
Hughes, W. Pneumocystis Carinii Pneumonia. New England Journal of Medicine 297:1381, 1977.
Stagno, S. Pneumocystic Carinii Pneumonia in Immunocompetent Infants. Pediatrics 66:56, 1980.
Boram, L. Strongyloidiasis in Immunosuppressed Patients. American Journal of Clinical Pathology 76:778, 1981.
Goldmann, D. Bacterial Colonization in the Neonate. American Journal of Medicine 70:417, 1981.
Ramamurthy, R. Nursery Epidemic Caused by . . . Staphylococcus. Pediatrics 51:608, 1973.
Allen, J. Administration Sets for IV Therapy. NITA 3:175, 1980.
Meyer, C. Linen in Newborn Intensive Care Units. Pediatrics 67:362, 1981.
Maki, D. Needle Sticks. American Journal of Medicine 70:928, 1981.
Brickman, A. Susceptibility of Medical Students to Mumps. Pediatrics 48:447, 1971.
Sampliner, R. Dilemma of Hepatitis B Carrier Physician. Archives of Internal Medicine 138:905, 1978.
Hall, C. Nosocomial Viral Respiratory Infections. American Journal of Medicine 70:670, 1981.
Hamoudi, A. Fatal Streptococcal Pneumonia. American Journal of Clinical Pathology 76:823, 1981.
Hughes, W. Nosocomial Infections in Immunocompromised Children. American Journal of Medicine 70:412, 1981.
Blaser, M. Fatal Salmonellosis. Journal of Clinical Microbiology 13:855, 1981.
Prosthetic Valve Endocarditis. Mayo Clinic Proceedings 57:109, 1982.
Kudsk, K. Pyogenic Arthritis Caused by TPN. Journal of the American Medical Association 240:1995, 1979.
Farber, B. Surgical Volume and Wound Infection. New England Journal of Medicine 305:200, 1981.
Goodpasture, H. Toxic Shock Syndrome. Journal of the American Medical Association 247:1464, 1982.
Morbidity and Mortality Weekly Report. Toxic-Shock Syndrome, U.S., 1970–1982. 31:201, 1982.
Marymont, J. Legionella . . . with Human Disease. Laboratory Medicine 11:665, 1980.
Stout, J. Legionnaires' Bacteria in VA Hospital Water Supply. New England Journal of Medicine 307:466, 1982.
Nova, Public Broadcasting System Telecast. Legionnaires' Disease Epidemics, January 31, 1982.
VanVorhis, L. Nosocomial Influenza B Virus. Annals of Internal Medicine 96:153, 1982.

Nail Dust Danger. Strides 19:2, 1982. (Pa. College of Podiatric Medicine)

Caplan, E. Nosocomial Sinusitis. Journal of the American Medical Association 247:639, 1982.

Morbidity and Mortality Weekly Report. Annual Summary, 1980, 29:12, 1981.

Eickhoff, T. Nosocomial Infections—A 1980 View. American Journal of Medicine 70:381, 1981.

Williams, R. Changing Perspectives in Hospital Infection. *In* Proceedings of the International Conference on Nosocomial Infections. Chicago, American Hospital Association, 1971, p. 1.

Stacey, J. Utilization Review. American Medical News. October 13, 1982, p. 1.

Chapter 7

Elnicki, R. Adverse Patient Incidents. Health Service Res. 15:379, 1980.

Latessa, P. Incident Data Compiled. Hospitals 53:53, 1979.

Lee, R. Health and Safety in Hospitals. Medical Science and Law 19:2, 1979.

Chambers, D. Accidental Death in Hospital. Journal of the Royal Society of Medicine 73:87, 1980.

Knaus, W. Range of Intensive Care Services. Journal of the American Medical Association 246:2711, 1981.

American Medical News. September 15, 1981.

Ibid. Less Use of the Intensive Care Unit Could Mean Better Medicine. February 6, 1982.

Relman, A. Intensive Care Units—Who Needs Them? New England Journal of Medicine 302:965, 1981.

Thibault, G. Medical Intensive Care Units. *Ibid.* 938.

Martin, F. Heartsounds. Diagnostic Medicine: 21, June, 1981.

Abramson, N. Adverse Occurrences in Intensive Care Units. Journal of the American Medical Association 244:1582, 1980.

Driver, A. Iatrogenic Malnutrition in Patients Receiving Ventilatory Support. Journal of the American Medical Association 244:2, 1980.

Trunet, P. The Role of Iatrogenic Disease in Admissions to Intensive Care. *Ibid.* 244:2617, 1980.

Shaw, J. Medication Errors a "Great Hidden Problem." American Medical News, January 8, 1982.

Ibid. Lidocaine in Three Deaths. November 5, 1981.

Ibid. Improper Drug Substitution. October 10, 1981.

Pettinger, W. Medication Multiplicity. Journal of the American Medical Association 242:2800, 1979.

Wear, J. Toxicity of Ingested Hexachlorophene. *Ibid.* 181:587, 1962.

Mullick, F. Hexachlorophene Toxicity. Pediatrics 51:395, 1973.

Check. W. Hexachlorophene Teratogenic in Humans. Journal of the American Medical Association 240:513, 1978.

Martin-Boyer, G. Hexachlorophene Poisoning. Lancet January 9, 1982.

Morbidity and Mortality Weekly Report. Neonatal Deaths Associated with Benzyl Alcohol. 31:290, 1982.

Chicago Sun-Times. Air-Oxygen Mixup Cited in 7 Hospital Deaths. February 2, 1982.

Mroczek, W. "I'm Sorry Mrs. Jones, But You Don't Have Hypertension." Journal of the American Medical Association 240:1991, 1978.

Chicago-Tribune. Public Ambulances Safer. January 11, 1981.

Wolf, W. Closed Chest Cardiac Massage. Archives of Surgery, 96:123, 1968.

Chin, S. Cardiopulmonary Resuscitation. New England Journal of Medicine 306:1057, 1982.

Roberts, A. Complications among CPR Trainees. Journal of the American Medical Association 246:1302, 1981.

American Medical News. Licensure Revision. October 10, 1981.

Nelso, R. Walt Whitman. New England Journal of Medicine 305:110, 1981.

(Ed.) An Error is an Error is an Error. Southern Medical Journal 74:650, 1981.

Davis, R. Sleep Deprivation in Medical Education. Illustrated Medical Journal, September, 1981.

American Medical News. M.D. Linked to Death Rate. October 30, 1981. (TIME, Feb. 1, 1982)

Brown, D. Environmental Health and Safety . . . In the Health Care Setting. Journal of Environmental Health. 43:11, 1980.

Medical Laboratory Observer. OSHA Eyes Safety Deregulation for Labs. November, 1981.

Yodaiken, R. The Uncertain Consequences of Formaldehyde Toxicity. Journal of the American Medical Association 246:1677, 1981.

Greenberg, S. Formaldehyde, Medical Ally or Adversary? Proceedings of the Institute of Medicine of Chicago 34:105, 1981.

Keller, J. "Hazardous" Wastes of the Clinical Chemistry Laboratory. Pathologist: 15, January, 1982.

Thomas, J. A Raped Nurse and Three Jailed Doctors. Chicago Sun-Times, October 3, 1981.

Shaw, J. Dealing with Violence in the E.R. American Medical News, October 29, 1982, p. 13.

McNeill-Lehrer Report. Nursing Homes. Public Broadcasting System, February 13, 1982.

American Medical News. Hospitalization Found Preventable. April 24, 1981.

Shaw, J. Emergency Centers. AMN *op. cit.*, p. 15.

Chapter 8

Vaisrub, S. Probing for Causes. Journal of the American Medical Association 139:397, 1979.

Sheehan, M. Diagnostic Errors in Clinical Practice. Texas Medicine 74:92, 1978.

Flegel, K. Adverse Effects of Diagnostic Tests. Archives of Internal Medicine 142:883, 1982.

Autopsy Diagnosis. Scott Medical Journal. 26:271, 1981.

American Medical News. Medicine's Errors. August 28, 1981.

Fineberg, H. Evaluation of Medical Practices. New England Journal of Medicine 301:1086, 1979.

Faulkner, P. Many Diagnostic Tests May be Unnecessary. Hospitals, April 16, 1981.

Zauel, D. Stroke After Carotid Compression. American Journal of Ophthalmology 95:510, 1977.

Bolsen, B. CAT Scan of Brain. Journal of the American Medical Association 246:2667, 1981.
Holder, A. Misdiagnosis of Appendicitis. Journal of the American Medical Association 212:1763, 1970.
American Cancer Society. Socioeconomic Factbook for Surgery. 1981.
Check, W. More Tests Not Always the Answer. Journal of the American Medical Association 244:1886, 1980.
Turkington, R. Physicians Disclaim Blood Glucose Test. Journal of the American Medical Association 240:833, 1978.
Forrest, J. Radiologic Errors in Lung Cancer. Western Journal of Medicine 134:485, 1981.
Randall, D. Leukemia-Like Syndromes. Journal of the American Medical Association 110:479, 1965.
Geboes, K. Is the Elderly Patient Accurately Diagnosed? Geriatrics 34:91, 1979.
Chicago Tribune. Wrong Operation on Groom. April 11, 1979.
Dahlin, D. Seventy-Five Years of Frozen Sections. Mayo Clinic Proceedings 55:721, 1980.
Fechner, R. Frozen Sections. *Ibid.* 56:135, 1981.
Umiker, W. Second Opinions. Medical Laboratory Observer, January, 1982.
American Medical News. Late Diagnosis of Melanoma. February 2, 1982.
Ibid. Pap Tests Misread. March 6, 1981.
Berkely, A. Pap Test Errors. Lancet, October 18, 1980.
Koss, L. Pitfalls in Cytological Diagnosis of Lung Cancer. Cancer 8:937, 1955.
Rosenzweig, A. Iatrogenic Anemia. Journal of the American Medical Association 240: March 5, 1978.
Medical Laboratory Observer. Plans to Probe Laboratories. February, 1982.
American Medical News. CDC's Lab Testing Program Criticized. October 10, 1981.
Barclay, W. Human Senses Exceed Technology. Journal of the American Medical Association 246:1709, 1981.
Scott, J. Simple Tests are Often Best. Journal of the American Medical Association 247:2110, 1982.
Akwari, A. Spuriously Elevated Platelet Counts. American Journal of Clinical Pathology 77:220, 1982.
Dale, N. Spurious Results with Automation. Laboratory Medicine 13:300, 1981.
Marymount, J. Rubella Testing. Laboratory Medicine. 13:83, 1982.
American Medical News. Genetic Test's False Negative. January 5, 1981.
Statland, B. Sources of Variation in Healthy Subjects. Diagnostic Dialog, January-February, 1982.
Clinical Chemistry Reviews. Iatrogenic Lab Errors. Bulletin of Pathology, August, 1969.
Chicago Sun-Times. Tests Sometimes Tell Too Much. October 28, 1981.
Chicago Sun-Times. February 11, 1982.
Rupani, M. Test Results Call for Sleuthing. Medical Laboratory Observer, March, 1982.
Somers, A. Moderating the Rise in Health-Care Costs. New England Journal of Medicine 307:944, 1982.
Koss, L. Cytologic evaluation of the Uterine Cervix. Pathologist 401: August, 1982.

Chapter 9

Mauldin, W. Population Trends and Prospects. Human Survival 6:3, 1980.
Chicago Sun-Times. Pill Leaves Her with Paralysis. August 24, 1981.
Stadel, B. Oral Contraceptives and Cardiovascular Disease. New England Journal of Medicine 305:607, 1981.
Slone, D. Risk of Myocardial Infarction in Current and Discontinued Use of Oral Contraceptives. *Ibid.*:420.
Rothman, K. Twinning After Discontinuing Oral Contraceptives. New England Journal of Medicine 297:468, 1977.
Linn, S. Delayed Conception for Former Pill Users. Journal of the American Medical Association 307:287, 1982.
Chicago Sun-Times. August 17, 1981.
Vana, J. Liver Tumors and Oral Contraceptives. Journal of the American Medical Association 238:2154, 1977.
American Cancer Society. Liver Tumors with Oral Contraceptives. Cancer 28:21, 1978.
Moses, A. Secondary Hyperparathyroidism Caused by Oral Contraceptives. Archives of Internal Medicine 142:128, 1982.
American Medical News. October 27, 1982, p. 12.
Cramer, D. Association of O.C. and Ovarian Cancer, NEJM 307:1047, 1982.
Jick, H. Vaginal Spermacides and Congenital Disorders. Journal of the American Medical Association 245:1329, 1981.
Oakley, G. Spermacides and Birth Defects. *Ibid.*:247; 2405, 1982.
Loomis, L. Toxic-Shock Syndrome with Diaphragm. New England Journal of Medicine 305:1585, 1981.
Schaeffer, G. Complications in Obstetric and Gynecologic Surgery. New York, Harper and Row, 1981.
Cates, W. Sex and Spermacides. JAMA 248:1636, 1982.
Poma, P. Pregnant Uterine Rupture with IUD. Illustrated Medical Journal, June, 1981.
Zakin, D. Perforated and Embedded IUDs. Journal of the American Medical Association 247:2144, 1982.
Case and Comment. Tresemer vs Burke, California Court of Appeals, 1978.
Home, J. IUDs and Pelvic Inflammatory Disease. Journal of the American Medical Association 247:1321, 1982.
Sobel, R. Pseudosulfur granules. American Journal of Clinical Pathology 77:230, 1982.
Valicenti, J. IUD Associated Actinomyces Colonization. Journal of the American Medical Association 247:1149, 1982.
American Medical News. Condom Manufacturer Sued. October 9, 1981.
Crowley, W. Male Contraceptive. New England Journal of Medicine 305:695, 1981.
Time. Doubts About Vasectomies. February 9, 1981.
Walker, A. Vasectomy and Non-Fatal Myocardial Infarction. Lancet 13: January 3, 1981.
Hussey, H. Complications of Vasectomy. Journal of the American Medical Association 245:2333, 1981.

American Medical News. Wrongful Birth. March 12, 1982.
Ibid. MDs Cleared in Vasectomy Suit. April 2, 1982.
Georgia Court of Appeals. April 14, 1981.
Pennsylvania Superior Court. April 16, 1981.
American Medical News. American College of Obstetrics and Gynecology Warns of Sterilization Failures. January 8, 1982.
Brown, H. Tubal Sterilization. Journal of the American Medical Association 245:714, 1981.
Cunanan, R. Complications of Laparoscopic Tubal Sterilization. Obstetrics and Gynecology 55:501, 1980.
Chicago Sun-Times. Simple Plug As Contraceptive. November 13, 1981.
Ryan, G. CBS's "Sixty Minutes." September 4, 1981.
Rubin, G. Fatal Ectopic Pregnancy After Attempted Legal Abortion. Journal of the American Medical Association 244:1706, 1980.
Bolsen, B. Human Life Proposals Assailed. American Medical News, May 8, 1981.
American Medical News. Thirty Percent of Pregnancies End in Abortion. May 8, 1981.
Harman, C. Morbidity in Termination of Pregnancy. American Journal of Obstetrics and Gynecology 139:333, 1981.
LeBolt, A. Mortality from Abortion and Childbirth. JAMA 248:188, 1982. *Ibid.*, p. 192, 1982.
Rovner, S. Natural Family Planning. Chicago Sun-Times, October 4, 1981.
Reed, J. The New Baby Boom. TIME, February 22, 1982.
Wallis, C. The Medical Risks of Waiting. *Ibid.*:59.
Schwartz, D. Fecundity as a Function of Age. New England Journal of Medicine 306:404, 1982.
Staples, B. The Baby Chain. Chicago Reader, June 25, 1982.
Brookings Institute Report. June 28, 1982.
Pierce, N. Teen Pregnancy. Chicago Tribune, June 28, 1982.
Morbidity and Mortality Weekly Report (CDC), 31:137, 1982

Chapter 10

Teele, D. Meningitis After Lumbar Puncture. New England Journal of Medicine 305:1079, 1981.
Batnitsky, S. Iatrogenic Intraspinal Tumors. Journal of the American Medical Association 237:148, 1977.
Dunn, D. Spinal Subdural Hematoma. *Ibid.* 241:1712, 1979.
Schroeder, S. Frequency and Morbidity of Invasive Procedures. Archives of Internal Medicine 138:1809, 1978.
Kline, T. Fine Needle Aspiration of the Breast. Cancer 44:1458, 1979.
Oertel, Y. Fine Needle Aspiration. Laboratory Medicine. 13:345, 1982.
Durkee, C. Sepsis Following Transperineal Needle Biopsy of the Prostate. Journal of Urology 125:752, 1981.
Fitts, C. Complications of Thoracentesis. *In* Hardy, J. Management of Surgical Complications. Philadelphia, W.B. Saunders, 1981.
Gerzof, S. Percutaneous Catheter Drainage of Abdominal Abscess. New England Journal of Medicine 305:695, 1981.

Schein, M. Penile Tumescence. South African Medical Journal 58:834, 1980.
Duma, R. Hazards of IV Therapy. New England Journal of Medicine 94:1178, 1976.
Maki, D. Endemic Rate of Fluid Contamination in Arterial Pressure Monitoring. American Journal of Medicine 70:733, 1981.
Medical News. Infusion Catheters a Poorly Recognized Septicemia Cause. January 12, 1981.
Abrams, H. Coronary Arteriography. Amer. Journal Radiology 139:1, 1982.
Vliestra. R. A New Image for Angiographers. Mayo Clinic Proceedings 56:715, 1981.
Istre, G. Amebiasis Spread by Colonic Irrigation. NEJM 307:339, 1982.
McDaniel, D. Catheter-Induced Pulmonary Artery Hemorrhage. Journal of Thoracic and Cardiovascular Surgery. 82:1, 1981.
Chastre, J. Thrombosis as a Complication of Pulmonary Artery Catheter. New England Journal of Medicine 306:278, 1982.
Chase, A. Balloon Angioplasties. Medical News, November 17, 1980.
Smith, C. Pediatric Vascular Injuries. Surgery 90:20, 1981.
Greenblatt, D. Intramuscular Injection-Site Complications. Journal of the American Medical Association 240:542, 1978.
Neustadt, D. Complications of Local Corticosteroid Injections. Journal of the American Medical Association 246:835, 1981.
Myers, M. and G. Ghahremani. Iatrogenic Gastrointestinal Complications. New York, Springer-Verlag, 1981.
Myers, M. Complications of Gastrointestinal Endoscopy. Mount Sinai Journal of Medicine 48:191, 1981.
Beecham, W. Salmonella Transmitted by Upper Gastrointestinal Fiberoptic Endoscopy. Journal of the American Medical Association 241:1013, 1979.
Erlangen Symposium, 1977.
Dubos, C. Esophageal Perforation. Journal of Thoracic and Cardiovascular Surgery 78:44, 1979.
Shamir, M. Complications of Fiberoptic Endoscopy. Gastrointestinal Endoscopy. 26:86, 1980.
Alexander, W. Bacteremia and Meningitis Following Fiberoptic Bronchoscopy. Archives of Internal Medicine 139:580, 1979.
Khan, M. Deaths Associated with Flexible Bronchoscopy. Chest 70:200, 1976.
Lukomsky, G. Complications of Bronchoscopy. *Ibid.* 79:319, 1981.
Dreisin, R. Flexible Fiberoptic Bronchoscopy. *Ibid.* 74:144, 1978.
Zavala, D. Complications Following Fiberoptic Bronchoscopy. *Ibid.* 73:783, 1978.
Parewijck, W. Serious Complications of Laparoscopy. Medical Science and Law 19:199, 1979.
Chamberlain, G. Gynecological Laparoscopy. London, Royal College of Obstetrics and Gynecology, 1978.
Sutherland, A. Laparoscopy in Diagnosis of Pelvic Tuberculosis. Lancet July 14, 1979.
Cushieri, A. Laparoscopy in General Surgery and Gastroenterology. British Journal of Hospital Medicine 24:252, 1980.
Makanji, H. Rupture of Spleen at Laparoscopy. British Journal of Obstetrics and Gynecology 87:73, 1980.
Goodnough, J. Gonococcal Peritonitis Following Laparoscopy. American Journal of Obstetrics and Gynecology 130:218, 1981.

Chi, I. Uterine Perforation During Sterilization. *Ibid.* 735, 1981.
Herrer, J. Pneumopericardium. Endoscopy 12:254, 1980.
Paulson, G. Neurological Complications of Laparoscopy. American Journal of Obstetrics and Gynecology 40:470, 1981.
Foster, H. Interval Mini-Laparotomy. Journal of the National Medical Association 72:569, 1980.
Nelson, R. Hypothermia during Infant Cystoscopy. Journal of Urology 121:33, 1979.
Goodman, G. Electrosurgical Burns and the Urologist. Journal of Urology 116:218, 1976.
Segura, J. Percutaneous Removal of Kidney Stones. Mayo Clinic Proceedings 57:615, 1982.
Queenan, J. Amniocentesis. Obstetrics and Gynecology 25:302, 1965.
American Medical News. August 8, 1982, p. 18.
Council on Scientific Affairs: α-Fetoprotein Monitoring. Journal of the American Medical Association 247:1478, 1982.

Chapter 11

Hackler, T. Surgery and Second Opinions. American Medical News, February 12, 1982.
Kra, S. and Boltax, R. Is Surgery Necessary? New York, Macmillan, 1981.
Congressional Subcommittee Report on Surgery, 1977.
American Medical News. October 30, 1981.
Crile, G. Surgery; Your Choices, Your Alternatives. New York, Delacorte Press, 1978.
American Medical News. March 5, 1982.
American Cancer Society. Socioeconomic Factbook of Surgery. 1981.
Brown, R. Perchance to Dream. Chicago, Nelson-Hall, 1981.
Aronow, S. Electrosurgery. Anesthesiology 42:525, 1957.
Buckspan, G. Intra-arterial Drug Injury. Journal of Surgical Residency 24:294, 1978.
Raj, P. Techniques for Fiberoptic Laryngoscopy. Anesthesia and Analgesics 53:708, 1974.
Greene, D. Tracheostomy or Not? Journal of the American Medical Association 234:1150, 1975.
Stauffer, J. Endotracheal Intubation and Tracheotomy. American Journal of Medicine. 70:65, 1981.
Hardy, J. (Ed.): Complications in Surgery and their Management. Philadelphia, W.B. Saunders, 1981 (see Fitts, C. Complications of Tracheostomy).
Tsairis, P. Brachial Plexus Neuropathies. *In* Peripheral Neuropathy (P. Dyck). Philadelphia, W.B. Saunders, 1975.
Mawk, J. Postoperative Ulnar Neuropathy. Journal of the American Medical Association 246:2807, 1981.
Forestner, J. Complications of Anesthesia. *In* Hardy, J., *op. cit*, p. 151.
Altemeier, W. and Culbertson, W. Complications of Appendectomy. *In* Hardy, J., *op. cit.*, p. 606.
McCarthy, E. Surgical Utilization. Medical Care 18:883, 1980.

Louisiana Court of Appeals, May 26, 1981.
North Dakota Supreme Court, April 23, 1981.
Barnes, P. Anesthetic Complications. Anesthesia and Intensive Care 8:404, 1980.
Cullen, B. Drug Interactions and Anesthesia. Anesthetics and Analgesics 53:413, 1979.
Katz, J. Complications of Spinal and Epidural Anesthesia. Journal of Bone and Joint Surgery 62A:1219, 1980.
Owens, W. Anesthetic Side Effects and Complications. Intensive Anesthesia Clinics 18:1, 1981.
Inman, W. Jaundice After Repeated Exposure to Halothane. British Medical Journal 1:5, 1974.
American Medical Association Citation. *Op cit.*, 31:2, 1975.
Utting, J. Human Misadventures in Anesthesia. Canadian Anesthesiology Society Journal 26:472, 1979.
Hunt, T. Wound Complications. *In* Hardy, J. *op. cit.,* p. 20.
Greenfield, L. Shock. *In* Hardy, J., *op. cit.,* p. 33.
Glenn, F. and Cameron, J. Complications Following Operations on the Biliary Tract. *In* Hardy, J., *op. cit.*, p. 512.
Payne, W. Complications of Esophageal and Diaphragmatic Surgery. *In* Hardy, J., *op. cit.*, p. 330.
Hardy, J. Complications of Gastric Surgery. *In* Hardy, J., *op. cit.*, p. 462.
Dainko, E. Gastric Wrap Surgery. ABC telecast, February 17, 1982.
Kocok, M. Gastroplasty for Morbid Obesity. Journal of the American Medical Association 246:2420, 1981.
Haid, R. Encephalopathy after Gastric Plication. *Ibid.* 247:2566, 1982.
Gourlay, R. Complications of Surgery for Morbid Obesity. American Journal of Surgery 126:154, 1978.
Check, W. Gastroplasty. JAMA 248:277, 1982.
Breuer, R. The Ileoptomists of Chicago. Ill. Medical Journal 131:313, 1967.
Gamble, C. Glomerulonephritis and Vasculitis Following Intestinal Bypass. American Journal of Clinical Pathology 77:347, 1982.
Kings County, New York, Index No. 24212/76, May 21, 1981.
Booth, B. Postmastectomy Venous Thrombosis. New England Journal of Medicine 305:170, 1981.
Kuhn, J. Treating Breast Cancer Conservatively. JAMA 248:1793, 1982.
Robbins, G. Complications Following Surgical Treatment of Potentially Curable Cancer of the Breast. *In* Hardy, J., *op. cit.,* p. 698.
Lepley, D. Heart and Great Vessels, *Ibid.*, p. 367.
Kalb, M. and Kalb, B. Kissinger. Boston, Little, Brown and Co., 1974.
TIME. Shuttle Fatigue. April 26, 1982.
Technology Assessment Forum. Coronary Artery Bypass Surgery. Journal of the American Medical Association 246:1645, 1981.
Technology Assessment Forum: Coronary Artery Bypass Surgery. New England Journal of Medicine 304:680, 1981.
Sanz, G. Prognosis in Survivors of Myocardial Infarction. *Ibid.* 306:1065, 1982.
Moore, G. Coronary Artery Bypass Grafts in 109 Autopsied Patients. Journal of the American Medical Association 246:1785, 1981.

Gould, K. Coronary Reperfusion: Medical, Surgical or not at all? JAMA 248:1362, 1982.
Tector, A. The Internal Mammary Artery Graft. Journal of the American Medical Association 246:2181, 1981.
Rich, N. Complications of Surgery of the Abdominal Aorta and Aortic Branches. *In* Hardy, J., *op. cit.,* p. 422.
Wilson, W. Prosthetic Valve Endocarditis. Mayo Clinic Proceedings 57:155, 1982.
Morbidity and Mortality Weekly Report. Bacteremia Among Aortic Valve Surgery Patients. February 26, 1982.
Chokshi, A. Peer Review in Reduction of Pacemaker Implantation. Journal of the American Medical Association 246:754, 1981.
American Medical News. September 24, 1982, p. 7.
Sundt, T. Carotid Endarterectomy. Mayo Clinic Proceedings 56:533, 1981.
Check, W. Value Still Unproven. Journal of the American Medical Association 247:1802, 1982.
Resnikov, L. Post-Pericardiectomy Syndrome. Journal of the American Medical Association 247:84, 1982.
Leaf, A. Massachusetts General Hospital Trustees Say NO to Heart Transplants. New England Journal of Medicine 302:1087, 1980.
Pluth, J. Cardiac Transplantation. Mayo Clinic Proceedings 56:202, 1981.
American Medical News. Heart-Lung Transplants. December 4, 1981.
Chicago Sun-Times. New Heart Transplant Method. April 18, 1982.
Reitz, B. Cardiac Transplantation—1982. JAMA 248:1225, 1982.
American Medical News. Plastic Surgeons Respond to Survey. January 15, 1982.
Goldwyn, R. The Unfavorable Result in Plastic Surgery. Boston, Little, Brown and Co., 1972.
Baker, D. Avoiding Facial Nerve Injuries in Rhydidectomy. Plastic and Reconstructive Surgery 64:781, 1979.
Thomas, S. Toxic Shock Syndrome Following Submucous Resection and Rhinoplasty. Journal of the American Medical Association 247:2402, 1982.
Courtiss, E. Aesthetic Surgery. St. Louis, C.V. Mosby, 1978.
Parkes, M. Functional Sequelae of Rhinoplasty. Annals of Plastic Surgery 4:116, 1980.
Ungar, W. The Intelligent Man's Guide to Hair Transplants. Chicago, Contemporary Books, 1979.
Iatrogenic False Aneurysm Following Punch Hair Grafting. Journal of the American Medical Association, 1982.
Hanke, C. Hair Implant Complications. Journal of the American Medical Association. 245:1344, 1981.
Parulkar, S. Iatrogenic Ureteral Injuries. Proceedings of the Institute of Medicine of Chicago. 34:59, 1981.
Ridley, J. Gynecologic Surgery. Baltimore, Williams and Wilkins, 1981.
Miyazawa, K. Urologic Injuries in Gynecological Surgery. Hawaii Medical Journal 39:11, 1980.
Dickey, R. Hysterectomy. JAMA 248:323, 1982. (From CDC)
Mumford, S. Laparoscopy and Mini-Laparotomy. Lancet 11:1066, 1980.

Kauppila, A. Endometrial Jet Washing. Journal of the American Medical Association 239:2446, 1978.

Poma, P. Tubal Surgery. Proceedings of the Institute of Medicine of Chicago. 34:99, 1981.

Goodwin, W. Perineal Prostatectomy. *In* Smith, R., Complications of Urologic Surgery. Philadelphia, W.B. Saunders, 1976, p. 252.

Thompson, I. *Ibid.*, p. 205.

Montague, D. *Ibid.*, p. 54.

Boyce, W. Complications of Renal Stone Surgery. *Ibid.*

Bass, R. Radical Retropubic Prostatectomy. Journal of Urology 134:495, 1980.

Rosen, R. Obstructed Ureteroileal Conduits. American Journal of Radiology 135:1201, 1980.

Malgieri, J. Ileal Loop in Treatment of Radiation Treated Pelvic Malignancies. Journal of Urology 120:32, 1978.

Dade, G. Complications of Scrotal Surgery. *In* Smith, R.: Complications of Urologic Surgery, W.B. Saunders, 1976, p. 395.

Peters, P. Complications of Penile Surgery. *Ibid.*, p. 414.

Management of Neurogenic Impotence with Inflatable Penile Prostheses. Urology 17:341, 1981.

Donahue, J. Complication of Retroperitoneal Lymph Node Dissections. Journal of Urology 125:338, 1981.

Preston, E. Whither the Foreskin? JAMA 213:1853, 1980.

Tushnet, L. Uncircumcision. Medical Times 93:588, 1965.

Perley, J. and Shapiro, S. Complications of Circumcision. *In* DeVries, P. and Shapiro, S., Complications of Pediatric Surgery. John Wiley & Sons, New York, 1982.

Report of Ad Hoc Task Force on Circumcision. Pediatrics 610: October, 1975.

Nyhus, L. Complications of Hernia Repair. *In* Hardy, J., *op. cit.*, p. 685.

Taylor, G. Sex in History. New York, Vanguard Press, 1954.

Kukora, J. Complications of Thyroid and Parathyroid Surgery. *In* Hardy, J., *op. cit.*, p. 295.

Beahres, O. Complications of Surgery for Cancer of the Head and Neck. *In* Hardy, J., *op. cit.*, p. 280.

Strohman, D. The Quick Knife. Post Washington, N.Y., The Kennicott Press, 1979.

Conway, W. Adverse Effects of Tracheostomy for Sleep Apnea. Journal of the American Medical Association 246:347, 1981.

Total Hip-Joint Replacement in the U.S. JAMA 248:1817, 1982.

Michel, R. Air Embolism in Hip Surgery. Anesthesia 35:858, 1980.

Alterbarmakian, V. Ureteral Injury Associated with Lumbar Disc Surgery. Urology 17:462, 1981.

Chicago Tribune. September 10, 1981.

Krueger, B. Infarction Following Chiropractic Cervical Manipulation. Mayo Clinic Proceedings 55:322, 1980.

Freeland, A. Complications Following Treatment of Common Fractures and Dislocations. *In* Hardy, J., *op. cit.*, p. 776.

American Cancer Society. Cancer Facts and Figures, 1982.

Putnam, C. Complications of Transplants. *In* Hardy, J., *op. cit.*, p. 783.

Koene, R. Renal Decapsulation After Transplantation. New England Journal of Medicine 300:1030, 1979.
American Society of Transplantation Surgery. Results and Expectations of Renal Transplantation. Journal of the American Medical Association 241:1330, 1981.
Adkins, P. Complications of Pulmonary Resection. *In* Hardy, J. *op. cit.*, p. 313.

Chapter 12

Hein, H.A. Secrets from Sweden. Journal of the American Medical Association 247:985, 1982.
Erikson, J.D. Fetal and Infant Mortality in Norway. *Ibid.*, p. 987.
Newton, M. and Lurain, J.R. Obstetric Operations. In Hardy, J.: Complications in Surgery and Their Management. Philadelphia, W.B. Saunders, 1981.
American Medical News. October 2, 1981.
Ibid., February 12, 1982.
California Court of Appeals. September 29, 1981.
Bellin, H. ABC telecast, May 3, 1982.
Check, W. Hexachlorophene Teratogenic in Humans. Journal of the American Medical Association 240:513, 1978.
National Institutes of Health: Breast Milk and Risk of Cytomegalovirus. Journal of the American Medical Association 246:2659, 1981.
Chicago Sun-Times. April 20, 1978.
American Medical News. February 26, 1982.
Chicago Reader. November 6, 1981.
Adamson, G.D. Home or Hospital Births? Journal of the American Medical Association 243:1732, 1980.
Thornton, R.R. Home Delivery. South Dakota Journal of Medicine 3412:17, 1981.
New Hampshire Supreme Court, May 27, 1981.
American Cancer Society. Socio-Economic Fact Book for Surgery, 1981.

Chapter 13

Mendelsohn, R.S. Confessions of a Medical Heretic. Chicago, Contemporary Books, 1979.
Peery, T.M. The New and Old Diseases. American Journal of Clinical Pathology 263:453, 1965.
Kaufman, B. Vaccine Roulette. NBC telecast, April 21, 1982.
Iber, F.L. Hepatitis B Vaccine. Journal of the American Medical Association 247:2272, 1982.
Krugman, S. Hepatitis B Vaccine. American Medical News, April 9, 1982.
CDC: Streptococcus Abscesses after DPT Immunization. MNWR 31:519, 1982.
Mullen, A. Indications for Use of HB Vaccine. NEJM 307:644, 1982.
CDC: HB Vaccine Safety. MMWR 31:465, 1982.
Goodman, R.A. et al. Influenza in a Nursing Home. Journal of the American Medical Association 247:1451, 1982.
American Medical News, August 21, 1981.
Ibid; February 19, 1982.

Kramer, P. Influenza Vaccine. New England Journal of Medicine 305:1262, 1981.

Horwitz, E.S. Influenza Vaccine. *Ibid.* 304:1557, 1981.

Smith, C.I. Hepatitis B Infection. Journal of the American Medical Association 247:2261, 1982.

Center for Disease Control. Influenza Update. Morbidity and Mortality Weekly Report 31:104, 1982.

Schwartz, J.S. Pneumococcal Vaccine. Annals of Internal Medicine 96:208, 1982.

Hirshmann, J.V. Pneumovax. Journal of the American Medical Association 246: 1428, 1981.

Center for Disease Control. Measles Cases. Morbidity and Mortality Weekly Report 31:211, 1982.

Center for Disease Control. Measles Prevention. *Ibid.*:217, 1982.

Orenstein, W.A. Congenital Rubella. Journal of the American Medical Association 247:1174, 1982.

American Medical News. Rubella. March 6, 1982.

Center for Disease Control. Poliomyelitis. Morbidity and Mortality Weekly Report 31:23, 1982.

Center for Disease Control. Vaccine Poliomyelitis. *Ibid.*:97, 1982.

Center for Disease Control. Smallpox. *Ibid.*:159, 1982.

Internal Medicine News. Smallpox Vaccine. January 21, 1982.

Kiernan, L.A. Chicago Sun-Times. November 1, 1981.

Physicians' Desk Reference. Rabies Vaccine: 1091, Oradell, N. J., Medical Economics Co., 1981.

Illinois Department of Public Health. Rabies Control, 1981.

Berlin, B.S. A New Rabies Vaccine. Journal of the American Medical Association 247:1726, 1982.

Center for Disease Control. Human Rabies. Mortality and Morbidity Weekly Report. 31:135, 1982.

Jacobs, R.C. Tetanus Toxoid. Journal of the American Medical Association 247:41, 1982.

American Medical News. March 5, 1982.

Jane, M. Hazards of Smallpox Vaccination. Journal of the American Medical Association 247:2709, 1982.

Center for Disease Control. Morbidity and Mortality Weekly Report 31:279, 1982.

Kaplan, J. GBS in the United States. JAMA 248:698, 1982.

CDC. Influenza vaccines. MMWR, 1982-83, 31:249, 1982.

Citron, M. Pneumoccal-Vaccine-induced Thrombocytopcnia. JAMA 248:1178, 1982.

AMN. November 19, 1982, p. 16.

CDC. Rubella Vaccination During Pregnancy. MMWR 31:478, 1982.

CDC. Vaccinia Necrosum after Smallpox Vaccination. MMWR 31:501, 1982.

Chapter 14

Mollison, P.L. Blood Transfusion in Clinical Medicine. London, Blackwell Scientific Publications, 1979.

Lefton, D. American Medical News, November 27, 1981.

Guy, L.R. Transfusion Patient Identification. Laboratory Medicine 12:542, 1981.

Citation. Volume 34, No. 8 (Feb.), 1977.
Barnes, A. Moving Cautiously—Fast. Diagnostic Medicine: 51, December, 1981.
American Association of Blood Banks' Believe It or Not. Bulletin of the American Association of Blood Banks: 4, July, 1968.
Guy, L.R. Identification of the Patient. *In* Adverse Reactions to Transfusion. Chicago, American Society of Clinical Pathologists, 1975.
Pineda, A.A. Hemolytic Transfusion Reaction. Mayo Clinic Proceedings 53:378, 1978.
Mayer, J.E. Transfusion Disasters. Lancet 824:618, 1981.
Yarrish, R.L. Transfusion Malaria. Archives of Internal Medicine 142:187, January, 1982.
New York Times. Malaria in Baby. February 18, 1982.
Man Dies After Transfusion. Chicago Sun-Times, November 12, 1981.
Smith, T.F. Cytomegalovirus Infections. Mayo Clinic Proceedings 56:769, 1981.
Drew, W.L. Transfusion Related Cytomegalovirus Infection. Journal of the American Medical Association 247:2389, 1982.
Silvergleid, A.J. Autologous Transfusion. Diagnostic Medicine: 29, December, 1981.
Valeri, C.R. Frozen Blood. Transfusion 21:138, 1981.
Perkins, H.A. The Blood Donor: Benefit vs Risk. Journal of the American Medical Association November, 1978.
Pollner, F. Donor Safety in Leukapheresis. American Medical News, January 5, 1981.
Granulocyte Transfusion. Laboratory Medicine 12:553, 1981.
Rosenshein, M.S. Leucocyte Transfusion. New England Journal of Medicine 302:1058, 1980.
Pineda, A.A. Granulocyte and Platelet Transfusion. Mayo Clinic Proceedings 56:645, 1981.
Thomas, E.D. Marrow Transplantation. American Society of Clinical Pathology 32:887, 1979.
Johnson, F.L. Marrow Transplants. New England Journal of Medicine 305:845, 1981.
Sarma, D.B. Blood in Elective Surgery. Journal of the American Medical Association 243:1536, 1980.
Rosenshein, D. Chicago Sun-Times, April 9, 1982.
Artificial Blood. American Medical News, March 5, 1982.
Greenberg, A.G. Hemoglobin Solutions. Diagnostic Medicine, December, 1981.
Grindon, A.J. The Decision to Transfuse. Laboratory Medicine 13:272, 1982.
Schmidt, W. RBC Destruction Caused by a Micropore Blood Filter. JAMA 248:1629, 1982.
Czaja, A. Hepatitis Non A, Non B. Mayo Clinic Proc. 57:639, 1982.
Hoagland, C. Bone Marrow Transplantation. Mayo Clinic Proc. 57:668, 1982.

Chapter 15

Kolata, G.B. Dialysis After Nearly a Decade. Science 208:473, 1980.
Wall Street Journal. December 22, 1981.
Relman, A.S. Treatment of End Stage Renal Disease. New England Journal of Medicine 303:996, 1980.

Gutman, R. Kidney Dialysis. *Ibid.* (Quoted in Chicago Sun-Times, February 6, 1981.)
Adelson, B.H. Ethical Considerations on Life Support Systems. Chicago Institute of Medicine: 4, October 19, 1979.
Friedman, E. Environmental and Iatrogenic Obstacles to Long Life on Hemodialysis. New England Journal of Medicine 306:169, 1982.
Vaisrub, S. Dangerous Waters. Journal of the American Medical Association 240:1630, 1978.
Gunby, P. Dialysis Encephalopathy. Journal of the American Medical Association 241:1875, 1979.
American Medical News. Liver Damage. February 3, 1982.
Najem, G.R. Hepatitis B Infection. Journal of the American Medical Association 245:153, 1981.
Deane, N. Hepatitis and Hemodialysis. *Ibid.*:171.
Kiernan, T.W. Hepatitis B Virus in Hemodialysis. Archives of Internal Medicine 142:51, 1982.
Osanloo, E. Viral Pericarditis in Hemodialysis. *Ibid.* 139:301, 1979.
Ellison, R.T. Spontaneous Mediastinal Hemorrhage. Annals of Internal Medicine 95:704, 1981.
Potter, D.E. End Stage Renal Disease in Children. Kidney International 18:103, 1980.
Denniston, D.J. Home Peritoneal Dialysis. American Journal of Nursing: 2022, November, 1981.
Johnson, R.S. Home Dialysis. Journal of the American Medical Association 245:1511, 1981.
Roberts, S.D. Home Hemodialysis Aides. Annals of Internal Medicine 141:855, 1981.
Prior, J. Dialysis Encephalopathy and Osteomalacic Bone Disease. American Journal of Medicine 72:33, 1982.
Scheff, R. Colonic Disease in Patients Receiving Hemodialysis. Archives of Internal Medicine 142:235, 1982.
Robinson, D. Kidney Dialysis: A Taxpayers' Nightmare. Readers' Digest, October, 1982, p. 149.
American Medical News. Nov. 12, 1982, p. 25.

Chapter 16

Myers, J. Preventing Iatrogenic Complications. New England Journal of Medicine 304:664, 1981.
Zook, C. High Cost Users of Medical Care *Ibid.* 302:996, 1980.
Drummond, R. Consensus Statements. *Ibid.* 304:665, 1981.
Kulata, C. Coronary Artery Bypass. Science 211:42, 1981.
Harrison, M. A Woman in Residence. New York, Random House, 1982.
Kolata, G. Hypertension Study Produces Surprising Result. Science 218:31, October, 1982.
Kass, L. Ethical Dilemmas in the Care of the Ill. Journal of the American Medical Association 244:1946, 1980.
Waltz, J. Seminar, Northwestern University, April 26, 1975.
Meisel, A. Informed Consent. Journal of the American Medical Association 246:2473, 1981.

Cousins, N. A Layman Looks at Truth Telling in Medicine. Journal of the American Medical Association 244:1929, 1980.
Veatch, R. Voluntary Risks to Health. Journal of the American Medical Association 243:50, 1980.
Relman, A. The New Medical-Industrial Complex. New England Journal of Medicine 303:963, 1980.

Index